Integrated Mental Health Services

Integrated Mental Health Services

Modern Community Psychiatry

Edited by

William R. Breakey

New York   Oxford
OXFORD UNIVERSITY PRESS
1996

Oxford University Press

Oxford   New York
Athens   Auckland   Bangkok   Bombay
Calcutta   Cape Town   Dar es Salaam   Delhi
Florence   Hong Kong   Istanbul   Karachi
Kuala Lumpur   Madras   Madrid   Melbourne
Mexico City   Nairobi   Paris   Singapore
Taipei   Tokyo   Toronto

and associated companies in
Berlin   Ibadan

Copyright © 1996 by Oxford University Press, Inc.

Published by Oxford University Press, Inc.,
198 Madison Avenue, New York, New York 10016

Oxford is a registered trademark of Oxford University Press

Library of Congress Cataloging-in-Publication Data
Integrated mental health services : modern community psychiatry /
edited by William R. Breakey.
p.   cm. Includes bibliographical
references and index.
ISBN 0-19-507421-1
1. Community mental health services
I. Breakey, William R.
RA790.55.I53 1996
362.2'2—dc20   95-47821

1 2 3 4 5 6 7 8 9

Printed in the United States of America
on acid-free paper

To the people
of East Baltimore,
from whom so many
have learned so much.

PREFACE

This book, written for psychiatrists and psychiatrists in training, traces the history of modern community psychiatry, reviews its basic sciences and fundamental principles, and proceeds to a discussion of current community psychiatric practice. It is concerned with the integrated system of services needed to meet the mental health needs of a population such as that of a mental health catchment area or the covered population in a managed mental health program. Each chapter stands on its own, but together they represent the coordinated elements of a system of care.

The volume encapsulates what has been learned over two decades at the Johns Hopkins Hospital in Baltimore and at other centers in the United States, the United Kingdom, and Canada and indicates where there are gaps in knowledge, and need for research and development. The authors, drawn from a wide circle, are not only in many cases distinguished scientists, but experienced clinicians who have practised what they preach. They have acquired their skills and insights as they have struggled with the practical problems of treating patients in the community and building integrated systems of community mental health services. Each chapter provides an historical introduction to its theme and describes current concepts and practice and has a bibliography that will guide the reader in further exploration of the topic.

In the United States, as this book goes to press, there is considerable uncertainty as to the shape of public mental health services in the years ahead. Indeed, the distinction between public and private may cease to have much meaning as managed care organizations increasingly take on the role of managing health care resources for everyone. However events unfold, integrated systems of mental health services will continue to be needed and the concepts contained in this book will continue to be applied in their organization.

ACKNOWLEDGMENTS

I am deeply appreciative of the work and expertise invested in the preparation of this book by all of the chapter authors and for their patience through a long and arduous process. Not only did they willingly write and rewrite various drafts of their chapters, but in many cases they contributed their time and expertise to review and critique each other's chapters.

Other colleagues also assisted the editorial process by reviewing individual chapters: Larry Alessi, Paula U. Hamburger, Sheppard Kellam, Paul R. McHugh, Everett Siegel, John C. Urbaitis and Jane Wells. Jeffrey House, at Oxford University Press, unfailingly provided good counsel a every stage of the process. Angela Breakey, Sandy Hensley and Dorothy Pumphry provided expert assistance with the preparation of the manuscript.

I am particularly indebted to Angela for her loving support, encouragement and forbearance throughout the seemingly interminable gestation period of this volume.

William R. Breakey

CONTENTS

CONTRIBUTORS

Thomas E. Arthur
Executive Director, Changing Directions, Inc.

Stephen J. Bartels, M.D.
Associate Professor of Psychiatry
Research Associate, New Hampshire-Dartmouth Psychiatric Research Center, Dartmouth Medical School.

Paul Bebbington, M.A., Ph.D., F.R.C.P., F.R.C.Psych.
Hon. Reader in Social and Epidemiological Psychiatry at the Institute of Psychiatry
Hon. Consultant Psychiatrist at the Bethlem/Maudsley Hospital.

Michael A. Bogrov, M.D.
Instructor, Division of Child Psychiatry, Johns Hopkins University School of Medicine.

William R. Breakey, M.B., F.R.C. Psych.
Professor and Deputy Director, Department of Psychiatry and Behavioral Sciences, Johns Hopkins University School of Medicine.

Paul Colson, Ph.D.
Department of Psychiatry, College of Physicians and Surgeons of Columbia University.

Raymond L. Crowel, Psy.D.
Director, East Baltimore Mental Health Partnership.

Ronald J. Diamond, M.D.
Associate Professor, Department of Psychiatry, University of Wisconsin-Madison Medical School.

Robert E. Drake, M.D., Ph.D.
Professor of Psychiatry
Director, New Hampshire-Dartmouth Psychiatric Research Center, Dartmouth Medical School.

Mary C. Eaton, Ph.D.
Senior Psychiatric Therapist, Johns Hopkins Community Psychiatry Program.

Pamela J. Fischer, Ph.D.
Associate Professor, Department of Psychiatry and Behavioral Sciences, Johns Hopkins University School of Medicine.

Marc Fishman, M.D.
Instructor, Department of Psychiatry and Behavioral Sciences, Johns Hopkins University School of Medicine.

Laurie Flynn
Executive Director, National Alliance for the Mentally Ill.

Hugh L. Freeman, D.M., F.R.C.Psych.
Honorary Visiting Fellow, Green College, Oxford.

Gerard Gallucci, M.D., M.H.S.
Assistant Professor, Department of Psychiatry and Behavioral Sciences, Johns Hopkins University of School of Medicine
Medical Director, Community Psychiatry Program, Johns Hopkins Bayview Medical Center.

Paula N. Goering, R.N., Ph.D.
Associate Professor, Department of Psychiatry and Faculty of Nursing, University of Toronto
Director, Health Systems Research Unit, Clarke Institute of Psychiatry.

Howard H. Goldman, M.D., Ph.D.
Professor, Department of Psychiatry, University of Maryland School of Medicine.

Ruth A. Hughes, Ph.D.
Executive Director, International Association of Psychosocial Rehabilitation Services, Columbia, Maryland.

Jeffrey S. Janofsky, M.D.
Associate Professor and Director, Psychiatry and Law Program, Department of Psychiatry and Behavioral Sciences, Johns Hopkins University School of Medicine.

Geetha Jayaram, M.D.
Assistant Professor and Physician Advisor, Department of Psychiatry and Behavioral Sciences, Johns Hopkins University School of Medicine.

Michael J. Kaminsky, M.D.
Associate Professor and Clinical Director, Department of Psychiatry and Behavioral Sciences, Johns Hopkins University School of Medicine.

Anthony F. Lehman, M.D., M.S.P.H.
Professor of Psychiatry, Department of Psychiatry and Human Behavior, University of Maryland at Baltimore.

Susan W. Lehmann, M.D.
Assistant Professor, Department of Psychiatry and Behavioral Sciences, Johns Hopkins University School of Medicine.

Bruno R. Lima, M.D.
Associate Professor, Department of Psychiatry and Behavioral Sciences, Johns Hopkins University School of Medicine (Deceased).

Constantine G. Lyketsos, M.D.
Assistant Professor, Department of Psychiatry and Behavioral Sciences, Johns Hopkins University School of Medicine.

Mark N. Mollenhauer, M.D.
Instructor, Department of Psychiatry and Behavioral Sciences
Director, Psychiatric Emergency Services; Director, Intensive Treatment Unit, Johns Hopkins University School of Medicine.

Gerald Nestadt, M.B., B.Ch., M.P.H.
Associate Professor, Department of Psychiatry and Behavioral Sciences, Johns Hopkins University School of Medicine
Director, Psychiatric Day Hospital.

Sandra J. Newman, Ph.D.
Associate Director for Research, Institute For Policy Studies, Johns Hopkins University.

Mark Olfson, M.D., M.P.H.
Assistant Professor of Clinical Psychiatry, College of Physicians & Surgeons of Columbia University.

Fred C. Osher, M.D.
Associate Professor; Director, Division of Community Psychiatry, University of Maryland School of Medicine.

Annelle B. Primm, M.D., M.P.H.
Assistant Professor, Department of Psychiatry and Behavioral Sciences
Director, Community Psychiatry Program, Johns Hopkins University School of Medicine.

Peter V. Rabins, M.D., M.P.H.
Professor, Department of Psychiatry and Behavioral Sciences, Johns Hopkins University School of Medicine.

Cyprian L. Rowe, M.S.W., P.H.D.
Assistant Dean for Student Services and Multicultural Affairs, School of Social Work, University of Maryland at Baltimore.

Jack F. Samuels, Ph.D.
Instructor, Department of Psychiatry and Behavioral Sciences, Johns Hopkins University School of Medicine.

Kathleen Schneider-Braus, M.D.
Clinical Assistant Professor, Department of Psychiatry, University of Wisconsin, Madison.

Steven S. Sharfstein, M.D.
Chief Executive Officer and Medical Director, Sheppard Pratt Health System.

Leonard I. Stein, M.D.
Professor, Department of Psychiatry, University of Wisconsin Medical School.

Ezra Susser, M.D.
Department of Psychiatry, College of Physicians and Surgeons of Columbia University.

Graham Thornicroft, M.A., M.Sc., M.R.C.Psych.,
Reader, PRiSM, Institute of Psychiatry, London.

Glenn J. Treisman, M.D., Ph.D.
Associate Professor, Department of Psychiatry and Behavioral Sciences
Director of Residency Education
Director of AIDS Psychiatric Service, Johns Hopkins University School of Medicine.

Laura Van Tosh
Technical Assistance Specialist, National Association of State Mental Health Program Directors, Alexandria, Virginia.

Donald Wasylenki, M.D., F.R.C.P.(C)
Psychiatrist-in-Chief, Department of Psychiatry
Wellesley/St. Michael's Mental Health Services, Toronto, Canada.

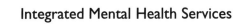

Integrated Mental Health Services

Modern
Community Psychiatry

WILLIAM R. BREAKEY

Community psychiatry has evolved over half a century. Its central premises have changed, and its emphasis has shifted with changes in philosophy, perspective, and public policy. In the 1950s and 1960s the term *community psychiatry* was used to define a theory-driven approach that focused on the social psychology of groups and social networks, the function of these relationships in promoting health, and the collective rather than individualistic aspects of human experience. This view emphasized the place of the person in the community and the influence of the social environment on the development of the individual and his or her capacity to adapt and be healthy. From these ideas came the concepts of mental hygiene and preventive psychiatry, based on the public health premise that disorders can be prevented or chronicity avoided by creating a healthy environment and providing the correct early interventions. The target for intervention was the community, and community psychiatry sought to understand the role of the community itself in promoting and enhancing mental health. Consultation and education became central functions for the community psychiatrist who adopted this perspective, with the goal that the community and its members should act in more healthful ways, benefitting individuals and the community as a whole.

Community has also been used in a more pragmatic sense, to refer to a target population for service provision—a usage that has come to predominate in the 1980s and 1990s. This approach views a community epidemiologically and addresses the clinical and administrative issues involved in providing services to the population. Interventions and treatments focus on individuals or small groups, but the service system is planned and organized with the aim of meeting the needs of a target population. This requires setting priorities for deployment of resources and concentrating in particular on the most severely ill. Working in the public sector, subject to the fluctuations in public budget-setting priorities, programs have often had to confront, and deal creatively with, the harsh realities of inadequate resources in government-funded programs. It is this approach that we have characterized as "modern community psychiatry."

Some prefer the term *community mental health.* Social workers and psychologists, in particular, but also nurses and people with training in counseling and related fields, have made important contributions both in theory and in practice. Community mental health emphasizes that many professionals, in addition to physicians, have important contributions to make in this field, and suggests that the emphasis should be on health rather than on disease. It has seemed to some critics of psychiatry that what was (inaccurately) described as "the medical model" is stultifying to a broader view of people in their social contexts. This book is written primarily for psychiatrists, however, so *community psychiatry* is used here, placing this field within the compass of psychiatry and establishing it as an integral part of the broad scope of the practice of medicine.

The methods of community psychiatry have evolved in the latter part of the twentieth century as the philosophy of caring for the mentally ill has shifted away from institution-based systems of care. To some extent, therefore, the field has been defined as a more humane and cost-effective alternative to older or outmoded ways of treating people with mental illness. This practical view is complemented by the central conceptual theme in community psychiatry that acknowledges the community as the place where people live and work, the place where their systems of social support are to be found, and the place where disorders of behavior, affect, or cognition originate and manifest themselves. Thus solutions should be sought in the community and therapeutic interventions applied there. In this view, institutional care is the least desirable of several options, only to be resorted to when other options are clearly inadequate.

At times, in recent years, it has seemed as if the efforts to provide better services for the mentally ill in the community were failing, as the public has become more and more outraged by the spectacle of mentally ill homeless people in the streets and by the tragedies striking some individuals whose illness ended in suicide or resulted in attacks on other people. This conclusion is premature, for bad outcomes are greatly outweighed by the many successes. The treatment of the mentally ill has been radically transformed over three decades from a situation where a chronically ill person could expect to spend the rest of his or her days in a barren and counter-therapeutic institution, in some cases subject to neglect and abuse. Today, a similar patient can expect to live closer to home and family, in a more normal environment, receiving a range of mental health services in accordance with his or her particular needs. The move of the locus of care for the mentally ill from institutions to the community has had advantages for patients and a number of benefits for psychiatry. A whole new range of methods has been developed, including the multidisciplinary team model of providing outpatient care, home-based care, case management, rehabilitation programming, and innovative strategies for housing.

Providing a comprehensive and integrated range of mental health services such as these presents major challenges, particularly in major cities or in sparsely inhabited rural areas. There are still too many places where a complete and responsive range of services does not exist, and there are still too many people who do not receive the services they need. This is not, however, because the methods of community psychiatry are inadequate to the task. We have learned over three decades most of what needs to be done. The reason that adequate service systems are not in place everywhere is that the political will does not exist to provide sufficient resources so that good systems of care can be developed everywhere.

Modern community psychiatry is concerned with organized systems of care and the development of cost-effective service models. In this sense, it holds the key to the future of psychiatric services in general. More and more, the solo practitioner and the psychiatric hospital are ceasing to be the focal points of psychiatric care; vertically organized and integrated systems of interconnected services are increasingly the norm. Medical priorities are balanced against consumer preferences and the dictates of the customers (government payers, insurance companies, and care managers); and approaches that are hallowed by tradition must give way under the pressure to demonstrate cost-effectiveness. The skills required to bring this about are precisely the skills that have been developed over several decades in the public sector as community mental health agencies designed and staffed integrated systems of care for the severely mentally ill.

The Public-Private Dichotomy

In the United States a public-private dichotomy in health services has persisted to a more marked degree than in other developed countries. Until recently, the private sector, comprising private physicians and hospitals, has depended largely on private insurance policies to make payment for services, and has only provided limited amounts of "charity care" to persons without the capacity to pay. Public sector mental health services have in most places been quite separate from the private hospitals and practitioners. In the mental health arena, public sector services (other than the federally funded services provided by the Department of Veterans' Affairs) have included the state and county hospitals and the community mental health networks, organized under state auspices since the demise of the federal Community Mental Health Centers in 1981.

Medicaid and Medicare, both federal programs, provide funds for indigent, disabled, or elderly people in certain circumstances to obtain services in the private sector, so that the public-private distinction begins to blur. An element of competition between levels of government exists, however, each having a powerful incentive to deflect costs to the budgets of the other. States have tried to use Medicaid funds to the maximum, hoping to relieve the burden on state mental health service budgets, while the federal government attempts to "return power to the states" by reducing the federal responsibility for local services and placing pressure on states to assume the burden.

Community psychiatry expertise has developed and been practiced within the public sector, and community psychiatrists have generally worked with people who are in the lower socioeconomic segments of the society. Community psychiatrists have been supporters of the public role in health service provision and believers in the government's responsibility for the health of the citizens. In the United States in the 1990s there is a national policy trend in the opposite direction, toward diminishing the role of government. The future looks bleak to those who rely on governmental funds for support, and it is not clear if and how the private sector will respond to fill the gaps left by government cut-backs.

In the United States in the 1990s, *managed care* is the predominant strategy to co-ordinate and control the supply of health care. Its premises are in one sense directly contrary to the traditional values of community psychiatry. Managed care seeks to control the supply of health care by erecting a variety of barriers or mechanisms to direct patients to less intensive treatment settings. This is accomplished, for example, through pre-admission screening of hospital admissions or pre-authorization of outpatient treatment. Managed care aims to reduce the amount of ''unnecessary'' or ''extravagant'' care through utilization review. Community psychiatry, on the other hand, has worked to minimize barriers to mental health services for people who might not otherwise have access, or might not seek help for a variety of reasons, on the principle that access to services and quality of care should not depend on capacity to pay.

Ultimately both systems are designed to promote efficient use of resources, and thus have much to learn from each other. New forms of service delivery in the private sector increasingly draw from methods developed in the public sector. Integrated systems of psychiatric services are being implemented to provide the array of services that an insured population needs. Inpatient care is being avoided where possible, largely on grounds of cost, and case management methods are being used to ensure that people are directed to the most effective and cost-effective treatment settings. As the government's role in providing health services changes, private managed care organizations are assuming responsibility for public mental health services in some states. Psychiatrists are going to have to learn how to work under these changed financial arrangements and must continue to contribute their insights into the treatment of populations in need.

In Britain, where the public-private distinction has been essentially eliminated for almost half a century, business principles and marketplace approaches from private industry are now being introduced with the aim of bringing greater efficiency to what was a bureaucratically controlled system. There, also, integrated systems of community-based care, governed by contracts between purchasers and providers, are replacing old systems of care for the severely mentally ill which were based on using mental hospitals and funded out of mental hospital and local health authority budgets.

Population Focus

Community psychiatry concerns itself with populations. Generally the target population is in a specific geographic area–the catchment or service area–although specialized programs may be targeted toward special populations, such as homeless people, AIDS victims, or children. This is an epidemiological perspective, which is why community psychiatrists should be familiar with the principles of psychiatric epidemiology. Epidemiology provides information about the extent of morbidity in the population, identifying subgroups at particular risk; it also provides methods for testing the effectiveness of interventions. While the traditional clinical approach confines its attention to those who present themselves for treatment, adopting an epidemiological perspective leads a service provider to be concerned also about those persons in the population who may have a psychiatric disorder but who do not spontaneously seek treatment.

The population focus of community psychiatry also includes a concern with cultural issues. A community psychiatrist must understand the ethnic composition and culture of the community served. This is important not only so that psychopathology can be correctly understood and therapy can be offered in a way that is meaningful to patients, but also so that services can be provided in a way that minimizes barriers to seeking help.

Community psychiatrists must listen to the voices of the populations they serve. This includes not only the formation of advisory boards and governing boards that include members of the community served, but also being receptive to, and learning from, the input from patients and their families, individually and through the advocacy organizations they form.

The Community Psychiatrist

In the 1960s and 1970s, most community mental health centers were directed by psychiatrists who were not necessarily trained for this role and often lacked administrative experience or expertise. Psychiatrists were also highly paid, relative to managers drawn from other professions. For these reasons, psychiatrists were increasingly moved out of the top administrative positions in community mental health centers (CMHCs), their places being taken by people who were from other mental health professions, or by professional administrators. Psychiatrists in such centers were assigned a purely clinical role, answerable to the executive director, without having ultimate authority over center policies. In the worst cases they were reduced to being prescription-signers, the primary clinical functions being assumed by therapists from other professions. Where decision making was controlled by professionals whose main skills and experience were in social intervention and psychotherapy, the centers tended to find most satisfaction in dealing with these issues. The "medical model" was devalued and the role of the psychiatrist diminished. Many psychiatrists found this situation intolerable, and they began to disappear from the CMHCs.

As deinstitutionalization proceeded, however, community programs were increasingly compelled to address the needs of the seriously ill. At the same time, effective medical treatments for major mental illnesses became available, and the utility of the disease perspective was recognized by more and more clinicians. The dangers of unskilled or reckless use of powerful psychoactive drugs also became apparent. Realizing that this is a challenging and satisfying area of practice, psychiatrists began to reassert the importance of psychiatry in community programs. The American Association of Community Psychiatrists was founded in 1984. Its most important initial goal was to establish and define the role of psychiatrists in community programs and to establish community psychiatry as a field with its own special skills and orientation.

Above all else, a community psychiatrist must be an excellent clinician. He or she must deal with extremely ill and disabled patients, often in circumstances where teams of psychiatric colleagues are not immediately available to give advice or assistance. A community psychiatrist must be skillful in the use of psychopharmacological agents, must understand family dynamics, must have an appreciation of the culture of different ethnic groups, and must understand the principles of rehabilitation. He or she also needs public health skills to understand the distribution of disorders within the community and to employ principles of primary, secondary, and tertiary prevention. He or she must also be able to function as a member of a multidisciplinary team.

Multidisciplinary Teamwork

Community psychiatry is a team effort, involving a variety of professionals working together to provide an array of support, treatment, and rehabilitative services. The role of the psychiatrist is central, but a psychiatrist alone is very limited in what he or she can do. The contributions of other professionals, such as social workers, nurses, psychologists, counselors, case managers, rehabilitation specialists, housing specialists, administrators, and support staff are vital if an adequate service system is to be developed. The psychiatrist is the team leader in planning treatment and supervising the execution of the plan. Part of the role is to draw out from other team members their particular skills, to train them in psychopathology and therapeutic methods, and to develop the whole team into a unit that provides state-of-the-art services to its patient population. This is not always as easy as it may seem. Resource limitations and time constraints burden everyone. Case loads get bigger and bigger and schedules get tighter and tighter, so that having time to develop the group's skill level and cohesion gets harder and harder. Interprofessional rivalries can breed conflict that militates against effective teamwork and presents a challenge to the team leader.

Integrated Systems of Services

A wide range of community service methods has been developed and is described in the later sections of this book. With the increasing numbers of programs and services, system integration is of central importance. The first aftercare clinics, established when patients started to leave the mental hospitals, were apparently believed to be adequate to meet the needs of deinstitutionalized patients. Hospital emergency rooms provided whatever other care was needed (Fig. 1–1). This simple view soon gave way, as the complexity of the needs of people with mental illnesses became apparent, to the twelve

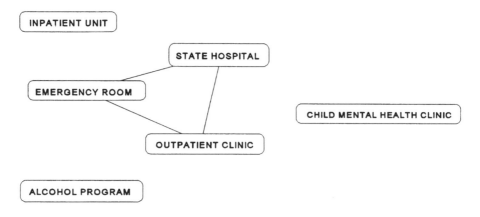

Figure 1–1 Mental Health Services in East Baltimore, 1975.

core services that were to be provided in federally funded CMHCs: inpatient treatment, outpatient treatment, partial hospitalization, emergency services, education and consultation, services for children and adolescents, services for the elderly, transitional living programs, substance abuse services, aftercare for patients being discharged from hospitals, screening of patients for admission to state hospitals, and program evaluation. The later CMHC legislation moved beyond the idea of a center as necessarily a single location to the idea of a center as a network of interconnected services provided under a series of contracts and agreements. The early 1980s produced the concept of *linkage,* encouraging mental health programs to develop formal working relationships with other health and social agencies. As methods of service provision became more and more sophisticated, increasingly complex service networks were needed, but as the networks became larger and more diffuse, patients or clients more easily became lost in them, so that *case management* developed to ensure that a person received the needed services and received them in a coordinated fashion.

Modern community psychiatry networks thus are complex systems of interconnected services (Fig. 1–2). In some cases, different programs are provided under the same management, but more often several public and private organizations provide services of different sorts. *Core service agencies,* or *lead agencies,* serve the function of coordinating the several groups that provide services in the area, ensuring that services are well integrated and that gaps in the system are identified and filled.

The Financing of Mental Health Services

Funding issues are vitally important, particularly in public programs. Community psychiatrists, perhaps more than psychiatrists in general, should be informed about developments in fiscal policies and must be active in responding to the challenges that new policies present in providing services in their own area. Despite its fundamental

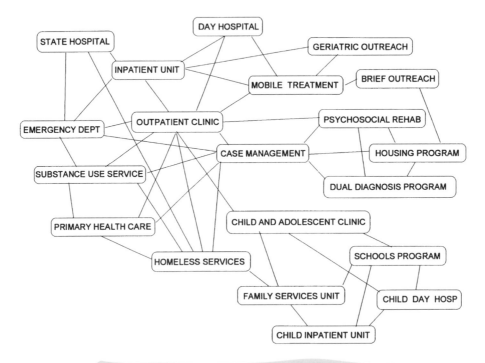

Figure 1–2 Mental Health Services in East Baltimore, 1995.

importance, the financing of mental health services is not addressed in this volume for two reasons. First, there is a great diversity of funding mechanisms. Each country has its own funding mechanisms, and in the United States, each state has its own variation. Adequately addressing all of these would be a herculean task. Second, this book is written in an era of dramatic change in funding mechanisms, particularly in the United States and United Kingdom. In the United States, where the public-private dichotomy has so far been preserved, the effects of managed care and utilization review are felt in both sectors; privatization of public services and capitation contracts are being experimented with, and the nation is struggling to understand and respond to the soaring cost of the Medicaid and Medicare programs and to address the problem of large numbers of uninsured and underinsured individuals. There is strong pressure for a national health care plan, but it is difficult to come up with one that is politically acceptable. In the United Kingdom, concepts from the business world have been introduced into the National Health Service, separating purchasing authorities from provider agencies, who must now compete with other providers for business in the internal market. Everywhere the emphasis is on efficiency and profitability. Every few months, it seems, there are new developments and new proposals.

Whatever the funding environment, however, the community psychiatrist's tasks remain those of providing high quality care to groups of people, seeking out and being responsive to the community's priorities, being creative in the use of whatever funding mechanisms are in place, making effective and efficient use of resources, and working collaboratively with the many other individuals and agencies who have roles in the prevention of disease, the promotion of health, and the care of those who are sick or disabled.

History and Context

I

2

The Rise and Fall
of the State Hospital

WILLIAM R. BREAKEY

The history of how mentally ill people have been cared for in America reflects not only changes in the scientific understanding of mental disorder, but also the political, social, and economic philosophies of the times (Grob, 1973). The seventeenth and eighteenth centuries viewed insanity as a problem with social, or spiritual, rather than medical implications, having much in common with other disruptive conditions such as criminality and pauperism. It was handled within the family or local community; as a last resort, an insane person could be confined in a jail or almshouse. In the nineteenth century, the concept of madness as illness began to be accepted, so that insanity came under the purview of physicians and the insane were treated in hospitals. However, the lack of real progress through science, and the abuses of hospitals in the twentieth century led to disillusionment with medical models and even to the idea on the part of some radicals that mental illness is a myth, developed for purposes of social control, and that mental patients should not be confined against their will (Foucault, 1971; Szasz, 1961). At the end of the twentieth century, science is at last beginning to unravel the biological and psychological bases of mental illness, and few people now believe that mental illness is a myth, although libertarian ideas continue to contribute to the movement away from institutional care in favor of less restrictive alternatives.

Progress in the care of the mentally ill is cyclical; history repeats itself (Armour, 1981; Goldman and Morrisey, 1985). The return of responsibility for the mentally ill to local communities in the latter half of the twentieth century, despite the benefits that have undoubtedly accrued for many patients, has for some meant a return to jails and homeless shelters, institutions intended not for care of the ill, but for custody of criminals and support of the poor. In some ways we appear to have come full circle since these words were written two centuries ago as a preamble to a petition for establishing the Pennsylvania Hospital:

THAT with the Numbers of People the Number of lunatics, or Persons distemper'd in Mind, and deprived of their rational Faculties, hath greatly increased in this province.

THAT some of them are going at large, are a Terror to their Neighbours, who are daily apprehensive of the Violences they may commit; and others are continually wasting their Substance, to the great Injury of themselves and Families, ill disposed Persons wickedly taking Advantage of their unhappy Condition, and drawing them into unreasonable bargains, &c.

(Benjamin Franklin, 1751, quoted by Grob, 1973)

These eighteenth-century observations echo very closely some of the concerns of modern-day mental health service providers, policy-makers, and the general public.

Several philosophical themes underlie this cyclical pattern: the general acceptance, enshrined in the English Poor Laws since Elizabethan times, of a public responsibility to care for those disabled by mental illness; the debate over which level of government should shoulder this responsibility; and the difficulty of obtaining sufficient public funds to support an adequate standard of service. These themes have recurred in each era up to the present day.

For two centuries, there was increasing reliance on institutional care for the mentally ill. The movement away from institutions is relatively recent, and the idea that care for large numbers of mentally ill people can be provided in the community in an urbanized society is still controversial. The history of public mental health services in the United States, therefore, is the history of the development and decline of state mental hospitals.*

The Colonial Period

During the early years of the American colonies, insanity was poorly understood and was often equated with demonic possession and witchcraft. These views of the origins of mental disorder, and the harsh responses arising from them, were exemplified by events in Salem, Massachusetts, in 1692. Several girls developed a pattern of what were probably dissociative symptoms (Veith, 1965), leading to accusations of witchcraft being made against them and against other people in the community. The outcome was communal uproar, a series of trials, severe punishments, and several executions.

The population was small and sparsely distributed in the colonies. If a person's behavior was disruptive or his ability to care for himself was severely impaired, responsibility to provide care rested first with the family and then with the local community. Some historians portray the treatment provided to the mentally ill in the colonial era as cruel and exploitive, citing cases where they were treated as servants, sold at auction like slaves, or expelled from towns and forced to travel to adjacent communities in search of shelter. Grob (1973) notes that in a frontier situation where

---

*Among those historians who have traced this history, none have done so with a level of scholarship to equal that of Gerald Grob, to whom the author is indebted for much of the information and many of the insights contained in this chapter.

the very survival of the family or community could be threatened by natural calamities or the burden of supporting unproductive individuals, in all likelihood the insane were accorded the best support that communities could afford.

The first hospital ward in the American Colonies for care of the sick and mentally deranged was established when the Pennsylvania Hospital opened in Philadelphia in 1752. The initial impetus came from Dr. Thomas Bond, who had visited the Bethlem Hospital in London. The effort was strongly supported by the Philadelphia Quakers, but many benefactors and the government of the colony were involved in raising the necessary funds, with Benjamin Franklin taking a central role.

The Era of Restraints

Benjamin Rush was the physician who some years later, in 1783, assumed charge of these patients. Sometimes described as the father of American psychiatry (Deutsch, 1937), he was a scientist, a physician, a reformer, and one of the signers of the Declaration of Independence. Rush attempted to integrate theories of constitutional and environmental influence on ethics and behavior. He believed that insanity was a brain disorder, and among his innovations was the ''tranquilizer'' chair, and a swinging centrifugal device by which the blood flow to a patient's brain would supposedly be increased, with anticipated therapeutic benefit. The example of the Pennsylvania Hospital was partly responsible for a movement to establish a hospital in New York. As in Philadelphia, a coalition of people with humanitarian and political interests attempted to gain support and funds. Dr. Samuel Bard, a friend of Benjamin Franklin and a medical graduate of Edinburgh University, led a campaign that resulted in the establishment of a medical school in New York at King's College (later Columbia University). The New York Hospital opened in 1791 with the intent of including the mentally ill among those served, although between 1792 and 1794 fewer than ten such patients were admitted (Grob, 1973).

The first public asylum was opened in 1773, at Williamsburg, Virginia. Conditions there during the early years were more custodial than therapeutic, the institution being run by lay keepers with little medical input. The hospital was very small and did little to influence the development of hospitals elsewhere (Grob, 1973). A similar venture was launched in neighboring Maryland in 1797. The effort failed initially, but the hospital was properly established under state auspices in 1836. Now known as Spring Grove Hospital Center, it has continued to have a major role in Maryland's mental health service system.

These early ventures into establishing hospital care for the mentally ill are notable as the starting points for an approach that would be central to care of the mentally ill for two centuries. Their primitiveness should not be overlooked. Small numbers of patients were cared for, and the methods for treatment were harsh and punitive. Patients were sometimes confined in very poor conditions; various forms of strait waistcoats and other restraints were standard; bleeding, emetics, and blisterings were among the medical treatments employed. For one short period, the Pennsylvania Hospital charged a fee for members of the public to view the lunatics.

Moral Treatment

Toward the end of the eighteenth century more enlightened approaches began to be introduced, associated most strongly with the names of Phillippe Pinel in Paris and William Tuke in England, and employing a set of principles that came to be known as Moral Treatment. Pinel was an empiricist, and he developed new ways of analyzing the phenomena of mental illness (Pinel, 1806). However, his claim to a place in history comes less from his scholarship than from his reformist approaches to care of the mentally ill. In this he was inspired by the work of several predecessors and by contemporary ideas of freedom and justice, in addition to his empirical observations on the futility of treatments employing cruelty and restraint. In 1793 Pinel became the medical superintendent of the Bicêtre and Salpetrière hospitals in Paris. The conditions he found there were miserable, with patients essentially chained and fettered in filthy cells. He removed their restraints and introduced treatment approaches based on firm but humane measures, relying on their higher instincts to mold their behavior in appropriate and acceptable patterns. He was able to demonstrate that when patients were treated in a more dignified and humane manner, they became less violent, less disturbed in their thoughts, and, in some cases, able to be rehabilitated.

Independent of Pinel's work in Paris, the Society of Friends in York, England, established a hospital for those of their members who suffered from mental disorders. William Tuke became the director of the York Retreat, which opened in 1792. The principles employed were very like those of Pinel; there was a similar lack of reliance on restraint and physical treatments and an emphasis on the patient's ability to gain control over his own thought and behavior through rigorous discipline. The task was seen as analogous to that of raising children, and the method sought to induce improved motivations or morals in the patient, which gave the method its name. Like many other reformers of mental health services, neither William Tuke nor his son Samuel, who succeeded him in his work, was a physician. Samuel Tuke's publication of the *Description of the Retreat* in 1813 was instrumental in the wide dissemination of their ideas, as far as the United States. Through the efforts of American Quakers a number of hospitals were developed in the United States in the early nineteenth century, including the Friends Asylum in Philadelphia, the Bloomingdale Asylum in New York, the McLean Asylum in Massachusetts, and the Hartford Retreat in Connecticut.

It should be noted that while these hospitals constituted a base from which psychiatry as a profession could emerge (Grob, 1973), they had a limited role in the development of public mental health services. They provided valuable services in their communities and were established with the aim of serving all economic classes. However, they were not large institutions, and they were unable to cope with the growing numbers of patients who needed care. Insane paupers still had to make do with the poorhouses, the jails, the streets, and the hedgerows. The enlightened new approaches were not yet available for them.

The Role of the State

Eighteenth-century America was largely rural and sparsely populated. The nineteenth century was characterized by enormous immigration and population growth, urbanization, industrialization, mobility, and the growth of the institutions of a modern state. In the early decades of the century a movement began to establish that states had a responsibility for care of the growing numbers of the insane, particularly those who were indigent. Massachusetts took the lead. The reformer Horace Mann was largely responsible for legislation to establish a state institution at Worcester in 1833. Its first superintendent, Samuel B. Woodward, was also elected the first president of the Association of Medical Superintendents of American Institutions for the Insane in 1844. His annual reports, which spoke enthusiastically of the benefits of a well-run hospital, contributed to the growing impetus for establishment of mental hospitals in every state.

This movement for establishing state hospitals was associated above all with the name of Dorothea Lynd Dix, a prosperous Boston Unitarian and former teacher who devoted her life to social reform. In 1841 she agreed to teach a Sunday school class for women in the East Cambridge Jail, and in the course of her visits she became aware of the conditions in which the inmates were living. In particular, she noted that along with criminals, a number of mentally ill people were confined there, living in squalid conditions, with little care and attention and no heat in the New England winter. Appalled by what she had found, Dorothea Lynd Dix surveyed other jails and poorhouses in Massachusetts and found similar conditions. Dix had some knowledge of enlightened approaches, having earlier visited the York Retreat and being familiar with the Worcester State Hospital. She began a vigorous campaign in Massachusetts to improve conditions for the mentally ill. She encountered much opposition in these efforts, but eventually her advocacy led to the enlarging of the overcrowded Worcester hospital. Encouraged by this success in Massachusetts, she turned her attention first to other Northeastern states, and then further south. In each state she documented the poor conditions in which insane persons were confined and persuaded legislatures to establish hospitals. Proceeding in this way, Dix and her supporters crusaded for 40 years. They provided energy and direction for one expression of a growing national sense of the need to support the expanding and increasingly complex society with institutions for education, culture, health care, and philanthropy.

Dix was one of the first of many advocates from outside the mental health professions who have played vital roles in the development of American public mental health systems. She and her collaborators not only spurred the widespread development of new facilities but, more important, they ensured the acceptance of the principle that the care of the poor and mentally ill cannot be left to the local community and is a responsibility of the state. These victories were not easily won. In every state, years of advocacy, political maneuvering, and searching for funds were required before hospitals could be established. Taxpayers and decision makers were not easily convinced that the mentally ill deserved better treatment.

The middle decades of the nineteenth century marked what was perhaps the greatest period of expansion of mental health services that this country has ever seen. Between 1825 and 1865 the number of mental hospitals grew from nine to sixty-two. The need for an organization to support the physicians working in these hospitals led to the formation in 1844 of the Association of Medical Superintendents of American Institutions for the Insane, which later became The American Medico-Psychological Association and ultimately The American Psychiatric Association.

After its initial period of growth, carried along by the enthusiasm and dedication of its founders, the momentum slowed, and the ideals of moral treatment gradually were obscured. Several factors contributed to a decline in quality of treatment. One was that while advocates had been successful in having funds appropriated for the building of hospitals, states had much greater difficulty in making funds available on a long-term basis for operating budgets to staff, equip, and extend the facilities as needs continued. Also, almost from the start, overcrowding became a problem. Soon after hospitals opened, they filled up, an early example of the now well-known principle in health services that "supply creates demand." As early as 1854, the Superintendent of Worcester State Hospital was complaining that the demand for treatment and the consequent overcrowding were such that they had to resort excessively to confining and restraining patients, rather than involving them in therapeutic activities (quoted in Grob, 1973). The increase in demand also arose to some extent from the enormous expansion of population that took place in the nineteenth century and continued into the twentieth. The population of the United States in 1820 was 9.6 million; by 1900 it had multiplied eight-fold to 76 million; and by 1980 had tripled again to 222 million. The number of asylums grew to 62 by 1865 and to approximately 200 by the middle of the twentieth century. This expansion was insufficient, however, to keep up with the needs of the population.

The effects of having to deal with large numbers of immigrants also contributed to the decline in the standards of care in the state hospitals. Many immigrants had great difficulty in adjusting to life in the United States, and the prevalence of psychiatric disorders among them was high. One way of coping with large numbers of immigrant patients was by recruiting immigrant employees who might, in theory, be more understanding of these patients' needs. In many cases, unfortunately, these employees had very limited understanding of enlightened principles of mental health care, had difficulty communicating with colleagues and patients, and were able only to provide elementary custodial treatment.

The accumulation of chronic patients in the twentieth century contributed further to overcrowding and deterioration in quality of care. Patients in state hospitals in the nineteenth century were not, by and large, those who today would be described as "chronic." The nineteenth-century hospital psychiatrists were therapeutic optimists who expected patients to be substantially cured in a matter of months (Deutsch, 1937).

The care of patients in state hospitals was paid for by the local community. It was therefore to the community's financial advantage that a patient who appeared to be incurable would be transferred back to his or her local community, to be kept in an almshouse or other local facility at lower cost, although often in very poor conditions. Toward the end of the nineteenth century, because of the conditions in which many of the "incurable insane" were kept, states took over responsibility for these people too. After 1900 the proportion of chronic patients in state hospitals increased rapidly. New York established an asylum specifically for incurables, but generally the preferred approach was to keep the incurables in the same institution as the curables. One consequence, which may not have been anticipated, was that local communities perceived an opportunity to shift the care of the elderly infirm from their almshouses to the state-run institutions, by redefining them as insane, on the basis of poor memory or inability to care for themselves. Thus a new trend was started: The indigent elderly were cared for in state hospitals. By mid-century the hospitals were swamped with chronic and geriatric patients (Grob, 1991).

Changes taking place within psychiatry around the turn of the century were also significant. Partly because of the frustration experienced in dealing with overwhelming numbers of patients, and partly because moral treatment had been oversold by the early enthusiasts, psychiatrists tended to move away from their earlier emphasis on the therapeutic environment and became more interested in the scientific advances that were being reported, especially from Germany, in understanding the topographical and functional organization of the brain. They came to concentrate on the understanding of mental illness as resulting from incurable brain disorders and to seek advances in its treatment through the study of brain pathology. Medicine was establishing its own scientific foundations in the early years of the twentieth century. In 1910, the Flexner Report stressed the fundamental importance of science in the training of physicians. Psychiatry, however, had no empirical scientific basis at this stage and was unable to share in the growth of twentieth-century scientific medicine—at least until the second half of the century. Instead, American psychiatry looked to the emerging theories of psychoanalysis for an understanding of the phenomena of mental life. Psychiatrists and certain of their patients found in the new models some hope that the abnormalities of mental life could be understood. As a consequence, the intellectual excitement of psychiatry moved out of the mental hospital wards into private offices. It became the goal of psychiatrists to practice psychotherapy with those patients who could participate in such therapy, and many of them abandoned the hospitals, especially those that provided asylum to the poor.

Public mental hospitals in the twentieth century came to be viewed as the backwaters of psychiatry. Vast numbers of patients were confined in them and were provided with treatment that was mediocre or worse. Staffs were inadequate in number and poorly trained; wards were often overcrowded; and it was commonly assumed that admission to a state hospital was a life sentence. Nevertheless, these institutions were the sole source of treatment for most mentally ill people. Since the mid-nineteenth century, the numbers of people in American state and county mental hospitals had been increasing year by year until 1955, when the number peaked at 550,000 (Fig. 2–1). This increase occurred not only because of increasing tendencies to institutionalize patients, but also because of increases in the population of the United States and increasing prevalence of disabling mental illnesses due to increased longevity of psychiatric patients (Gruenberg, 1977). Until the introduction of electric convulsive therapy in the 1940s, there were no specific medical treatments available for treating mental illnesses. The moral treatment approaches were impractical in the overcrowded and understaffed institutions. Although many fine and dedicated professionals worked in the state hospitals under very difficult circumstances, conditions for patients were often demeaning and dehumanizing, and abuse of patients occurred in many places. It is not surprising that the fear and stigma associated with mental illness increased and that admission to the mental hospital was dreaded as much as, or more than, being sentenced to prison.

Hospitals varied greatly in size, and some were enormous. In the 1950s there were eighteen hospitals in the United States housing more than 5,000 patients and several with close to 20,000 patients. They were worlds unto themselves, often remote from urban centers. In many cases staff lived on the hospital campus, in a culture with its own norms, its own systems of exchange, and its own hierarchy (Goffman, 1962). As early as 1894, mental hospital superintendents had been rebuked for their isolationism and shortsightedness. The noted neurologist Weir Mitchell, at the fiftieth anniversary of the American Psychiatric Association, criticized psychiatrists and the culture of the mental hospitals:

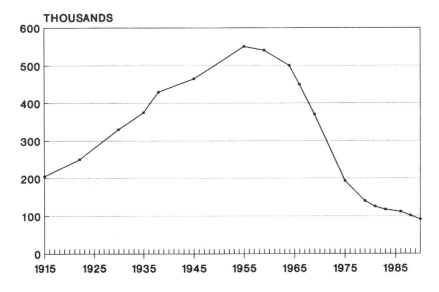

Figure 2–1 Year End Census, U.S. State and County Mental Hospitals.

It is the system which is most to blame, (but) my fear is that some of you would not change your organization if you could. . . . You live alone, uncriticized, unquestioned, out of the healthy conflicts and honest rivalries which keep most of us up to the mark of the fullest possible competence. The whole system has been let to harden into organized shapes which are difficult to reform.

You ought not to live and sleep in your hospitals at all; you ought to be in contact with the world of sane men, having consultations outside, seeing us and our societies. A good deal of this can never be had in your hospitals, for incredible folly has put most of them remote from cities. . . .

I may be wrong as to some men and some hospitals, but fifty years hence another will possibly stand in my place and tell your history, and to him and the beautiful wisdom of time I leave it to be declared whether I was right or wrong.

Obviously, events showed that Weir Mitchell was right, and indeed it did take 50 years before the mainstream of psychiatry was willing to acknowledge that what he said was true.

Seeking New Approaches

Clifford Beers was a remarkable figure in advocacy for renewal and reform in the early part of the twentieth century (Dain, 1980). Beers, a Yale graduate who was starting a business career, suffered from bipolar disorder and was hospitalized on a number of occasions in public and private institutions in New England. In 1907, in *A Mind That Found Itself,* he vividly described his experiences in the hospitals, the ill treatment to which he had been subjected, and the harsh conditions to which psychiatric patients were exposed (Beers, 1981). His book was a clarion call for reform in the treatment of the mentally ill. Perhaps carried along by hypomanic energy, he launched a movement that resulted, in 1908, in the founding of the Connecticut Association for Mental Hygiene, and in 1909 the National Committee for Mental Hygiene, now known as the Mental Health Association, an organization which, over the years, partly through its numerous local chapters, has played a major role in advocacy for improved mental health services. In spite of these promptings, however, little changed in the early decades of the century. The state hospital continued in its unchallenged position as virtually the sole provider of services for the severely mentally ill.

The deterioration of conditions in mental hospitals accelerated in the 1930s with the Great Depression. The need for public services increased as poverty increased, but the public funds available to meet the need were shrinking. In the early 1940s national energies were focused on fighting World War II and little progress was made, but when the war ended, there was an increasing demand for change. A number of important ideas and concepts that emerged from the experiences of the two World Wars contributed significantly to developing improved methods for treating the mentally ill. Psychiatrists had been impressed during World War I by the number of soldiers with psychiatric disorders, including those who developed "shell shock," a condition that would now be described as post-traumatic stress disorder. This awareness of the importance of psychological factors in the military led to the development of new screening methods for recruits in World War II. The large numbers of individuals who were found to have some degree of impairment aroused considerable concern and contributed to a new wave of interest in methods of psychiatric treatment. William C. Menninger, who was chief of psychiatric services for the military during World War II, observed that psychiatric casualties were most effectively treated if they remained close to the front rather than being evacuated to a military hospital remote from the firing line. After the war he applied this insight to work in the community and became an advocate for early intervention and keeping mentally ill patients close to their homes, families, and social environment.

The impetus for change was increased by new understandings of the importance of social factors in the psychiatric hospital. Stanton and Schwartz (1954) published a sociological analysis of the workings of the mental hospital. They emphasized that a mental hospital is different from a medical hospital in that its social structure has an impact on the psychiatric status of its patients that may be as great as that of any treatment prescribed. In 1961 Irving Goffman published a popular exposé of the peculiar relationships that exist within a "total institution" and how its social structure fosters the development of a special culture that can work against expected goals of rehabilitation. One of the clinical innovations that emerged from the social psychiatric studies in that period was the concept of the "therapeutic community," which originated with Maxwell Jones in London (Jones, 1953). This concept holds that the hospital community, if properly organized, is in itself a therapeutic agent; patients and staff together form a social system with therapeutic potential.

In 1961 Wing and Brown published an important study of three English mental hospitals which, in the way they were managed, represented three points on a continuum of authoritarianism and routine deemphasis of patients' individuality. They demonstrated that in the hospital that had the highest degree of individual attention devoted to patients, with the greatest opportunities for them to exercise independent judgment and decision making, the likelihood of patients being discharged was significantly greater than in more restrictive settings.

Other important contributions were made by Ernest Gruenburg, who in the 1950s developed his concept of the "social breakdown syndrome," a pattern of disability that characterizes the behavior of the chronic psychiatric patient. Gruenberg visited England, under the sponsorship of the Milbank Memorial Fund, where he was impressed by the open, community-oriented English mental hospitals. He returned to New York and established an experiment designed to prevent the social breakdown syndrome by encouraging the treatment of individuals within the community and the establishment of strong linkages between the community, social and health services, and the state hospital (Gruenberg et al., 1969).

Prompted by new information and new ideas, movements were begun after the war to develop new patterns of caring for the mentally ill, using methods superior to those employed in the traditional hospitals. In 1946 the National Mental Health Act was passed, resulting in the establishment of The National Institute of Mental Health, a new federal agency to sponsor research and training in psychiatry and to encourage the development of improved methods of mental health care, with an emphasis on outpatient services. The Joint Commission on Mental Illness and Health, set up by Congress in 1955, echoed this emphasis. The Commission documented the sad state of American mental health services, describing mental hospitals that were outmoded, overcrowded, primitive, and anti-therapeutic. In their 1961 report, *Action for Mental Health,* the Commission advocated a shift for the mental health service system away from dependence on state hospitals and toward a new system of community-based mental health care (Joint Commission on Mental Illness and Health, 1961). In 1963 President Kennedy introduced new legislation to Congress. His address to both houses of Congress constituted a clarion call for a new era in mental health services in America (Kennedy, 1963). The Commission's plan, translated into legislation, called for the development of a network of community mental health centers around the country that would enable many mentally ill people, unnecessarily confined to hospitals, to return to the care of their families in their own communities. Kennedy accurately predicted that within a few decades the population of the hospitals would be reduced by 50 percent.

The decrease in hospital censuses, ending a century of increasing reliance on institutional care, began in 1955 and has continued year by year since that time. The introduction of neuroleptic drugs in 1956 was undoubtedly a factor in this revolutionary change in policy and practice, but it is generally agreed that social, philosophical, and political factors were at least of equal importance in bringing about the change. Kennedy's address to Congress and the passage of the Mental Retardation Facilities and Community Mental Health Centers Construction Act in 1963 officially marked the end of the preeminence of state hospitals in America's mental health system and the beginning of the era of deinstitutionalization.

Deinstitutionalization

The proposal for a federally funded system of community mental health centers in every part of the country was equal in importance and in magnitude to the revolution that had occurred with the establishment of state hospitals (Goldman and Morrissey, 1985). Responsibility for the care of the psychiatrically ill and disabled, which had shifted a century before from the local communities to the states, was being shared by the federal government. The principal locus of care for the mentally ill was moving away from the mental hospitals, into "the community."

The movement was reinforced by a series of social, political, and economic trends with broad significance for the entire population, which lent strong support to the initiatives for discarding the old system of care for the mentally ill. One was the renewed emphasis on civil rights, out of which grew the doctrine that patients should be treated in the least restrictive setting possible. Another was the pressure to reduce government spending, specifically the enormous expense of maintaining state hospitals.

Deinstitutionalization was greatly facilitated by the availability of federal funding

for support of the disabled through the Social Security legislation of the 1960s and
1970s. Supplemental Security Income (SSI), Social Security Disability Income (SSDI),
Medicare, and Medicaid made it financially possible for mentally disabled people to
survive outside hospitals and to receive essential medical care. Social Security and
Medicare also made it possible for many of the elderly patients in state hospitals to
be moved to nursing homes. This had the effect of reducing state hospital censuses,
but it did not reduce reliance on institutional models of care (Kramer, 1977). With
the development of federally funded community mental health centers in the 1960s
and 1970s, and new payment mechanisms for the indigent, access to a spectrum of
outpatient services began to be available in many places.

For a number of reasons, state hospitals have not been closed as rapidly as the
architects of deinstitutionalization had foreseen. In 1993 there were still 256 state-
operated psychiatric hospitals in the United States (Lutterman, 1994). Deinstitutionalization has been effected by downsizing rather than closure of hospitals. While
hospitals are being phased out or reduced in size, there is nonetheless a need for them
to maintain adequate standards of care. Indeed, as standards of care everywhere are
raised, it is necessary to make additional investment to keep hospitals in line with
current practice. This entails continuing investment of funds and the recruitment of
good staff. At the same time, additional funds are needed to establish and maintain a
system of community services to support the patients who are being discharged. These
services, if properly provided, are costly also. Thus both systems must be funded
while the transition is in progress, a type and scale of expenditure that state legislatures
are generally reluctant to approve. In many cases local political and business interests,
and the concerns of employees facing redundancy, have stood in the way of closing
hospitals. It was reported, for example, in 1992, that the State of New York was
keeping a large hospital open, caring for only fourteen patients, because of local
political pressure (Verhovek, 1992).

Apart from funding considerations, there was a dearth of community resources.
Suitably trained staff, facilities, and technology all take time to develop. The fiscal
and technical problems of developing sophisticated systems of community-based care
in a period of a few years were formidable. The ultimate problem, however, in downsizing the state hospitals has been an overall increase in the demand for psychiatric
inpatient services. In 1969 there were 1.3 million admissions to psychiatric inpatient
units of all sorts in the United States. In 1986 there were 1.8 million. This represents
an increase in admission rates from 644 to 760 per 100,000 civilian population. Hospital censuses were falling, but admission rates were rising, reflecting increased demand for more short-term treatment for acute problems. This greater demand for
psychiatric inpatient services was largely met by other types of hospitals: The share
of all psychiatric admissions accepted by state hospitals fell from 38 percent in 1969
to 18 percent in 1986, while the proportion being admitted to private psychiatric
hospitals and psychiatric units of general hospitals increased from 45 percent to 60
percent over the same period (National Institute of Mental Health, 1990). Considerable

pressure persists to retain state hospitals for people who lack the insurance coverage to finance admission elsewhere or for patients who are dangerous or very severely disabled. There has thus been a major change in the patient population of state hospitals. Most long-stay patients have been discharged to community-based care or transfered to nursing homes or similar facilities. The state hospital population now is made up of people who are uninsured or underinsured, and it includes a much higher proportion of acute and highly disturbed patients than in the 1960s (National Institute of Mental Health, 1990).

Thus, though their centrality has been diminished, state hospitals still play a major part in the provision of public mental health services, and the question of their future is unresolved. The cycles of neglect and deteriorating standards, reformers' zeal, exposés, and public outcry have a long history and continue at the end of the twentieth century.

The trends in health care in the early 1990s are in the direction of marketplace controls and privatization of public facilities, and it is not clear what the future holds for state hospitals in this climate. There is a small residual population of very disabled, very disturbed, or very dangerous individuals who will need institutional care for the rest of their lives. It is the opinion of most people that these individuals will need to remain in residential care indefinitely, but there is as yet no consensus as to the size of this group of patients, or as to the type of facility that can provide optimal care for them. To a large extent the future of state hospitals depends on the degree of success with which modern community psychiatry is able to meet the challenge of caring for the mentally ill in alternative settings.

References

Armour, P.K. (1981) *The Cycles of Social Reform.* Washington, D.C.: University Press of America.

Beers, C.W. (1907, 1981) *A Mind That Found Itself.* Pittsburgh: University of Pittsburgh Press.

Dain, N. (1980) *Clifford Beers: Advocate for the Insane.* Pittsburgh: University of Pittsburgh Press.

Deutsch, A. (1937) *The Mentally Ill in America.* New York: Columbia University Press.

Foucault, M. (1971) *Madness and Civilization: A History of Insanity in the Age of Reason.* New York: Plume Books.

Flexner, A. (1910) *Medical Education in the United States and Canada.* New York: Carnegie Foundation for the Advancement of Teaching.

Goffman, E. (1962) *Asylums.* Chicago: Aldine.

Goldman, H.H., and Morrisey, J.P. (1985) The Alchemy of Mental Health Policy: Homelessness and the Fourth Cycle of Reform. *American Journal of Public Health,* 75:727–731.

Grob, G. (1973) *Mental Institutions in America.* New York: The Free Press.

Grob, G. (1991) The chronically mentally ill in America: The historical context. In Fransen, V.E. (ed.), *Mental Health Services in the United States and England: Struggling for Change.* Princeton, N.J.: The Robert Wood Johnson Foundation.

Gruenberg, E.M. (1977) The Failures of Success. *Milbank Memorial Fund Quarterly: Health and Society,* 55:3–24.

Gruenberg, E.M., Snow, H.B., and Bennett, C.L. (1969) Preventing the social breakdown syndrome. In Redlich, F.C., *Social Psychiatry.* Baltimore: Williams and Wilkins.

Joint Commission on Mental Illness and Health (1961) *Action for Mental Health: Final Report of the Commission.* New York: Basic Books.

Jones, M. (1953) *The Therapeutic Community: A New Treatment Method.* New York: Basic Books.

Kennedy, J.F. (1963) "Message on Mental Illness and Mental Retardation," Feb. 5, 1963, *Congressional Record,* 88(1), CIX, Part 2, 1744–1749.

Kramer, M. (1977) *Psychiatric services and the changing institutional scene, 1959–1985.* NIMH Series B, No 12. Washington, D.C.: Alcohol, Drug Abuse and Mental Health Administration.

Lutterman, T.C. (1994) The State Mental Health Agency Profile System. In Manderscheid, R.W., and Sonnenschein M.A. (eds.), *Mental Health, United States, 1994.* DHHS Publication No. (SMA) 94-3000. Washington, D.C.: U.S. Department of Health and Human Services.

National Institute of Mental Health (1990) *Mental Health, United States, 1990.* Manderscheid, R.W. and Sonnenschein, M.A., eds. DHHS Publication No. (ADM) 90-1708. Washington, D.C.: Supt. of Docs., U.S. Govt. Printing Office.

Pinel, P. (1806, 1962) *A Treatise on Insanity.* Translated by D.D. Davis, Sheffield, England. Facsimile edition, New York: Hafner.

Stanton, A.H., and Schwartz, M.S. (1954) *The Mental Hospital.* London: Tavistock Press.

Szasz, T. (1961) *The Myth of Mental Illness.* New York: Harper and Row.

Tuke, S. (1813) *Description of the Retreat, an Institution near York for Insane Persons of the Society of Friends.* York: W. Alexander.

Veith, I. (1965) *Hysteria: The History of a Disease.* Chicago: University of Chicago Press.

Verhovek, S.H. (1992) Emptied mental hospital is still open, still costly. *New York Times,* October 4.

Wing, J.K., and Brown, G.W. (1961) Social treatment of chronic schizophrenia: A comprehensive survey of three mental hospitals. *Journal of Mental Science,* 107:847–861.

3

Developmental Milestones for Community Psychiatry

WILLIAM R. BREAKEY

Origins

Home-based or community-based care for the mentally ill has been practiced on a small scale in Europe and America for centuries. As early as the thirteenth century, in Gheel, Belgium, mentally ill people were brought for healing to the shrine of St. Dymphna. Dymphna was an Irish princess who was martyred there, having fled from the incestuous advances of her father. A tradition developed, which has persisted until today, of caring for mentally ill people in the homes of people in the surrounding community. In seventeenth-century New England, also, patients were boarded in people's homes in Massachusetts and Connecticut. In the modern era, state-sponsored arrangements for care of mental patients in families were instituted in Massachusetts in 1885 and in New York in 1935 (Caton, 1984). Nevertheless, these efforts were small in scale. For more than a century, the mentally ill were treated almost exclusively in institutions, and the main emphasis did not shift to community-based care until the latter half of the twentieth century.

There were, however, several influential developments in the preceding decades. One of the first effective challenges to the prevailing methods of hospital treatment came with Clifford Beers's *A Mind That Found Itself* (1907), and the foundation of the National Committee for Mental Hygiene (Dain, 1980). This organization, which later became the Mental Health Association, has constantly pressed for reform of the public mental health service system and continues as a foremost advocacy group for improved services.

Another important contribution to the shift in emphasis away from asylum-based psychiatry was the development of psychiatric units in association with medical schools and general hospitals. This advance was exemplified by the opening of a psychiatric unit at the Albany Hospital in New York in 1902 (Lipowski, 1981), the opening of the Boston Psychopathic Hospital in association with Harvard Medical

School in 1912, and the establishment of the Henry Phipps Psychiatric Clinic at The Johns Hopkins Hospital in 1913. The movement toward a community perspective can be discerned in remarks made at that time by Adolf Meyer, the first director of the Phipps Clinic and the first professor of psychiatry at The Johns Hopkins University School of Medicine:

> I consider it of the greatest importance that the clinic make itself responsible for the mental health work of a fairly well circumscribed unit of population, so as to make possible studies of the dynamic factors which lead to the occurrence of mental derangement which must be attacked for purposes of prevention.
>
> (Meyer, 1913)

He thus expressed his hope that the new approach to psychiatry that would be taught at the Phipps would have a clear epidemiological, community focus.

However, the most influential development in psychiatry in the first half of the twentieth century was psychoanalysis. Freud and his followers provided a theory that would enable disordered behavior and thinking to be explained in a way that had never been possible before. The incomprehensible could be comprehended. Psychoanalysis had two effects that may be considered to have helped prepare the way for community psychiatry. One was to emphasize psychological and social factors in determining human behavior. The other was to encourage the development of outpatient office practice, as opposed to hospital practice, for psychiatrists.

The Postwar Years

The movement away from the asylums thus began in the early decades of the twentieth century, but their central role in the treatment of mental illness was essentially unchallenged until the 1940s and World War II. Two aspects of the experience of military psychiatrists were very influential in developing an impetus for change. One was a new realization of the widespread occurrence of psychiatric disorder. This had been observed in military recruits in World War I, and it had been recognized that psychiatric disorders could be significantly disabling (Foley and Sharfstein, 1983). Improved methods to screen recruits were developed in World War II, and the large number of men who failed to pass the screen was all the more impressive. A second observation made in both wars was that otherwise stable individuals can develop significant psychiatric symptoms under conditions of extreme stress, emphasizing the etiological importance of environmental conditions and events.

In 1944, Erich Lindemann published his seminal findings describing the psychiatric consequences of a disaster, a fire at the Cocoanut Grove nightclub in Boston. He described the effects of the disaster on the survivors, as well as the evident effectiveness of early intervention. One development from this was the idea of crisis intervention, based on the premise that many disorders, or ''reactions,'' develop in response to a crisis in a person's life and that serious emotional problems can be avoided if there is a prompt and energetic intervention. This approach provided the promise of at least secondary prevention.

Several other new approaches were developed in the postwar years. One was partial hospitalization. Day hospitals were first introduced in Russia; from there the concept spread to England and Canada after World War II and then to the United States. The idea that psychiatric hospital treatment can be provided without the patient necessarily spending all 24 hours in the hospital does not now seem revolutionary. The principle has been tested many times and found to be highly effective and less costly than full inpatient care. It clearly represents a move away from the notion that psychiatric patients need total hospital-based care, but its acceptance has been extraordinarily slow (see Chapter 18).

A concept that contributed to the development of day hospitals, but also contributed to a better understanding of the importance of milieu, was that of the "therapeutic community" (Jones, 1953). This method, employed initially in inpatient settings, holds that the people on the unit, patients as well as all categories of staff, constitute a therapeutic community. Each person in the community has a contribution to make to the treatment of the others. Many therapeutic decisions are made by group process rather than professional prescription; the emphasis is on the ward community as the healing agency.

Similar principles were embodied in another new type of psychiatric facility, the "halfway house," first established in Boston in 1954. This model was to be widely replicated in many places in succeeding years. The halfway house is generally located in an ordinary neighborhood setting and provides residential accommodation for people with mental disorders who need a supportive and structured environment, but who are not sufficiently symptomatic or dysfunctional to need hospitalization. Generally such programs are designed to provide a temporary residence, an intermediate stage in a person's transition from hospital to home. They often expect residents to be out at work during the day and employ group therapy approaches in the evening to assist residents in their adjustment. Halfway houses of this sort were not designed to meet the needs of the severely mentally ill for long-term residential care, but may be considered to be forerunners of the modern residential programs that serve this population.

Another new development in this era which was to be very influential was mental health consultation. The underlying premise was that conflict, distress, or disorder generally occur as responses to anxiety or conflict-producing situations in the social environment. In a situation such as a school, a factory, or a human service agency, a mental health consultant could assist the organization to identify and eliminate stress-producing situations or dynamics. In this way noxious influences on the mental health of employees or members of the organization could be reduced or eliminated. Consultation could be client-centered, that is, aimed at producing change in a client or patient; or consultee-centered, aimed at producing change in the consultee that would indirectly affect the organization; or it could be program-centered, focusing more specifically on seeking system change (Caplan, 1970). Consultation was thus an indirect service, where the service-provider did not come in direct contact with the person or persons who were the targets of the intervention. It offered promise of spreading the effect of the mental health worker's intervention by influencing the mental health of a group through changes brought about in the consultee or the organization, and it held out promise of offering primary prevention. Mental health consultation in the 1960s and 1970s would come to be regarded by many as a core activity of community mental health practitioners, and of the CMHCs, although its effectiveness was never well demonstrated (Mannino and Shore, 1979).

The prevailing view in American psychiatry during this period continued to be that mental disorders had their origins not so much in the brain as in the social and emotional environment of the individual, especially during the developmental years. Psychoanalysis focused on early childhood, and Adolph Meyer stressed that a person's behavior and mental life were constantly being affected throughout life by events in the surrounding world. A central idea was that if the social and emotional environment could be ameliorated, mental health would be improved, and mental disorders would be prevented.

This model was incorporated and developed through the first half of the century in the child guidance movement (Harms, 1947; Stevenson and Smith, 1934). This movement received its initial impetus from concern about conditions in the slums of major cities and about the prevalence of juvenile delinquency. Juvenile courts were set up in the early 1900s, and in Chicago, William Healy set up a clinic in association with the court to study and treat the problems of children. The child guidance clinics developed a number of operating principles that would be very influential in the development of community psychiatry. One was an emphasis on the family and social environment of children as productive of psychopathology and maladaptive behavior. A second principle was the use of an interdisciplinary team. In particular, the role of the social worker was developed to work with the child's family. Another was collaboration with other community agencies, such as the juvenile courts, welfare agencies, and schools. The Commonwealth Fund had an important role in stimulating this development in major cities, and child guidance clinics were set up in many centers across the country. By 1930 there were more than 500 clinics in operation. The principal aims were for treatment of the child's problems, but also for the prevention of future delinquency. However, as time passed, many child guidance clinics departed somewhat from their original direction. They became more interested in dynamic, psychoanalytically oriented therapies that emphasized intrapsychic rather than environmental factors in childhood disorders, minimizing and even excluding the involvement of parents in treatment. In these clinics there came to be greater interest on treating the neuroses of middle-class children than in preventing delinquency in the inner-city slums.

The Federal Role

In 1929, the federal government had taken a first step in the direction of accepting responsibility for mental health by establishing within the Public Health Service a

Narcotics Division, which in 1931 was broadened and designated the Division of Mental Hygiene. However, in the 1940s the need for a separate neuropsychiatric institute to take a lead in developing better understanding of mental disorders and better approaches to their prevention and treatment was advanced by the American Psychiatric Association. The National Mental Health Act was passed in 1946. It authorized setting up the National Institute of Mental Health (NIMH) to conduct research and training and encouraged the states to establish mental health authorities. With a strong belief in the psychosocial etiology of mental disorders, the benefits of early intervention, and the value of outpatient treatment, and impressed by the perceived value of child guidance clinics, NIMH actively encouraged the establishment of outpatient clinics across the country. Funds were made available to assist local jurisdictions in establishing clinics, mainly for the provision of psychotherapy.

The movement for change in the mental health service system, which was gathering momentum in the post-war years, embraced two groups. The first group comprised those who might be said to view mental disorder from a "life story" perspective (McHugh and Slavney, 1983). This group, which included psychiatrists, psychologists, social workers, and others who were impressed with psychosocial approaches to understanding, preventing, and treating mental illness, wanted psychotherapeutic treatments and preventive interventions to be made more widely available. A second group comprised individuals who adopted a "disease" perspective on mental illness. They saw the need for renewal and reform of the public mental health system, particularly for chronic patients, but, impressed with the dramatic results obtained with electroconvulsive treatment and the new psychotropic medications, this group focused on improved biological treatment methods as the answer to the problems of mental illness, the social environment seeming of less importance. As will be seen, the failure to distinguish between these perspectives, to understand the usefulness of each and to integrate them in effective service models, had unfortunate consequences.

The first major move toward developing systematic governmental organizations for community psychiatry came in New York with the passage of its Community Mental Health Services Act in 1954. This legislation provided support for local governments to take responsibility for the care of the mentally ill. The state provided 50 percent funding for outpatient clinics and rehabilitation services, inpatient care in local hospitals, and consultation and education services. A number of other states followed New York's lead.

However, there continued to be pressure for a national response to the need for reform in the psychiatric service system. In 1955 a Joint Commission on Mental Illness and Health was established by the American Psychiatric Association and the American Medical Association to study the problem. At the same time, there was intense political activity to develop federal support for a national study of mental illness, and in 1955 the National Mental Health Study Act was passed by Congress. The Joint Commission was given the task of conducting this study and produced its report, *Action for Mental Health,* in 1961. The report called for a move away from reliance on mental hospitals and for the development of community-based treatment systems built on outpatient models.

By the time the report was released in 1961, John F. Kennedy was president. With the prevailing liberal view of that era, that states were generally conservative in social policy and that more progressive policies could only be introduced through federal initiatives (Grob, 1991), the administration prepared a plan, which was introduced to Congress by Kennedy in 1963, for "a wholly new national approach." The Community Mental Health Centers Construction Act of 1963 and additional legislation introduced during the 1960s and 1970s provided that the federal government would fund the construction and staffing of centers. The country was divided into 1,500 catchment areas, and in each of these a Community Mental Health Center (CMHC) was to be established, providing open access for the population of the area. NIMH would fund the operation of the centers for eight years, after which time their support would be taken over by state and local funding. Each CMHC was required to provide an array of services. The requirement initially was for five core services: inpatient treatment, outpatient treatment, partial hospitalization, emergency services, and education and consultation. By the late 1970s, the list had grown to twelve, to include services for children and adolescents, services for the elderly, transitional living programs, substance abuse services, aftercare for patients being discharged from hospitals, screening of patients prior to admission to state hospitals, and program evaluation. An additional feature was that, in contrast to the original concept, all services did not have to be provided under the same roof, or by the same agency. Services provided by a CMHC could be "scattered," or provided by contract with other agencies. Thus emerged the concept of a coordinated network of services within a catchment area.

With the view that the community should not only be the target of service provision, but also has the primary decision-making authority in matters concerning its own health, professionals were called on to abandon elitist and authoritarian stances, and to yield power within the CMHC to the community itself. Centers were to be governed by boards of community residents. This populist initiative met with varied success; in many places very effective collaborations were developed, although disastrous conflicts developed in others (Kaplan and Roman, 1973). However, the requirement for citizen participation served to emphasize several principles: that the community has a primary stake in its own health and in the way in which health services are provided, and that mental health professionals have an obligation to relate to members of the community in constructive ways, one of which is to educate lay people regarding mental health, mental disorders, and their treatment. In this way citizens can participate most effectively in planning and advocacy and can contribute to a lessening of the stigma surrounding mental illness.

However, the CMHCs did not adequately address the needs of the severely mentally ill; they did not help meet governmental policy goals of deinstitutionalization. The focus on social, psychological, and political issues contributed to the demedicalization of the centers, and community psychiatry became increasingly discredited within the psychiatric profession (Group for the Advancement of Psychiatry, 1983).

Refocusing Priorities

Several developments at the federal level contributed to changes in the role of the CMHCs. In 1965, Medicaid and Medicare were introduced as Title XVIII and Title XIX of the Social Security Act. Medicaid is a federal program to provide medical insurance for the poor, but funded jointly by the federal government and the states, who are responsible for its implementation. States have considerable latitude as to the extent to which they develop Medicaid programs in their own jurisdictions, and there is considerable variability in the range of services available. Medicare is a federally funded Social Security program, providing medical insurance for the elderly and the permanently disabled. In 1972, Supplemental Security Income (SSI) was introduced to provide financial support for disabled persons even though they had never worked, and thus had not paid into Social Security. With these entitlements it became more feasible for a severely mentally ill person to live in the community and obtain necessary health care. Through Medicaid and Medicare, community-based programs could obtain some level of fee-for-service reimbursement for clinical services provided to the indigent—the income category into which most severely mentally ill people fall.

Nevertheless, CMHCs were being established more slowly than expected. One problem was that developing and running a CMHC proved to be more costly than anticipated. When the initial eight-year federal funding ended, local groups had great difficulty in obtaining continuation funds from state or other local sources. Administrative problems were more complex than had been anticipated, and there was no cadre of administrators with experience in this field. Applying for a grant required a complicated planning process within the local community; not every community was equipped to do this, and not every state was able or willing to provide the necessary support or technical assistance.

The CMHCs were also being criticized increasingly for not addressing the need they were designed to meet. Clinicians were ill-prepared for the new era. Instead of providing community-based services for the severely mentally ill, thus facilitating the process of deinstitutionalization, they did what their training had best equipped them for: provided treatment to the less severely disordered. The staffs who manned the centers concentrated on psychological therapies, counseling approaches, and preventive interventions with a life-story perspective, approaches that are suitable for assisting troubled people but ineffective in addressing the needs of the severely disabled. As it became apparent that physicians were not only costly to employ, but could be replaced by other professionals such as psychotherapists, counselors, and managers, the centers became demedicalized; administrative roles were increasingly assumed by other professionals; and psychiatrists' functions were seen as merely the signing of prescriptions, certification of disability, and other tasks that are reserved by law to physicians. "The medical model" was a term used to refer disparagingly to the disease perspective and treatment approaches that emanate from it. Psychosocial interventions were most highly regarded, prevention was seen as a primary goal, and there was scant attention to the needs of the severely mentally ill, many of whom remained in institutional care.

By the mid-1970s only about one-fourth of the 1,500 catchment areas had a center. Disadvantaged and minority populations were underserved and centers were not ful-filling their responsibility to chronic patients, most of whom were still institutionalized in state hospitals. In 1977 President Carter appointed a President's Commission on Mental Health to reassess the progress. The report of the Commission was generally supportive of current policies but made a number of suggestions for improvement, including greater flexibility in the configuration of CMHCs, greater responsiveness to local circumstances, greater attention to the needs of minorities, and a stronger focus on the needs of the severely mentally ill. This report was generally welcomed by people in community psychiatry, and a series of reforms was embodied in the Mental Health Systems Act of 1980, which was signed into law by President Carter shortly before he left office.

The End of the Federal Role

Within weeks the administration of his successor, Ronald Reagan, developed an Omnibus Budget Reconciliation Act which effectively repealed the Mental Health Systems Act and signaled the end to federal support for CMHCs. Reagan, with this action, was reasserting the conviction that mental health care is not a federal responsibility, but a responsibility of the states, the same assertion that President Franklin Pierce had made in 1854 when he vetoed legislation to allow federal land sale revenues to be used for developing hospitals for the mentally ill. NIMH, in addition to its role in stimulating research, would have a reduced role, confined to assisting states in developing innovations in mental health services for the severely mentally ill, through its Community Support Program (Turner and TenHoor, 1978), but for all intents and purposes the federal role in providing community mental health service development came to an end after 15 years. Whatever small amounts of federal mental health service funds that were still available went to states in the form of block grants.

During the 1980s states struggled, with varying degrees of success in the face of reduced federal support, to provide mental health services for their citizens. The CMHC model continued to influence the form of service provision. However, because states could only support community mental health programs through money saved from the mental hospital sector, they accorded top priority to programs that would enable patients to be moved out of institutions. Community mental health programs that devoted more of their resources to helping people with troubles in their emotions and relationships than to those with major illnesses came under increasing criticism. State governments increasingly directed their service programs to focus on "target populations," defined as those with severe mental illnesses and histories of extensive inpatient treatment, although funds were scarce, skills in meeting the needs of the severely disabled were limited, and many of the community support systems were underdeveloped.

In spite of the difficulty of creating alternatives, states pressed ahead more rapidly than ever with reducing the censuses in their mental hospitals. State governments were motivated by the enormous costs of maintaining institutions and of bringing them up to minimal modern standards, necessary for accreditation by the Joint Commission on Accreditation of Hospitals (JCAH) or the Health Care Financing Administration (HCFA), prerequisites for Medicaid and Medicare reimbursement. Legislatures were also being implored by community mental health professionals and advocates for the mentally ill to redirect funds from the institutional to the community sector—for the funds to follow the patients into the community. It was generally claimed, without clear supporting evidence, that community care would be cheaper than institutional care. For these reasons, state legislatures generally supported moves to reduce hospital capacity and hospital censuses but found themselves unable to make major investments of resources in community programs. Large savings from mental hospitals did not materialize. Surpluses that might be expected to accrue from downsizing were eaten up by inflation, increasing salary demands of professional staff, essential improvements to physical plants, and other improvements needed to bring facilities up to acceptable minimal standards. Phasing out hospitals was opposed by institutional bureaucracies, by local commercial and community groups, by hospital employee unions, and by other vested interests so that, while hospitals generally reduced their censuses, very few actually closed. The notion that funds would follow patients into the community thus turned out to be unrealistic. States had to find "new money" to fund community services, including federal Medicaid and Medicare dollars.

The 1980s were years of struggling with resource constraints but also with the need to develop and implement new methods. Community psychiatrists sought to define the roles and methods of modern community psychiatry. They came to focus more and more on the needs of the severely mentally ill "target population." Less and less time was available to consider the needs of people with less severe problems, many of whom were directed elsewhere, to counseling or treatment programs of other sorts. Indirect services such as consultation and education were phased out to a considerable extent. Belatedly, the importance of integrating life-story and disease perspectives came to be recognized. The major benefits accruing from the application of biological treatments to mental illnesses were apparent, but the sterility of this approach in the absence of sensitivity to the personal and social dimensions of the experience of the ill person was made clear by those who developed psychosocial models of support and treatment.

There were a number of programmatic innovations of note, small in scale, but radical in their approach. These were programs focused on the needs of the seriously ill and disabled, which were not widely implemented at first and had little immediate impact on the national scene, but which with time would come to be influential.

Fountain House was one of these, established in New York City in the late 1940s, a day program in which former mental hospital inpatients worked together, shared with staff members in the governance and administration of the program, and participated in supported employment as they became increasingly independent. Described as a "clubhouse," Fountain House was established to be clearly separate from the treatment system, at times in opposition to the psychiatric establishment. The program focused on members' strengths rather than their pathology; normalization and empowerment were key concepts. Fountain House became one of the most influential models in modern psychiatric rehabilitation (see Chapter 21).

In California George Fairweather developed and tested a model described as a "lodge." The lodge was home for a group, or "society," of mentally ill people who together performed the various tasks and made the everyday decisions needed to maintain the household community (Fairweather, 1980). The model proved successful and was replicated in several other places, but many of its ideas have been adopted more widely.

Soteria was another residential, community-based program that represented a more radical departure from traditional psychiatric thinking. The model did not deny the validity of the disease perspective on mental illness, but deliberately deemphasized it in order to stress the uniqueness of each individual and to avoid the use of medications as far as possible. The staff and residents were more oriented toward "understanding" the needs or experiences of individuals than "treating" symptoms of illness (Mosher and Menn, 1979).

Training in Community Living was the name given to a new program in Madison, Wisconsin, in the early 1970s, one of several experiments in providing home-based psychiatric treatment for severely ill psychiatric patients (e.g., Pasamanick, Scarpitti, and Dinitz, 1967). The Madison experiment evolved from work that had been done at the Mendota Mental Health Institute. Their success with an in-hospital program of rehabilitation to prevent chronicity in schizophrenic patients prompted an effort to avoid hospitalization altogether. This plan involved relocating a team of hospital staff into the community to provide in-home care for patients who otherwise would have been admitted to hospital. This model, later to become more widely known as the Program for Assertive Community Treatment (PACT), was carefully evaluated by its developers and shown not only to be more acceptable to patients than conventional hospital treatment but to be cost-effective and to have certain clinical advantages (Stein and Test, 1985). This model, or slight modifications of it, has since been replicated widely in the United States and in other countries (Olfson 1990; see Chapter 16).

Another advance in patient care concepts that had an influence in the movement away from institutional care and long hospital stays derived from the finding that treatment programs offering shorter hospital stays were often as effective as those providing longer stays (Glick et al., 1977; Herz et al., 1977; Gordon and Breakey, 1983). Inpatient care thus could increasingly move into the inpatient units of general hospitals, offering short stays. People could be treated closer to their home communities, with less stigmatization, at lower cost per episode of care, and each bed could be used to provide care for a greater number of patients in a given time period.

In implementing new approaches such as these, a variety of services and skills were needed that heretofore psychiatrists had largely ignored. The importance of psychiatric rehabilitation became evident, and models such as the clubhouse began to be widely implemented. New cadres of professionals developed with the orientation and skills needed to manage and staff these programs. The need for special housing programs emerged. Somehow it had been assumed that President Kennedy was correct in predicting that patients could return home "without hardship to themselves or their families" (Kennedy, 1963). However, as deinstitutionalization proceeded, it soon became evident that in many places, finding suitable and supportive residential placements outside mental hospitals was difficult or impossible. The provision of special housing became top priority. However, resources and skills to develop residential programs were not in place, and there was a national shortage of low-income housing. As states forced the pace on deinstitutionalization, public concern about the numbers of homeless mentally ill people in America increased. Critics blamed the mental health service system (Torrey, 1989; Hope and Young, 1986). One reaction was to urge a return to greater use of institutional care (Gralnick, 1985), another was to encourage greater efforts to provide appropriate services and support for the severely mentally ill, in particular those who were homeless (Lamb, 1984; Institute of Medicine, 1988). The federal government, with the reluctant approval of President Reagan, enacted the McKinney Homeless Assistance Act in 1987 to make additional services available to homeless people, specifically including those with mental illnesses.

Other trends of the 1980s had important influences, notably the growth of consumerism. "Mental health consumers" were identified as people who were or had been patients, or their relatives and friends who had been affected by the illness and the service system. Associations of consumers developed to challenge the traditional assumptions and practices of the professionals and also to demand increased resources and the development of improved methods. National umbrella organizations of primary consumers came into being, including the National Mental Health Consumers Association, and the National Alliance of Psychiatric Survivors. Organizations of secondary consumers also developed, most notably The National Alliance for the Mentally Ill, an organization primarily of the families of mentally ill people; this group has come to have a major role at local, state, and federal levels for advocacy, policy development, and provision of alternative services (see Chapter 11).

Certain subgroups of patients came to be identified as presenting special sets of problems. One group, many of whom had never been hospitalized for lengthy periods, but were significantly disabled in terms of living a successful life in the community, provided major challenges for treatment providers. Known as the "young adult chronic patients," they were loath to be identified as "patients," reluctant to accept regular medication schedules, and prone to frequent relapses (Bachrach, 1981; Pepper and Ryglewicz, 1984). Struggling with this group first led to the concept of a case manager whose role it is to ensure that the person gets the services that he or she needs (Berzon and Lowenstein, 1984; see Chapter 23).

Another group that became evident in the 1990s as presenting special problems were the "dually diagnosed," in particular those patients with a major mental illness and concomitant substance dependence. This umbrella term included a variety of individuals with differing combinations of problems (see Chapter 25). Not only does each disorder complicate treatment of the other, but the interaction of two treatment systems with their own cultures and bureaucracies—for mental illness and for substance abuse—often proves difficult to manage.

Increasing scrutiny from consumers and from governmental and private funding agencies called into question the high cost and effectiveness of the new community approaches. By and large the new methods were based on commonsense approaches to perceived problems faced by mentally ill people in the community. There had been a number of carefully evaluated programs, but much of community psychiatry practice was based on clinical experience and anecdotal reports of successful programs. Increasing demands for accountability required better evidence of the effectiveness of new approaches, and a new field of mental health services research developed (see Chapter 8). Increasingly, new programs such as those sponsored by the Community Support Program had evaluation components built in from the outset, and new methods were developed for measuring variables such as *quality of life, family burden* and *needs for services* (see Chapter 9).

In the 1990s community psychiatry is at another crossroads. The high cost of health care in the United States and the United Kingdom has prompted radical reviews of the organization and funding of health services. When resources are limited and economies are necessary, psychiatric services are vulnerable. The principles that have guided the development of community psychiatry—emphasis on providing services for population groups, the use of multidisciplinary teams, public accountability, a belief that treatment provided close to a person's home with minimum disruption of family and social networks is preferable to treatment in institutional settings, and a concern with cost and cost-effectiveness—are the principles underlying the several approaches to health system reform being advocated in the United States. It is not clear how the policy debates will end, but there is little doubt that the concepts and methods developed by community psychiatrists over the previous half-century will provide the framework for whatever new system of mental health services emerges for the next half-century.

References

Bachrach, L.L. (1981) Young adult chronic patients: An analytical review of the literature. *Hospital and Community Psychiatry,* 33:189–197.
Beers, C.W. (1907, 1981) *A Mind that Found Itself.* Pittsburgh: University Press.

Berzon, P., and Lowenstein, B. (1984) A flexible model of case management. In Pepper, B. and Ryglewicz, H. (eds), *Advances in treating the young adult chronic patient.* San Francisco: Jossey-Bass.

Caplan, G. (1970) *The theory and practice of mental health consultation.* New York: Basic Books.

Caton, C.L.M. (1984) *Management of chronic schizophrenia.* New York: Oxford University Press.

Dain, N. (1980) *Clifford Beers: Advocate for the Insane.* Pittsburgh: University of Pittsburgh Press.

Fairweather, G.W. (ed.) (1980) *The Fairweather Lodge: A twenty-five year retrospective.* San Francisco: Jossey-Bass.

Foley, H.A., and Sharfstein, S.S. (1983) *Madness and Government: Who Cares for the Mentally Ill?.* Washington, D.C.: American Psychiatric Press.

Glick, I.D., Hargreaves, W.A., Drues, J., Showstack, J.A., and Katzow, J.J. (1977) Short vs long hospitalization: a prospective controlled study. VII. Two-year follow-up results for non-schizophrenics. *Archives of General Psychiatry,* 34:314–317.

Gordon, T., and Breakey, W.R. (1983) A comparison of the outcomes of short-and standard-stay patients at one year follow-up. *Hospital and Community Psychiatry,* 34:1054–1056.

Gralnick A. (1985) Build a better state hospital: deinstitutionalization has failed. *Hospital and Community Psychiatry,* 36:738–741.

Grob, G.N. (1991) *From Asylum to Community.* Princeton: Princeton University Press.

Group for the Advancement of Psychiatry (1983) *Community psychiatry: a reappraisal.* New York: Mental Health Materials Center.

Harms, E. (ed.) (1947) *Handbook of Child Guidance.* New York: Child Care Publications.

Herz, M.I., Endicott, J., and Spitzer, R.L. (1977) Brief Hospitalization: a two-year follow-up. *American Journal of Psychiatry,* 134:502–507.

Hope, M., and Young, J. (1986) *The Faces of Homelessness.* Lexington, Mass.: Lexington Books.

Institute of Medicine (1988) *Homelessness, health and human needs.* Washington, DC: National Academy Press.

Jones, M. (1953) *The Therapeutic Community.* New Haven, Connecticut: Yale University Press.

Kaplan, S.R., and Roman, M. (1973) *The organization and delivery of mental health services in the ghetto: The Lincoln Hospital experience.* New York: Praeger.

Kennedy, J.F. (1963) "Message on Mental Illness and Mental Retardation," Feb. 5 *Congressional Record,* 88(1), CIX, Part 2, 1744–1749.

Lamb, H.R. (ed.) (1984) *The homeless mentally ill.* Washington D.C.: American Psychiatric Association.

Lindemann, E. (1944) Symptomatology and management of acute grief. *American Journal of Psychiatry,* 101:141–148.

Lipowski, Z.J. (1981) Holistic-medical foundations of American psychiatry: A bicentennial. *American Journal of Psychiatry* 138:888–895.

Mannino, F.V., and Shore, M.F. (1979) Evaluation of consultation: problems and prospects. In Rogawski, A.S. (ed.), *Mental health consultation in community settings.* San Francisco: Jossey-Bass.

McHugh, P.R., and Slavney, P.R. (1983) *The Perspectives of Psychiatry.* Baltimore: The Johns Hopkins University Press.

Meyer, A. (1951) The aims of a psychiatric clinic. In Winters, E.E. (ed.), *The collected papers of Adolf Meyer.* Baltimore: The Johns Hopkins Press.

Mosher, L.R., and Menn, A. (1979) Soteria: an alternative to hospitalization for schizophrenia. In Lamb, H.R. (ed.), *Alternatives to Acute Hospitalization.* San Francisco: Jossey-Bass.

Olfson, M. (1990) Assertive Community Treatment: an evaluation of the evidence. *Hospital and Community Psychiatry,* 41:634–641.

Pasamanick, B., Scarpitti, F., and Dinitz, S. (1967) *Schizophrenics in the community: An experimental study in the prevention of hospitalization.* New York: Appleton Century-Crofts.

Pepper, B., and Ryglewicz, H. (1984) *Advances in treating the young adult chronic patient.* San Francisco: Jossey-Bass.

Stein, L.I., and Test, M.A. (1985) *The training in community living model: a decade of experience.* San Francisco: Jossey-Bass.

Stevenson, G.S., and Smith, G. (1934) *Child Guidance Clinics.* New York: The Commonwealth Fund. Facsimile edition, New York: Garland Publishing, 1987.

Torrey, E.F. (1989) *Nowhere to go: the tragic odyssey of the homeless mentally ill.* New York: Harper and Row.

Turner, J.C., and TenHoor, W.J. (1978) The NIMH Community Support Program: Pilot approaches to a needed social reform. *Schizophrenia Bulletin,* 4(3):319–349.

4

The Political and Social Context of Modern Community Psychiatry

STEVEN S. SHARFSTEIN

> We as a Nation have long neglected the mentally ill and the mentally retarded. This neglect must end, if our Nation is to live up to its own standards of compassion and dignity and achieve the maximum use of its manpower.
>
> This tradition of neglect must be replaced by forceful and far-reaching programs carried out at all levels of government, by private individuals and by State and local agencies in every part of the Union.
>
> We must act—
> to bestow the full benefits of our society on those who suffer from mental disabilities;
> to prevent the occurrence of mental illness and mental retardation wherever and whenever possible;
> to provide for early diagnosis and continuous and comprehensive care, in the community, of those suffering from these disorders;
> to stimulate improvements in the level of care given the mentally disabled in our State and private institutions, and to reorient those programs to a community-centered approach . . .
>
> (John F. Kennedy, The White House, *February 5, 1963*.)

Of the many influences that shape psychiatric care in the community in the 1990s, political and related social forces are among the most powerful (Sedgwick, 1982). Politics emerges from the attitudes and values of society, and powerful people, both elected and unelected, influence the social environment in which the treatment encounter takes place.

The saga of the treatment of the mentally ill in America over the past 150 years is a complex tale of successive cycles of reform with the pendulum swinging between social neglect and social concern, political inertia and political activism (Morrissey, Goldman, and Klerman, 1980). Underlying each era of reform is a particular political and social context; and with each successive wave, the old system of care becomes layered with the new. So like an archeological site, we can observe today the results of nineteenth- and early twentieth-century psychiatric reform through the levels of treatment provision, from public asylums to modern short-term units in general hospitals, from homeless shelters to community sheltered workshops, group homes, and day treatment programs. This chapter will focus on the historical sociopolitical roots of community psychiatry. It is a story of political and social reformers from Dorothea Dix to John F. Kennedy, from Adolph Meyer and the development of the Mental Hygiene Movement in the early 1900s to the founding of the National Alliance of the Mentally Ill in the 1980s.

Dorothea Dix and the Rise of the Asylum

A most instructive case of the power of the political and social context of community psychiatry is that of Dorothea Lynd Dix (1802–1887). Her method of political activism, which began in Massachusetts in the early 1840s, was to visit the jails, poorhouses, and other places that housed the insane. She would survey the state on the plight of the mentally ill, collecting copious statistics and developing case studies or extensive anecdotes, and compile and present them in the form of a "memorial." This memorial was a statement of facts addressed to the state legislature, accompanied by a petition for redress or correction. These were very powerful documents. Her memorial to the General Assembly in the State of Maryland in 1852 is one example:

> I have glanced at the inefficiency and cruelty of a poor-house and prison residence for the epileptic and the maniac. In imagination for a short time, place yourselves in their stead. Enter the horrid noisome cell; invest yourselves with the foul tattered garments which scantily serve the purposes of decent covering; cast yourself upon the loathsome pile of filthy straw, find companionship in your own cries and groans, or in the wailings and gibberings of wretches miserable like yourselves; call for help and release for blessed words of soothing and kind offices of care till the dull walls weary in sending back the echo of your moans; then, if your self-possession is not overwhelmed under the imagined miseries of what are the actual distresses of the insane, return to the consciousness of your sound intellectual health, and answer if you will longer refuse or delay to make adequate appropriation for the establishment of a hospital for the care and cure of those who are deprived of the use of their reasoning faculties. . . .
>
> (Dix, 1852)

This vivid language, appropriate for the social context of the time, certainly would capture the imagination and concern of many politicians. She would reside near the state capitol where she would intensively lobby influential politicians to support her proposed reforms. It should be noted that she focused on the evils of community care and neglect and the benefits of the well-run asylum. She successfully used this approach in over 20 state legislatures, resulting in the founding of some 32 state mental hospitals over a 20 year period.

All of Dorothea Dix's efforts did not succeed. She was not able to persuade the federal government to assume responsibility for the mentally ill and the development of mental hospitals. In the 1840s, the federal government raised revenues mostly through land sales. For seven years, from 1847 to 1854, Dix lobbied the Congress for a bill granting the proceeds of a federal land sale for the building of federal mental hospitals. She enlisted former President Millard Fillmore as a principal lobbyist in her cause. The "12,225,000 Acres Act" passed the Senate in 1851, the House in 1852, and both in 1854. It was then sent to President Franklin Pierce for his signature.

President Pierce chose to veto the bill, citing the limited powers of the federal government and stating that the care of the mentally ill was principally the responsibility of the states. Pierce feared that the bill might set a dangerous precedent by which "the whole field of public beneficence would be thrown open to the care and culture of the federal government." This would continue to be federal policy for 100 years until the development of Social Security and the Community Mental Health legislation of the 1960s (Foley and Sharfstein, 1983). The appropriate roles of the federal and state governments continued to be hotly debated. President Pierce's view in the 1850s was quite similar to that of President Reagan in the 1980s. Reagan's Block Grant legislation of 1981 (the Omnibus Reconciliation Act), returning responsibility for mental health services to the states, reversed several decades of federal leadership in community psychiatry.

Adolph Meyer, and the Mental Hygiene Movement

Dorothea Dix's vision of the well-ordered institution did not anticipate the harsh public health reality of chronic mental illness. When asylums were established under state auspices, local communities took the opportunity to transfer care of the chronically psychotic, addicted, and senile from local almshouses to the state hospital, thus beginning the saga of clinical and cost shifting which continues today (Gruenberg, 1979). State health care acts, beginning in 1890, began to require that all care of the mentally ill take place in centralized state-supported facilities. With tens of thousands of needy individuals requiring care and support, these fledgling institutions were rapidly overwhelmed. For example, in New York between 1890 and 1900, there was a four-fold increase in the population of patients in state hospitals with the passage of the State Care Act of 1890. The population increased from 5,400 to almost 22,000 as counties in New York reclassified their senile elderly as mentally ill, shifting their care and its cost to the state.* The net result was that in state after state, care became custodial and chronicity was reinforced by long hospital stays.

In the early 1900s, Adolph Meyer coined the phrase, "the Mental Hygiene Movement," and initiated this important reform that remains a forerunner of modern community psychiatry. Meyer realized that he needed to move psychiatry from the hopelessness of the back wards of state asylums to adopt a new credo of prevention

*Conversely, in 1984, Medicare issued an advisory which suggested that Alzheimer's Disease be classified with the neurologic rather than the psychiatric code in order to provide more payment for diagnosis and treatment. There could be no better example of economic power and the social and political context of psychiatric care influencing practice.

and cure. He promoted the notion of a short-term receiving hospital, the psychopathic hospital, affiliated with the medical school, which would provide the most modern diagnosis and treatment and a network of neighborhood-based aftercare services to treat a large number of those diagnosed. He promoted the new profession of psychiatric social work. Although he never intended to replace the custodial state institutions, the now entrenched bureaucracy of state superintendents effectively ignored the Mental Hygiene Movement, which then did little for the thousands of chronically mentally ill. It did begin, however, to move the field toward a remedicalization of psychiatry, a scientific and professional commitment to research and care, and a wedding of public health and clinical practice.

Public Asylum Psychiatry and Deinstitutionalization

The founding of the National Institute of Mental Health, a federal agency, in 1946 provided an important structural element in the reforms of the next four decades: Muckraking journalistic exposés of the excesses of the state hospitals started a search for alternatives to the custodial asylum (Deutsch, 1948). By the mid-1950s, the peak of public asylum psychiatry was reached in the United States with the number of persons hospitalized in these hospitals at almost 560,000. Half of all hospital beds in America were occupied by psychiatric patients. Over three-quarters of all patient-care episodes were in mental health facilities; inpatient care in the community was virtually nonexistent. Deinstitutionalization began in the mid-1950s. Since then, a major growth has occurred in the numbers of professionals and community-based programs, so that today three out of four patient-care episodes take place in the ambulatory sector, and four times as many patients are seen in the course of a year by mental health specialists. A principal factor in this expansion has been the rise of public and private financing for diagnosis and treatment of mental illness as diagnosis and treatment became more effective. The community mental health centers legislation of the 1960s and 1970s and a series of class-action lawsuits on right to treatment in state programs and right to treatment in least restrictive settings fueled the discharge of patients from state facilities.

Deinstitutionalization provides perhaps the best example of the influence of political and social factors in mental health policy and practice (Johnson, 1990). Although many observers attempt to attribute deinstitutionalization to the introduction of psychotropic medications, political and fiscal issues have been dominant in what has essentially been an unplanned process. In the late 1940s and early 1950s, hospitals were filled beyond capacity, and states began to recognize that they could not afford the ever-expanding custodial responsibilities. The states began to get together as early as 1949 (Council of State Governments, 1950) to discuss the chronically mentally ill and the need to develop community resources and alternatives to state programs. At the same time, there was an attitude shift led by psychiatry, which identified the custodial institution as part of the problem rather than as part of the solution and, once again, attempted to move psychiatry in a more medical direction. Accompanying the profound ambivalence of American psychiatry on the appropriate use of the psychiatric hospital, an ideological shift occurred, with an emphasis on the curability of mental illness and the potential of prevention. Sociology and law reinforced each other and helped shift the attitude of professionals and informed lay public on the appropriate role of the state hospital (Goffman, 1961; Isaac and Armat, 1990). Social thought pushed the notion of mental illness as a myth, and freedom as being more important than control of socially inappropriate behavior (Szasz, 1974).

One important factor in the decline of psychiatric beds in state mental hospitals is the growth of private nursing homes. Medicare and Medicaid especially began the cost shift of the burden of care for the aged mentally ill from the states to the federal treasury and the transfer of patients to these new facilities. From 1969 to 1973, the number of individuals aged 65 and over residing in nursing homes, with a primary diagnosis of mental disorder, doubled from 96,000 to 194,000. During the same period, the mentally ill aged 65 and over in psychiatric hospitals decreased by almost 40 percent.

Unfortunately, for many of the discharged patients, there was neither nursing home nor organized community setting. There was no adequate political or administration response to new needs. Community psychiatrists in those communities with large numbers of discharged patients had to work in an environment characterized by increasing neglect of needy individuals. The homelessness of thousands of mentally ill people is but one example, and perhaps the most tragic one, of the failure of social and political support for community psychiatry in the era of deinstitutionalization (Torrey, 1988).

Once the state hospital was no longer an affordable alternative and its custodial and therapeutic roles were discredited, community mental health care became the obvious compelling solution. The report, *Action for Mental Health,* was an important document that represented 5 years of study by the congressionally mandated Joint Commission on Mental Health and Illness with a wide constituency of mental health advocates and social policymakers (Joint Commission, 1961). Although it made a number of important recommendations designed to improve state hospitals, these were largely ignored in favor of its recommendation to develop an array of community services appropriate for patient care. In 1963, President John F. Kennedy signed Public Law 88-164. The scope of this act and the mission of community mental health centers was extremely large. It assumed that after a 51-month period of declining federal financial support, these centers would generate alternative sources of funding and become self-sufficient. It deliberately bypassed state programs but assumed that state monies as well as private third-party dollars would replace the declining federal "seed money" and still keep the basic mission of the mental health center intact. It was expected that the entire country would be blanketed with community mental health centers in 20 years. Money was appropriated successfully for construction and staffing and then for a variety of additional services so that by 1975, the essential services had moved from five to twelve. As of 1981, the year the federal program was repealed, 798 community mental health centers were operational—far short of the 2,000 envisioned by Congress in 1963. At the same time, there was a chorus of discontent about the ability and willingness of the mental health centers to care for the tens of thousands of patients discharged from state facilities or candidates for admission to those facilities (Sharfstein, 1978). The appearance of thousands of homeless mentally ill people in our public libraries, doorways, and streets, tattered and hallucinating, generated a public health crisis that today is only second to the AIDS epidemic (Lamb, 1984). That this happened during the decade of the 1980s, one of the most affluent periods in American history, is noteworthy and ironic, but fully explainable within the political and social realities of that decade. The repeal of the Mental Health Systems Act of 1980 by the passage of the Block Grant Program to states in 1981 ushered in an era of federal benign neglect and a progressive shortfall of funds for housing, psychosocial rehabilitation, and treatment for the thousands of patients with chronic mental illness (Foley and Sharfstein, 1983). Five key issues in the sociopolitical arena were not addressed during this time period. They include (1) the need for special living arrangements for this population; (2) the need for day-time rehabilitative and supportive programs; (3) the need for supportive work opportunities; (4) the need for coordination of multiple levels of support—local, federal, and state as well as private sector; and (5) the need for first-rate emergency care and treatment in the least restrictive setting (Sharfstein, 1983). The Community Support Program of the National Institute of Mental Health was an important effort to work with states in resolving these five sociopolitical issues through the provision of timely case management and a planned approach utilizing all sources of funding. The need to consider the clinical reality of the patients, however, exceeded the imagination of the planners and politicians who tried to address this particular population.

Shifting Cost and Clinical Responsibility

As one can see from the above discussion, many of the changes in mental health policy over the decades have been justified on the grounds of saving money. The cost issue especially was a driving force in depopulating the state hospitals, beginning in the mid-1950s and accelerating in the 1960s and 1970s. The original funding of state facilities through the prodigious work of Dorothea Dix and her allies compelled states to share with localities in the costs of care for indigent individuals with mental illness. The principle of state responsibility survived a hundred years and only began to be changed in the mid-1950s after it was discovered that the costs of maintaining patients for life in large institutions was threatening to bankrupt state governments. In a study published in the early 1950s, The National Governors' Conference described the increase in the median annual cost per patient in the nation's mental hospitals from $246 in 1939 to $636 in 1949. During that time period, the consumer price index increased 100.2 to 171.4—nowhere near the rise in mental health costs (Council of State Governments, 1950).

With the increase in life expectancy and the growing admission rate, the states faced a grim prospect in 1950. As one observer stated it, ''Based on their uniform experience over the past century, they could expect more admissions of more people who would stay longer at prices that could only rise, presumably by the same or even more enormous increments'' (Johnson, 1990, p. 91). Taxpayers resented the burden of providing ever-increasing custodial care for an intractable illness. Custodial care is labor intensive. It is essential to cover three shifts, 24 hours a day, every day of the year including holidays; and therefore, the drive to seek alternatives is compelling and obvious.

It was necessary for these sociopolitical reasons to recast the concept of long-term mental health care and cast out the patients from these expensive facilities (Moran, Freedman, Sharfstein, 1984). But this would not have happened except that the federal government began a process of reversing President Pierce's veto of 100 years before by providing funds for chronic care, especially if it took place outside the custodial state-supported institution. These new funding sources included Title II of the Social Security Act (the Disability Income Program) passed in 1954, but funding was truly accelerated by the passage in 1965 of Titles XVIII and XIX, Medicare and Medicaid, which began the process of moving the elderly out of the state hospitals into nursing homes and expanding the use of alternative institutions as indicated above. The switch from the mental hospital to the nursing home as a locus of care for the demented was fueled in large part by the cost shift from state-supported funds to the federal-state formula embodied in Medicaid. But all of the above would not have occurred except for the passage of Title XVI of the Social Security Act, the Social Security Amendments of 1972 (PL92-603). This program, Supplemental Security Income (SSI) for the aged, disabled, and blind, established national uniform eligibility requirements for people considered disabled enough to be rendered incapable of working and provided a floor of federal money to support these individuals. This important program had the unique characteristic of being a welfare program that patients could apply for prior to discharge from the state hospital; understandably, all took advantage of it, and state hospital populations declined by 11 percent between 1972 and 1974 in anticipation of the legislation. By 1974, the first year SSI was truly available, state hospitals saw an additional decrease in population of 13.3 percent, the largest decrease ever.

Therefore, in the 1960s and 1970s, the states recognized the new sociopolitical context for the treatment of mental illness and figured out how to move their chronic caseload from the state institution into a variety of community alternatives, thus shifting the financial burden from the state treasury to the federal. Most of the patients leaving with SSI benefits either returned to their families or lived in boarding care homes in the community.

What was not planned for at the time was the increased burden on the community and the need for treatment when discharged patients are better but not well. Lack of clarity about responsibility for these former patients compounded the lack of clarity as to the precise costs of care. If the total costs in the community paid from a variety of sources were calculated, the apparent cost savings disappeared. However, it became clear that the key policy parameter was not only the cost of community care, but also, with cost shifting, the question of who pays (Sharfstein, 1982).

Political and Economic Forces in the Passage of Federal Legislation

The specific roles of the Kennedy and Carter families in the passage of community mental health legislation in 1963 and 1980 are of particular interest. Presidential politics have been crucial ever since President Pierce's veto in 1854. That veto set the pattern for state-supported care for well over 100 years. It took presidential politics in the 1960s and 1970s to reverse an anti-federal perspective.

Within our federal system there is a strong national disinclination for the federal government to usurp or take over responsibilities traditionally delegated to states. Mental health care certainly has been a major state responsibility throughout the nineteenth and twentieth centuries. When we reached the peak of public asylum psychiatry in the United States in 1955, the process of change and the emergence of federal leadership began to take place. Title II of the Social Security Act was signed by President Eisenhower, and Social Security disability was the first milestone since President Pierce's veto of 100 years before in asserting a role for the federal government that had traditionally been left to states. The Mental Health Study Act was passed and a congressional commission established to review a variety of major concerns about the government-supported care and treatment of psychiatric patients. But it was a presidential family with the personal experience of mental illness in a family member that brought us the first major piece of federal legislation in 1963 and the strong federal leadership that was necessary to get this legislation through Congress.

Action for Mental Health initially recommended substantial investments to improve current deteriorating infrastructure in state hospitals and to provide a network of community mental health centers. It was this second recommendation that the Kennedy Administration pursued vigorously with Congress. One noteworthy feature of the testimony before Congress was the grand rhetoric from a wide array of witnesses, including the American Psychiatric Association and federal officials, on the effectiveness of community programs that had not been tested or researched to any significant extent. It was felt that these promises were necessary in order to secure passage by a reluctant Congress and over the opposition of powerful groups such as the American Medical Association.

The Community Mental Health Centers Act was amended no less than 13 times between 1965 and 1980, often adding more and more requirements and provisions without actually adding significant funds to cover new populations and new services. Some amendments were required to overcome the Nixon Administration's attempt to end the federal program. However, by the late 1970s a thorough review was in order as the program was coming under increasing financial and clinical pressure. Deinstitutionalization was exposing major problems in the delivery of community mental health care, and the gap between promise and reality became all too evident. The President's Commission on Mental Health under the leadership of the First Lady, Rosalyn Carter, produced landmark legislation in 1980, and again it was the leadership of a presidential family that helped carry the day in Congress to secure the passage of this important legislation.

The most significant aspects of this reform in the CMHC program were (1) focusing federal efforts on providing for services to the severely and chronically ill, adults and children, and (2) to beginning to repair the infrastructure of community care that was severely strained by the discharge of thousands of patients from state facilities. Once again, however, presidential politics intervened. With Ronald Reagan, the Mental Health Systems Act of 1980 was essentially repealed and the functions of that federal law devolved to the states. Ronald Reagan rearticulated the position of Franklin Pierce, that the appropriate role for the federal government was circumscribed severely and states must be given the authority, flexibility, and latitude to provide care. But no steps were taken to secure the funding base necessary to provide adequate systems of care and support.

Citizen and consumer activism, however, is even more critical in understanding the nature and pace of change in mental health care. From Dorothea Dix in the mid-nineteenth century to the National Alliance for the Mentally Ill in the late twentieth century, there is a story of agitation for change to improve the opportunities for the mentally ill (see Chapter 12).

Citizen Activists Reemerge

As community psychiatry emerges from the social policy successes and failures of the last two decades, there are a number of pressing public health issues that must be addressed. The social policy failures of deinstitutionalization are represented by the army of homeless mentally ill people in many of our cities and towns, and the pressure to further cut back both the public and private funds that provide care and support for individuals with severe mental illness creates a grim mood of retrenchment throughout the community care system. There has been, however, a fundamental change in the sociopolitical context of community psychiatry with the emergence of an effective advocacy movement embodied by the National Alliance for the Mentally Ill. This group, in concert with the American Psychiatric Association and other professional groups, has invigorated the funding for basic research in the neurosciences in an effort to come to grips with more fundamental solutions to the tragedy of severe mental illness. More recently, this group has turned to issues of private insurance coverage and public funding through state treasuries in an effort to expand their advocacy to those already under care. Other advocacy groups with special interests—manic-depressive illness, eating disorders, Alzheimer's disease, alcohol and substance abuse—lend increasing credibility to the sociopolitical environment in which a variety of pressing health and social needs can be debated. This movement is similar to the movement in the mid-nineteenth century spearheaded by Dorothea Dix. It has the force of moral suasion, reinforced by public health statistics and new clinical and scientific breakthroughs. It provides hope to tens of thousands of families who have found the patchwork quilt of community supports bewildering and demoralizing. For professionals, it provides a constituency that is necessary to get funding, whether public or private, for the provision of essential services. The consumer movement in our democratic system provides one of the most positive examples of how politics and social forces may influence opportunities for care and treatment in the community. It is the hope for the future.

References

Council of State Governments (1950) *The Mental Health Programs of the Forty-eight States.* Chicago: The Council.

Deutsch, A. (1948) *The Shame of the States.* New York: Harcourt, Brace.

Dix, D.L. (1852) Memorial of Miss D.L. Dix to the Honorable General Assembly in Behalf of the Insane of Maryland, February 25, 1852.

Foley, H.A., and Sharfstein, S.S. (1983) *Madness and Government: Who Cares for the Mentally Ill?* Washington, D.C.: American Psychiatric Press.

Goffman, E. (1961) *Asylums.* Garden City, N.Y.: Anchor Books.

Gruenberg, E.M., Archer, J. (1979) Abandonment of responsibility for the seriously mentally ill. *Milbank Memorial Fund Quarterly–Health and Society* 57:485–506.

Isaac, R.J., and Armat, V.C. (1990) *Madness in the Streets: How Psychiatry and the Law Abandoned the Mentally Ill.* New York: The Free Press.

Johnson, A.B. (1990) *Out of Bedlam: The Truth About Deinstitutionalization.* New York: Basic Books.

Joint Commission on Mental Illness and Health (1961) *Action for Mental Health.* New York: Basic Books Reprint, New York: Arno.

Lamb, H.R. (ed.) (1984) *The Homeless Mentally Ill. A Task Force Report of the American Psychiatric Association.* Washington, D.C.: American Psychiatric Press.

Meyer, A. (1952) Where should we attack the problem of the prevention of mental defect and mental disease? In Winters, E.E. (ed.), *The Collected Papers of Adolph Meyer.* Baltimore: Johns Hopkins Press.

Moran, A.E., Freedman, R.I., and Sharfstein, S.S. (1984) The journey of Sylvia Frumkin: A case study for policymakers. *Hospital and Community Psychiatry* 35:887–893.

Morrissey, J.P., Goldman, H.H., and Klerman, L.V. (1980) *The Enduring Asylum: Cycles of Institutional Reform at Worcester State Hospital.* New York: Grune & Stratton, Inc.

Sedgwick, P. (1982) *Psycho Politics.* London: Pluto Press.

Sharfstein, S.S. (1982) Medicaid cutbacks and block grants: Crisis or opportunity for community mental health? *American Journal of Psychiatry,* 139:466–470.

Sharfstein, S.S. (1983) Sociopolitical issues affecting patients with chronic schizophrenia. In Bellak, A. (ed.), *Treatment and Care of Schizophrenia.* New York: Grune & Stratton.

Sharfstein, S.S. (1978) Will community mental health survive in the 1980s? *American Journal of Psychiatry,* 135:1363–1365.

Szasz, T.S. (1974) *The Myth of Mental Illness.* New York: Perennial Library.

Torrey, E.F. (1988) *Nowhere To Go: The Tragic Odyssey of the Homeless Mentally Ill.* New York: Harper & Row.

5

The Evolution of Community Psychiatry in Britain

HUGH L. FREEMAN

It is characteristic of some historical processes that they follow not a linear, but rather a circular—or more precisely, an elliptical—form. So far as the mentally ill in Britain are concerned, they came under the aegis of "community care" in premodern times, as they still do today in most developing countries, where public responsibility is limited to confining those cases who present a physical danger to others. Recent trends in British mental health services—particularly the large-scale transfer of those with chronic disorders from the public to the private sector—provoke disquieting echoes of earlier periods.

Asylums

Before the early eighteenth century, there was only one institution in England for the care of the insane, and none in the other countries of the British Isles. This was the Bethlem (or more familiarly, Bedlam) Hospital in London which—particularly through Hogarth's pictures—became an exemplar of neglect, cruelty, and professional incompetence. It was a reputation, though, that was not fully deserved (Allderidge, 1985). During the eighteenth century, the growth of humanitarianism, particularly associated with nonconformist religious groups, led to the opening of a number of hospitals for the insane, either as independent institutions or associated with general hospitals. These were supported by subscriptions from the wealthier classes, but others were operated for profit, initiating the "trade in lunacy" (Parry Jones, 1972). In many of them, care was little better than at Bethlem, and it was concern over this state of affairs that led the Quakers to establish a new type of institution at York, The Retreat, where the principle of Moral Treatment was first developed by William Tuke (Digby, 1985). This new approach was to be an influential force in psychiatric care, not only in Britain but also particularly in the United States.

For complex reasons, the psychiatric annexes to voluntary general hospitals in England were all closed by the early 1800s (Mayou, 1989). The consequence was that for well into the next century most institutional care of the mentally ill would be in specialized hospitals, set apart from the mainstream of medicine and nursing. However, the unfortunate state of lunatics confined in poorhouses, prisons, private madhouses, or family homes—as well as those who were homeless or wandering—continued to be a humanitarian issue. An Act of Parliament in 1808 gave permissive powers to the administrative authorities for the counties to build asylums, which would be supported by local revenues, but during the next 40 years, this process continued very slowly. Since many of those admitted were destitute, the responsibility for their costs came under the Poor Law. This legislation, however, was amended in 1834 to require that relief was to be provided only within institutions—primarily work-houses—which were then constructed throughout the United Kingdom.

The ideology underlying this change, which was strongly influenced by the views of Malthus, continued to regard Britain as an agrarian and mercantile society, though in fact, it had already become the world's first industrialized nation. As a result, the size of towns and cities exploded on a hitherto unknown scale, with mass migration into them both from the countryside and from Ireland. Their unregulated growth produced enormous public health problems, one of which was the aggregation of large numbers of people disturbed by psychosis (Cooper and Sartorius, 1975). In 1845, the provision of asylums by counties became mandatory; most of Britain's mental hospitals were constructed during the next quarter-century (with a second wave in the 1880s), representing—like the workhouses—an enormous volume of capital investment.

The workhouses, though, became filled not with work-shy adults, as the 1834 Act had feared, but with abandoned children, infirm elderly, and those disabled by physical or mental illness. The intention of the law was that all those identified as mentally ill should be transferred to asylums, but since care in the workhouses was cheaper, such moves were often resisted by the local Poor Law Guardians. However, neither this reluctance nor a high death rate prevented the asylums from growing steadily in size, mainly through the accumulation of incurable cases. For their part, the workhouses became obliged to build large infirmary annexes, which were in fact embryonic general hospitals—a process that gathered momentum from the 1860s. In 1890, the law regulating asylums and compulsory care was codified, in a "triumph of legalism" (Jones, 1972); the rigid procedures and criteria this imposed meant that only people suffering from severe psychosis were likely to be admitted. The mental hospital system then remained largely unchanged for 40 years, and was very similar in its institutional culture to that in the United States and other industrialized countries.

In the development of British social policy, it is very significant that in 1874, the government began to pay a subsidy to county authorities of up to 25% of the cost of maintaining pauper lunatics in asylums. This was the first direct involvement of the central government in responsibility for the financing of any social or welfare service. Combined with the enormous scale of asylum construction, relative to the more modest building of general hospitals at that time, it indicates that mental illness was a special case. Historians such as Foucault (1963) and Scull (1977), with a Marxist orientation, have seen this phenomenon purely in terms of social control and the removal of unproductive members from the industrial proletariat. The threat to public order posed by the mentally ill must certainly have been relevant, but humanitarian concern was at least as important, and detailed studies of the early asylum records (e.g., Walton, 1986) show that people were admitted there only when those outside were unable to care for them any longer. Furthermore, many of these cases also involved serious physical illness or neglect; often, they were in fact failures of community care. The mental hospital system began on a wave of optimism and idealism, but before long it was overwhelmed by the tide of then untreatable disorder. As a result, the principles of Moral Treatment were mostly lost, but it would be wrong to accuse the system of failure at that time by applying the criteria of today (Berrios and Freeman, 1991).

World War I and Its Aftermath

One of the outstanding features of World War I was the large number of psychiatric casualties—a phenomenon that had never been recognized before. In the British Army, the term "shell shock" came to subsume most of these problems, after punitive methods had failed to control them and attempts to find organic lesions had proved fruitless (Merskey, 1991). Methods of combined physical and psychological rehabilitation were then developed, and a few psychiatrists who had become aware of Freudian theories were involved in these. This wartime experience had some effect subsequently. Nineteenth-century concepts such as "degeneration" became discredited and the management of neurosis was seen as a legitimate part of psychiatry. A few outpatient clinics were opened, mainly in London, at which psychotherapy was available for neurotic disorders, and the Cassel Hospital provided the same for inpatients (Pines, 1991). In 1923 the Maudsley Hospital was opened by the London County Council as the first public psychiatric hospital operating outside the restrictions of the Lunacy Act, while a few years later, the Tavistock Clinic was founded as a center for psychotherapeutic training and treatment. These developments were all on a small scale, but they represented the beginnings of an approach to psychiatric disorder that was not centered on the mental hospitals.

Those institutions, however, had returned to operating much as they did before 1914, and dissatisfaction with them led to the appointment of a Royal Commission, which reported in 1926. Its views were progressive for the time, and it recommended that mental illness should be dealt with on modern public health lines. The legislation of 1930, though, was a compromise; voluntary admission to mental hospitals was made possible, offensive terms such as "pauper lunatic" were abolished, and outpatient work by the medical staff of public mental hospitals was permitted. By 1936, 143 such clinics were operating; there is little information as to what actually went on in them, though some had social workers attached (Freeman and Bennett, 1991).

A number of mental hospitals also established admission units, where voluntary patients in particular were segregated from the mass of chronic cases.

Meanwhile, reform of the Poor Law had brought the workhouse infirmaries under
the control of city and county local authorities, and during the 1930s more of these
institutions progressed toward becoming general hospitals in a modern sense. Many
had observation wards to which acutely ill patients were admitted under the Lunacy
Act and then transferred to mental hospitals, unless they recovered very quickly. Some
also had long-stay mental wards, which contained a mixture of chronic psychotics,
the mentally retarded, epileptics, and patients with dementia.

World War II and After

With the approach of World War II and expectations of mass civilian casualties, a
national survey of all hospital facilities in Britain revealed an alarming picture of
incoordination, neglect, and under-provided populations. In response to this, a
government-funded Emergency Medical Service rapidly established new hospital
units, run by salaried specialists. The need to improve morale in both the armed forces
and civilians, through hope of a better future, led to planning for a National Health
Service (NHS), but this at first excluded mental hospitals, on the grounds that there
would have to be reform of the mental illness law before they could be merged with
others. However, in 1945 the new Minister of Health, Aneurin Bevan, decided that
the only way out of the morass into which negotiations had sunk was to nationalize
all hospitals within a single administrative system (Webster, 1987). This would provide the secondary (specialist) level of health care, while primary care was the responsibility of general practitioners, who remained independent contractors to the
NHS; access to specialists would normally be through them. Local authorities were
to provide accommodation for infirm old people, mainly in the former workhouses,
as well as (non-medical) staff who arranged compulsory admissions to mental hospitals—representing an embryonic social work service. The NHS, however, was only
one of a number of measures (including social security, public housing, and child
welfare) that constituted the Welfare State. This meant that it was no longer necessary
for people to remain in mental hospitals—as they had often done—mainly to receive
free medical care, shelter, and maintenance; such provision was now available to them
in the general community. In the post-war period of full employment, all but the most
seriously disabled could find work. Subsequent developments in community psychiatry are best understood in relation to this background.

By the late 1940s, the first effective physical treatments—principally electric convulsive treatment (ECT) and leucotomy—had come into general use in Britain. Their
main effect in mental hospitals was to increase the rate of turnover, but admissions
began to rise ever more rapidly, leading to serious overcrowding. A significant number
of new doctors had come into psychiatry through the war, and these tended to have
a more active approach to the management of patients than had been usual among
established mental hospital staff. At the same time, the evolution of the Therapeutic

Community concepts from the wartime work of Main (1946) and Maxwell Jones (1952) was one of a number of ideological changes that challenged the traditional habits and thinking of institutional psychiatry. Out-patient ECT was also an important development, in that it allowed some people with quite serious psychiatric disorders to be treated while continuing to live at home.

However, it was the arrival from France in the mid-1950s of neuroleptic drugs that provided an impetus for more fundamental changes. In 1955, the number of occupied psychiatric beds in England and Wales which, except for falls during the two World Wars, had been rising for over a century, showed a reduction for the first time—as it did in the USA, but not in other industrialized countries. Most likely, this represented a combination of pharmacological effects, greater confidence among psychiatrists that people suffering from psychosis could be discharged earlier, and the new possibilities of treating patients with medication in extramural settings. By 1960, this steady fall in bed numbers had reached striking proportions (Tooth and Brooke, 1961), so that two years later, a national Hospital Plan envisioned a rapid run-down of the mental hospitals and the replacement of this accommodation—though at a much reduced level—in district general hospitals (DGHs). By then, the introduction of antidepressants and tranquilizers had further increased the scope of pharmacological treatment, both in primary care and in extramural psychiatry. The latter was seen particularly in the rapid growth of out-patient attendances, in spite of serious recruitment difficulties for psychiatry, which had been an area of medical work with very low prestige. Psychiatrists, even more than most other specialists in the NHS, began to see increasing numbers of patients first at home, on domiciliary visits. This arrangement had been designed for people who could not readily attend hospital out-patient clinics, and it was assumed that the family doctor would normally be present, so that he could continue treatment at home. In practice, psychiatrists found that initial evaluation of a case was often more effective in a patient's familiar surroundings, with relatives present, than in a hospital clinic, though the attendance of the family doctors varied greatly. However, their place was taken increasingly by a social worker or psychiatric nurse. Visits to patients' homes by mental health professionals later evolved in various ways, particularly in the work of crisis-intervention teams.

Other developments that were to be important for community psychiatry occurred during the 1950s. Day hospitals began to be established, increasing the flexibility with which psychiatric treatment could be offered and further reducing the use of hospital beds, though in an opposite trend the aging of the population caused a greater demand for the inpatient care of dementia. The Mental Health Act of 1959 swept away a jungle of old restrictive legislation, allowing most psychiatric admissions to occur informally. The first hostels and therapeutic social clubs provided support particularly for discharged patients. In the northwest of England, some district psychiatric services developed from general hospital bases—former workhouse infirmaries—and ceased to use beds in the region's mental hospitals, thus providing a model for future changes (Freeman, 1960). Psychiatric nurses, who in Britain had become a specialized and fairly large (though ill-paid) profession, started to work with patients outside hospitals.

By the end of the decade, locked doors were disappearing from psychiatric hospitals and wards, and traditional restrictive habits were being abandoned. The effect of all these changes, which probably occurred earlier in Britain than anywhere else, was to attenuate the rigid separation that had always existed between psychiatric inpatient care and the outside world. In spite of shortages of all resources (except mental hospital beds), there were widespread feelings of optimism about the way ahead. This began to be spoken of as "community psychiatry," though the term did not represent any change in theoretical models. As with most developments in Britain, it consisted of a series of pragmatic responses to changes that mostly originated outside the mental health care system. The thought of this decade about community-based psychiatry was also largely in line with the recommendations of the World Health Organization's Expert Committee on Mental Health in its report of 1953, though not with their view that specialist psychiatric hospitals should continue to provide most inpatient care.

The 1960s and After

The 1960s was mainly a period of consolidating these same trends. Unlike the United States or West Germany, nearly all Britain's modest number of psychiatrists worked wholly or primarily within NHS hospitals, and because of the remarkable autonomy of the consultant's role, they could pursue innovative schemes, provided these did not require spending much extra money. Since hardly any new hospitals were being constructed at this time, the small amounts of capital available were used for alterations to the largely Victorian building stock. Where progress occurred locally toward a more comprehensive service, this was achieved mainly by better integration between hospital-based psychiatry, local authority community services, and general practitioners (Freeman, 1963). Within the mental hospitals, rehabilitation and industrial therapy developed steadily, together with the beginnings of specialized services for the elderly, children and adolescents, forensic cases, and misusers of alcohol or drugs. All these in turn were to form their own links, as time went on, with community-based provision, such as local authority facilities for old people or disturbed children. Home visits by all the professions, psychiatry, social work and nursing, became increasingly common, especially to evaluate patients before possible admission to hospital. There was growing emphasis on continuity of care for people from defined populations, whatever the nature or severity of their psychiatric disorder, thus avoiding wasteful bargaining between services or the passing of responsibility from one to another. Apart from overall shortage of resources, the main problem, though, was the autonomy of local authorities in their level of provision of community services, which resulted in enormous variations from one area to another. Also, by the end of the decade, the Western "cultural revolution," beginning in Paris, saw the growth of anti-psychiatry, which exposed some mental health services, particularly in large cities, to unaccustomed hostility.

The 1960s were additionally marked by a strong divergence between the interpretation and implementation of community psychiatry in Britain and the United States respectively (Bennett and Freeman, 1991). As described above, the British version was one of developing services for defined communities, with emphasis on the needs of those most severely ill or disabled, and integration of hospital with extramural care. On the other hand, American policy, seen in the Kennedy legislation of 1963 and subsequent construction of comprehensive community mental health centers, focused on the goals of primary prevention and "positive mental health," mainly through psychotherapeutic intervention in less severe conditions. In this latter case, the new form of care was not integrated with the work of state mental hospitals, where bed numbers were drastically reduced (Grob, 1991). The American approach is more accurately described as "community mental health" than "community psychiatry."

The 1970s began in Britain with a rapid growth in public expenditure, though this was brought to a halt, first by the oil crisis of 1973 and then by International Monetary Fund restrictions in 1976. However, the building of new district general hospitals had at last gathered some momentum, and this resulted in a growing contribution to psychiatric inpatient care; in 1970, these had accounted for only 15.5% of admissions. In the first half of the decade, managerial reorganization was seen as the key to efficiency in every major service. The nursing and social work professions, local government, and the NHS all experienced this in turn, with very mixed results. In social work a generic formula was imposed, virtually ending the special skills of psychiatric social workers; at the same time, all were made employees of the local authorities, with whom hospital psychiatric units now had to negotiate for a social work service. This "integration" of the profession meant in practice the disintegration of mental health teams, where these had been established (Jones, 1979). The changes were carried out without any preliminary research or any serious inquiry as to whether they were likely to achieve the benefits claimed (Martin, 1984); this situation was repeated in the NHS "reforms" of the 1990s. The view of most psychiatrists was that the consequences of reorganizing social work on a generic basis were disastrous, and it is likely that the overall quality of mental health care suffered permanently as a result. The NHS reorganization did not affect psychiatry significantly more than other specialties, but the new managerial structure was seriously flawed and had to be changed again in 1982.

Although the officially approved direction of change for British mental health services had been clear since the late 1950s, there had so far been no comprehensive statement of national policy. However, after a preliminary publication in 1971, this eventually emerged as *Better Services for the Mentally Ill* (Department of Health and Social Services, 1975). Its declared aim was to establish a comprehensive service for each Health District (averaging 250,000 population in urban areas), based on a DGH psychiatric unit. The running down or closure of mental hospitals was said to be not a primary objective, but only a consequence of better services being provided, though the number of occupied psychiatric beds had in fact already fallen by 60,000. The NHS would continue to depend on local authority social services for such community-based facilities as sheltered accommodation and day centers. Target norms were laid down for each form of provision, including 0.5 hospital beds per 1,000 population for general psychiatry, though reaching most of these norms would clearly have to be a very long process. Another significant development during the decade was the establishment of the Royal College of Psychiatrists in 1971, especially because of the highly organized national system of specialist training and examination which it instituted. The number of psychiatrists in post was already increasing rapidly, but it was now guaranteed that they would be of steadily improving quality, which would in turn be reflected eventually in better national standards of mental health care.

Other professional cadres also grew significantly in number during this decade, including general practitioners, who continued to be responsible for managing the great bulk of less severe psychiatric morbidity. As psychiatry was starting to assume an important place in the undergraduate medical curriculum, it could be expected that the younger doctors at least would be better equipped to undertake this function. The universal coverage of the population by primary medical care, carried out by independent practitioners who enter into contract with the NHS to provide this to patients registered with them, is unique to the United Kingdom. Compared with similar European countries, people in Britain consult their doctors fairly infrequently and are referred to specialists at a relatively low rate—in spite of the absence of financial constraints. Depression is the most common psychiatric disorder, both in the community and in the general practitioner's surgery, though anxiety-related symptoms often predominate in new episodes of illness. If these symptoms persist, however, it is usual for depressive features to be present also (Tantam and Goldberg, 1991). About two-thirds of these disorders remit within 6 months, but the remainder, which are often associated with adverse social circumstances, have a tendency to chronicity. In Britain, most depressed people are seen by their GP during the illness, though their complaints are often somatic and the psychiatric disorder may not be diagnosed; family doctors still vary widely in their ability to detect these conditions.

The most common method of management in primary care is by psychotropic medication, particularly antidepressants; until the mid-1980s, benzodiazepines were widely prescribed for anxiety, but their use is now restricted to short-term treatment. Psychological treatments such as counseling and cognitive therapy have become more prominent in recent years, but are largely dependent on the availability of clinical psychologists or specially trained community psychiatric nurses (CPNs) or social workers. Though GPs are well placed to provide a continuous service to people in the community with severe, chronic disorders—particularly schizophrenia—up to now this has not happened effectively on any large scale; this responsibility has nearly always remained directly with the specialist (secondary) psychiatric services. In spite of the development of alternative service models, such as crisis intervention, most initial contacts for psychiatric care are still with the GP, who refers directly to a psychiatrist when necessary. Apart from the presenting severity of the patient's condition, the most common criterion for referral to a specialist is probably failure of response to the initial treatment.

Whereas at the beginning of the NHS most GPs were either in single practice or small partnerships, usually working in their own homes or converted accommodation (such as old shops), the trend since then has been strongly toward larger groups and practice in purpose-built health centers. There has also been a considerable growth in the activities of other health professions within primary care; these include several (CPNs, clinical psychologists, social workers) that are wholly or partly concerned with the care of psychiatric patients.

Community Psychiatric Nursing

Finally, the 1970s saw the emergence of community psychiatric nursing as a specialty with its own training; it grew rapidly, partly because of the general disappearance of psychiatric social workers following the reorganization of their profession. The first outpatient nurses had been appointed in 1954 at the psychiatric hospital in Croydon, at the southern edge of London. Their duties included visiting outpatients who had failed to attend or who needed to be seen between attendances, supporting inpatients who had been discharged, helping to find jobs or accommodation for them, and giving support and advice at outpatient clinics or therapeutic social clubs. One of the reasons for this development was a very severe national shortage of mental health social workers. Subsequently, as the inpatient sector began to shrink, psychiatric nurses began to be appointed to work entirely outside hospitals, though from a variety of bases and with differing sources of referral. These numbers began to grow in the 1970s, and then even more sharply in the 1980s; although largely unplanned, this increase outstripped the growth of all other groups of mental health personnel. CPNs came to fall into one of two main groups: those working within a psychiatric multidisciplinary team (which could be based in a psychiatric hospital, a general hospital's psychiatric unit, or a mental health center), and those working in a primary health care setting. The second of these arrangements was encouraged by the fact that many psychiatrists also began to spend part of their time in primary care facilities, but this had the effect of breaking up the mental health team. Views have varied greatly about the optimal way for community nursing to be organized, and this has been associated with increasing ambiguity about how the responsibility for patients should be shared and about the respective acceptability of CPNs to doctors and to their own professional managers (Rawlinson and Brown, 1991).

The first phase of growth of community psychiatric nursing was associated with the trend to extramural management of schizophrenia, which itself was encouraged by the extensive use of depot neuroleptics (Freeman, 1981). CPNs came to take on an essential role in ensuring that those schizophrenic patients who could not be relied on to attend a hospital clinic regularly would in fact continue to receive regular injections; this could be in their own homes, at primary medical care centers, at day centers, in hostels, in group homes, etc. The growth of the service was also associated with the development of special training courses (post-qualification), which mostly last one year; health authorities pay both the fees and the nurses' salaries during training.

After community nursing had been in existence for a few years, specialized CPNs

began to work exclusively with one type of patient—psychogeriatric, mentally retarded, forensic, those requiring behavioural therapy, etc. Specialization greatly improved the quality of care that could be offered to each group, but at the same time
increased costs in a way that became alarming, when real resources for the mental
health services were scarcely growing overall. Community psychiatric nursing by
trained staff exists on a small scale in some other countries, such as Australia, but as
a national service it seems to be unique to Britain. Nevertheless, provision is still at
a very varying level in different parts of the country, though less so than that of social
workers.

The Current Era

For Britain, the 1980s may be said to have begun in 1979, with the return of a radical
right-wing government and dissolution of the ''liberal consensus'' that had governed
social policy since World War II. Although the framework of mental health objectives
remained outwardly unchanged, major differences of emphasis soon emerged. There
was certainly a policy dilemma, in that over 70 percent of mental health expenditure—
which in turn was some 20 percent of NHS expenditure (Office of Health Economics,
1989)—was taken up by hospital costs. While this limited the growth of community-
based services, mental hospitals were supposedly not to be closed until a better service
was available to replace them. In fact, a notable acceleration in the process of hospital
run-down and closure could be observed in the early 1980s, and this often aroused
alarm both among mental health professionals and among the relatives of patients with
more severe disorders, particularly schizophrenia. It was not so much the resettlement
of long-stay hospital residents that caused this concern (though these arrangements
were not always what might have been expected from government statements), but
rather the inadequacy of resources to care for patients already living in the general
community who had long-term disabilities or recurrent episodes of decompensation.
At the same time, structural unemployment was rising to levels not known since the
1930s, so that the chance of paid work for anyone with a psychiatric handicap virtually
disappeared.

As a proportion of Gross Domestic Product, U.K. health expenditure remained the
lowest among advanced industrial countries during the decade, while NHS funding
persistently failed to increase in line with the true rate of inflation. Circumstances,
therefore, were not propitious for a major reorientation of mental health services—as
was required by the rapid shrinking of mental hospital resources—and these material
problems were compounded by disagreement over objectives. Whereas psychiatrists
saw ''community psychiatry'' as the provision of high-quality professional care on a
local basis, with the least possible disruption to patients' normal lives, some other
professionals, ''user'' representatives, and local politicians—in a rerun of 1960s anti-
psychiatry—sought to deny the existence of psychiatric illness altogether, and particularly the need for anyone to be in a hospital on that account.

The decade (if one may expand it, at the other end, to the early 1990s) was one in which administrative changes, policy statements, and proposals for reorganization (some implemented and some not) came thick and fast. A new Mental Health Act in 1983 was to some extent a "lawyers' revenge" for that of 1959; it had no relevance to the overwhelming majority of people with psychiatric disorders (Jones, 1988). A report by the independent Audit Commission (1986) was strongly critical of the state of "community care," as had been the House of Commons Social Services Committee (1985). They had recommended that no psychiatric patient should leave the hospital without a comprehensive care plan that had been agreed among the various services involved. The Griffiths Report on community care (1988) advised that local authorities should have the primary responsibility for all such care, but was unclear about the distinction between this and "treatment," which remained the province of the NHS. The NHS and Community Care Act of 1990 implemented some of the Griffiths proposals, but others were postponed until 1993 because of their implications for local authority budgets. Beginning in 1991, individual care plans became mandatory for patients discharged from a hospital, and a Mental Illness Specific Grant was the first direct subvention from the government to local authorities that could be used only for community mental health services, though the case for it had been strongly argued 30 years earlier (Titmuss, 1961). Also in 1991, the most fundamental reorganization of the NHS since its inception in 1948 seemed to make financial considerations paramount, while the separation of many hospitals or other services into independent trusts posed a threat to the planning and integrative efforts that had patiently been pursued over many years. Both these trends seem likely to have unfavorable implications for the development of community-based psychiatry.

The 1980s also saw a rapid increase in the number of mental health centers operating in Britain; while there was much diversity between these—and some were not very different from DGH units, except for the absence of beds—indications emerged that many were following American trends of the 1970s (Good Practices in Mental Health, 1991). In other words, they were tending to concentrate on patients with less severe neurotic, personality, or situational problems, at the expense of those with serious, long-term disorders. Firm evidence was also discovered that community psychiatric nurses were affected by the same tendency to move away from the care of severe, chronic disorders (Wooff et al., 1988)—an ironical development, since this service had partly come into being because of the abandonment of these clients by social workers.

Both the "key worker" and "case manager" concepts gained some popularity, with both roles being taken at times by the same individual, but an unresolved issue was how to reconcile the needs identified by such a person with the constraints of limited (and sometimes shrinking) resources. Similarly, the "multi-disciplinary team" has often been seen as fundamental to community-based work, but without clarifying the way in which the special skills, status, and legal responsibilities of the consultant psychiatrist fit into that framework. Crisis intervention by such teams has been advocated as a more effective alternative to conventional methods of providing psychiatric services; it might be particularly suitable for areas with high rates of psychiatric morbidity.

Unresolved Issues

Freeman and Bennett (1991) described the British view of community psychiatry as "an eclectic, non-ideological, and largely atheoretical discipline . . . open to and capable of absorbing ideas or data from any school, provided that these are found pragmatically to be capable of reducing disease, distress, or disability." While this national understanding of the term owes more to the biological model than any other single one, "it is equally open to psychodynamic concepts or to such sociological ones as social support and social networks."

In this development, since the end of World War II, such pragmatic questions as how the needs of the relatively small number of people who have severe psychiatric disabilities can be managed have tended to be converted by some into an ideological issue—all care within a hospital by professional staff being labeled as "oppressive." From a different point of view, the need to protect the community from the few mentally disordered individuals who show disruptive or dangerous behavior is often denied by those responsible for planning or managing services, mainly because the facilities required to deal with these cases are expensive, particularly in staff time. British community psychiatry has shown that it can replace many but perhaps not all of the functions of the traditional mental hospital, which was often the place of last resort for individuals with multiple and undifferentiated problems. Meanwhile, there has been steadily growing public concern over incidents of violence and even murder caused by mentally ill people whose treatment and care has been inadequate.

Grob (1991) pointed out that in the United States, a reform movement that began with concern about the condition of people in mental hospitals suffering from long-term disorders ended by setting up a completely new care system, which in fact offered nothing to that group; with the run-down of state hospitals, they were left worse off than ever. In Britain, the possibility remains that the same process could occur, though a well-evaluated solution for those who need constant nursing care is the hospital-hostel. The first unit of this kind was established in a large old house, adjacent to the Maudsley Hospital in south London. An uncontrolled study (Wykes and Wing, 1982) showed that patients attained a better social adjustment there, compared with those of similar clinical status who had remained in hospital wards, while the cost was somewhat lower. In south Manchester, there has been detailed evaluation of a similar unit, also in an old house but quite separate from the hospital campus. There, two groups of patients were matched for chronicity, clinical features, and problem behavior; they had been ill for an average of 12 years, had prominent florid symptoms, and needed 24-hour nursing care. After two years, those in the hospital-hostel had fewer defect symptoms, had acquired more skills, and spent their time more usefully; they much preferred life in this setting to being in hospital. Nursing costs were higher in the hostel unit, but its "hotel-type" maintenance costs were much lower (Hyde et al., 1987). It would seem feasible to establish several such units for any population, forming a network around a hospital base, with each caring for a different kind of patient needing long-term care. So far, however, no such comprehensive arrangement exists, either in Britain or elsewhere. At present, there are still only three units of this kind operating in England, although the model has been recommended in official statements.

Although a unit of this kind can operate very well in ordinary domestic accommodation, it needs permanent staffing at the level of an acute hospital ward; managers whose performance is measured by a financial balance-sheet tend to be unable or unwilling to accept this. At a more modest level, larger numbers of those chronically disabled by psychiatric disorder need long-term asylum: shelter, protection from exploitation, and whatever degree of rehabilitation is possible. The care of this group requires a coordinated policy between the NHS, social services, and voluntary organizations, but little attention has been given to the problem, and virtually no controlled comparison has been made of possible facilities that might replace the mental hospital in this respect (Wing, 1990).

Voluntary Effort and the Views of Users

Another problem that has emerged in more recent years is how to accommodate the views of consumers or "users" of community psychiatric services. The British tradition in these matters has been a paternalistic one, starting with the aristocratic patrons of charitable hospitals and followed by the work of public health pioneers in the nineteenth century. The service developments after World War II followed a similar direction, in which psychiatrists and medical civil servants played the leading roles. With the growth of consumerism and of more egalitarian trends in British society, however, it was to be expected that professional views of this kind would become less prevailing, and this has indeed been the case.

Britain has had a long tradition of voluntary effort in the mental health field, beginning with the establishment in 1863 of the Mental After-Care Association, which has continued to provide a number of residential homes for discharged patients in the Greater London area, with a limited period of stay. In 1948, it was the only one of the existing voluntary organizations that did not amalgamate to form the National Association for Mental Health (NAMH). Essentially an alliance of professionals and interested volunteers at the national level, NAMH lobbied for better services, offered pilot training services (e.g., for social workers and residential care staff), published information on both facilities and general issues, and provided advice to members of the public. At a local level, relatives of the mentally ill were more active, and the emphasis was mainly on providing care facilities, such as day centers and hostels. In 1972, the organization changed its name to MIND and took on a much more "radical" philosophy, resulting in the eventual departure of most of the mental health professionals from its councils.

Partly as a consequence of this change—in which hostility to psychiatric hospitals became increasingly strident—but also through a feeling that the problems caused by schizophrenia were not adequately recognized, a new organization was set up by relatives of people suffering from that disorder. The National Schizophrenia Fellowship (NSF) has provided both a means of mutual support for these families and a strong voice against the premature running down of hospital facilities, when the community-based service that is supposed to replace them still remains very incomplete. NSF probably corresponds most closely to the National Alliance for the Mentally Ill in the United States, though it has not had the same success in obtaining government funding for psychiatric research. Two British organizations—the Mental Health Foundation and Schizophrenia–A National Emergency (SANE)—have been primarily concerned with this latter objective. The Wellcome Trust has also supported research on a very large scale, making up for some of the increasing inadequacies of official funding during the 1980s. In addition, there are groups consisting mostly of ex-patients, such as Survivors Speak Out, which have a specifically anti-psychiatric purpose.

A Department of Health discussion paper on planning district mental health services (1990) urged health authorities to obtain views from the main users of services, particularly as to which activities they regard as key indicators of good performance. It is far from clear, though, how this can be done or how those who claim to be the representatives of users have obtained their legitimacy. Community-based mental health services, including the contribution of primary care, may have contacts with over 20 percent of the population, and within these millions of people, there are likely to be very diverse views. So far, no method has been devised by which the views of these very many users of services could be genuinely represented.

Conclusion

At the mid-point of the 1990s, more than 90 of the 130 mental hospitals that were functioning in England 40 years earlier have already closed, and the number of psychiatric beds has fallen to under 50,000 (Kingdon and Freeman, 1995). The official view is that the total number of places available for people with mental health problems has remained unchanged, because of the growth of private facilities or of housing schemes with some degree of supervision. To equate beds in fully staffed hospitals, though, with accommodations in "bed and breakfast" hostels, operated for profit by unqualified individuals, represents either ignorance of the problem or questionable honesty. Both health and social services now remain in a constant state of turmoil, with constantly increasing numbers of independent facilities engaged in endless bargaining and confrontation, a scenario that British mental health professionals did not have to face before. Since most national information systems for mental health have been disbanded, the precise picture is very difficult to elicit, but it does seem clear that the movement away from hospital care has left the overall service with an institutional base that cannot meet even essential demands (Hollander and Slater, 1994). This deficiency is particularly marked in London and other large cities, where psychiatric hospital units have descended into a perpetual state of crisis. As Rossi and Freeman (1993) wrote of an earlier situation in the United States, organizational changes have been "hurriedly put into place . . . poorly conceived, improperly implemented, and ineffectively administered, without any systematic attempt to assess their impact."

Perhaps the overwhelming lesson of the evolution of community psychiatry in Britain is that public policy is "the art of the possible"—the manifold functions of the asylum *can* be reproduced in community settings, but this will only happen with adequate services and an unvarying commitment to high standards of treatment and care. Regrettably, this is not what has happened. Though the radical critics of conventional services, such as MIND, have lobbied for much more rapid changes from institutions, real-life experience seems to point to an opposite conclusion. The positive aspects of "community psychiatry" would have been better achieved by a much slower process of evolution, which could also have avoided some of the deplorable consequences of recent changes.

References

Allderidge, P. (1985) Bedlam: fact or fantasy? In Bynum, W.F., Porter, R., Shepherd, M. (eds.), *The Anatomy of Madness, Vol. II.* London: Tavistock.

Audit Commission (1986) *Making a Reality of Community Care.* London: HMSO.

Bennett, D.H., and Freeman, H.L. (1991) *Community Psychiatry.* London: Churchill Livingstone.

Berrios, G.E., and Freeman, H.L. (1991) *150 Years of British Psychiatry.* London: Gaskell.

Cooper, J.E., and Sartorius, N. (1975) Cultural and temporal variations in schizophrenia: a speculation of the importance of industrialisation. *British Journal of Psychiatry,* 130: 50–57.

Department of Health (1990) *Planning Distinct Mental Health Services.* London: HMSO.

Department of Health and Social Services (1975) *Better Services for the Mentally Ill* (Command 623). London: HMSO.

Digby, A.L. (1985) *Madness, Mortality and Medicine: a History of the York Retreat.* Cambridge: Cambridge University Press.

Foucault, M. (1963) *Madness and Civilization.* New York: Vintage.

Freeman, H.L. (1960) Oldham and district psychiatric service. *Lancet,* 2:218–221.

Freeman, H.L. (1963) Community mental health services: some general and practical considerations. *Comprehensive Psychiatry,* 4:417–425.

Freeman, H.L. (1981) Long-term treatment of schizophrenia. *Comprehensive Psychiatry,* 22: 94–102.

Freeman, H.L., and Bennett, D.H. (1991) Origins and development. In Bennett, D.H., Freeman, H.L. (eds.) *Community Psychiatry.* London: Churchill Livingstone.

Good Practices in Mental Health (1991) *Community Mental Health Teams.* London: Good Practices in Mental Health.

Griffiths Report (1988) *Community Care: Agenda for Action.* London: HMSO.

Grob, G.N. (1991) *From Asylum to Community.* Princeton: Princeton University Press.

Hollander, D., and Slater, M.S. (1994) "Sorry, no beds": a problem for acute psychiatric admissions. *Psychiatric Bulletin,* 18:532–534.

House of Commons Social Services Committee (1985) *Community care, with special reference to the adult mentally ill and mentally hadicapped.* London: HMSO.

Hyde, C., Bridges, K., Goldberg, D.P., Lowson, K., Sterling, C., and Faragher, B. (1987) The evaluation of a hostel ward: a controlled study using modified cost-benefit analysis. *British Journal of Psychiatry,* 151:805–812.

Jones, K. (1972) *A History of the Mental Health Services.* London: Routledge and Kegan Paul.

Jones, K. (1979) Integration or disintegration of the mental health service. In Meacher, M. (ed.), *New Methods of Mental Health Care.* Oxford: Pergamon Press.

Jones, K. (1988) *Experience in Mental Health: Community Care and Social Policy.* London: Sage.

Jones, Maxwell (1952) *Social Psychiatry.* London: Tavistock.

Kingdon, D., and Freeman, H.L. (1995) Personnel options in the treatment of schizophrenia. In Moscarelli, M., Sartorius, N. (eds.), *The Economics of Schizophrenia.* Chichester: Wiley.

Main, T.F. (1946) The hospital as a therapeutic community. *Bulletin of the Menninger Clinic,* 10:24–30.

Martin, F.M. (1984) *Between the Acts.* London: Nuffield Provincial Hospitals Trust.

Mayou, R. (1989) The history of general hospital psychiatry. *British Journal of Psychiatry,* 155:764–776.

Merskey, H. (1991) Shell-Shock. In, Berrios, G.E., Freeman, H.L. (eds.), *150 Years of British Psychiatry.*

Office of Health Economics (1989) *Mental Health in the 1990s.* London: OHE.

Parry Jones, W.L. (1972) *The Trade in Lunacy.* London: Routledge and Kegan Paul.

Pines, M.L. (1991) The development of the psychodynamic movement. In Berrios, G.E., Freeman, H.L. (eds.), *150 Years of British Psychiatry.* London: Gaskell.

Rawlinson, J.W., and Brown, A.C. (1991) Community psychiatric nursing in Britain. In Bennett, D.H., Freeman, H.L. (eds.), *Community Psychiatry.* London: Churchill Livingstone.

Rossi, P.H., and Freeman, H.E. (1993) *Evaluation: A Systematic Approach* (5th edition). London: Sage.

Scull, A.T. (1977) *Decarceration: Community Treatment and the Deviant—A Radical View.* Englewood Cliffs, NJ: Prentice-Hall.

Tantam, D., and Goldberg, D.P. (1991) Primary health care. In Bennett, D.H., Freeman, H.L. (eds.), *Community Psychiatry.* London: Churchill Livingstone.

Titmuss, R. (1961) Community Care: fact or fiction. In *Proceedings of the Annual Conference of the National Association for Mental Health.* London: NAMH.

Tooth, G.C., and Brooke, E.M. (1961) Trends in the mental hospital population and their effect on future planning. *Lancet,* i:710–713.

Walton, J.K. (1986) Casting out and bringing back in Victorian England: pauper lunatics. In, Bynum, W.F., Potter, R., Shepherd, M. (eds.), *The Anatomy of Madness, Vol. II.* London: Tavistock.

Webster, C. (1987) *The Health Services Since the War, Vol. I. Problems of Health Care: The National Health Service Before 1957.* London: HMSO.

Wing, J.K. (1990) The functions of asylum. *British Journal of Psychiatry,* 157:822–827.

Wooff, K., Goldberg, D.P., and Fryers, T. (1988) The practice of community psychiatric nursing and mental health social work in Salford: some implications for community care. *British Journal of Psychiatry,* 152:783–792.

Wykes, T., and Wing, J.K. (1982) A ward in a house: accommodation for "new" long-stay patients. *Acta Psychiatrica Scandinavica,* 63:315–330.

II

The Foundations

6

Epidemiology:
The Distribution of Mental
Disorders in the Community

JACK F. SAMUELS
GERALD NESTADT

Psychiatric epidemiology is concerned with describing and explaining the patterns of psychiatric disorders in populations. The discipline comprises a set of principles, a collection of methods, and a body of knowledge for measuring frequency and elucidating patterns of psychiatric disorders in the community. Epidemiological methods provide clues to the etiology and prevention of these disorders and provide a rational basis for planning and evaluating community mental health services. This chapter presents an overview of epidemiological methods useful for gaining information about the frequency and patterns of occurrence of psychiatric disorders in the community and for investigating the relationship of these disorders to sociodemographic and other factors.

Descriptive Epidemiology: Quantification of Psychiatric Disorders in the Community

Rates

Epidemiologists use *rates* to quantify the occurrence of psychiatric disorders in the community and to compare the occurrence between subgroups within communities. A rate is a quantity defined as the number of ''events'' in a population in a specified time period, divided by the number of persons in the population.

There are three essential components of a rate. The first component, the numerator, is the number of cases or events. Some examples of psychiatric events include a new case of schizophrenia, relapse of psychotic symptoms in a previously treated schizophrenic patient, adverse consequences of psychiatric disorders such as suicide attempts, and hospitalization or utilization of other psychiatric services.

The second component, in the denominator, is the size of the population out of which the cases or events arise; for instance, the entire community, or subsets of the community specified by age, sex, and race or ethnicity; or persons receiving a specific intervention. The third essential component, also in the denominator, is a period of time, such as a year. A rate might be conceived as the change in the number of events, relative to the population size, over the specified time period.

Rates inform us about the frequency and dynamics of psychiatric disorders in the community. Thus, 100 new cases of a disorder over a year in a population of one thousand people suggests a much more dynamic situation than 100 new cases of a disorder in a population of one million. In addition, properly estimated rates are useful for approximating the number of cases of a specific psychiatric disorder in the community. For instance, if a representative sample of 1,000 subjects is drawn from a community with 100,000 members, and seven of the sampled subjects have schizophrenia (i.e., an estimated rate of current schizophrenia of 7 per thousand), then we would estimate that there are approximately 700 cases of schizophrenia in the entire community of 100,000 at this point in time, within a certain sampling margin. This is an example of a *point prevalence* rate, which measures the number of existing cases of a disorder at a point in time.

Other types of rates also are used in psychiatric epidemiology. A *period prevalence* rate measures the number of cases of a disorder that are present in a population during all or part of a specified time period. The *lifetime prevalence* rate measures the number of cases of the disorder ever occurring in the lifetimes of the members of the community up to the current point in time. An *incidence* rate measures the number of new cases of a disorder in a population during a specified time period.

A census of the community, with interpolation for inter-censal years, provides an approximation of the number of individuals in the population and the denominator for calculation of rates. Data on the frequency of psychiatric events, to provide numerators, come from two major sources: treated cases and community surveys.

Treated Cases

Treatment records.   As far back as the early nineteenth century, psychiatrists have collected statistical information about cases treated in psychiatric hospitals (Grob, 1985). Surveys of cases receiving inpatient and outpatient psychiatric services continue to provide valuable information about those who utilize mental health services and about the services provided. For example, the NIMH National Reporting Program collects information about resident patients in state and county psychiatric hospitals (Census of State and County Mental Hospitals) (Manderscheid and Sonnenschein, 1992) and patients receiving psychiatric care from a sample of office-based physicians (National Ambulatory Medical Care Survey) (Regier and Burke, 1989). A census of mental health facilities and a sample of providers of mental health services at the local level could provide similar information for any geographically defined community.

Information about treated cases has several advantages for quantifying psychiatric disorders in the community. First, it is useful in describing the demographic and clinical features of patients, such as diagnosis, length of stay, and treatment received, as well as the patterns of utilization of psychiatric services. Second, the information is routinely collected and readily available. Third, information about clinical features of the disorder is provided by physicians involved in treatment of the cases. The use of this type of information has demonstrated, for example, the dramatic decline since 1955 in the number of resident patients in psychiatric hospitals and the corresponding dramatic shift toward nursing home care for geriatric patients. It also has revealed that most treatment for mental disorders is provided by the primary care/outpatient medical sector (Regier et al., 1978).

Case registers and record linkage.   A *case registry* contains basic information about cases of a disorder coming to treatment in the community. A *record linkage system* is defined by Woogh (1987a,b) as ''a systematic standardized collection [and integration] of data about contacts made by unduplicated individuals with specified facilities over time.'' In such a system, all cases of a disorder coming to the attention of psychiatrists, other mental health professionals, and even criminal justice, legal, and social service agencies, are recorded on a data form containing demographic, diagnostic, and other information. These data are transmitted on paper or electronically to a central registry and stored in a computerized data base. All subsequent contacts of the individual with the mental health system are linked, on the basis of a unique patient identifier, such as name or Social Security number.

There are several advantages to such a system, relative to using routinely collected information about cases coming to treatment. First, all information about mental services utilization is collated for each individual, rather than duplicated for each patient contact. Second, broader coverage of information can be included in data collection forms than is possible for routinely collected information on psychiatric cases. Third, more rigorous diagnostic standards can be implemented, so that only cases meeting certain clearly specified diagnostic criteria are included in the registry. Fourth, collecting information about individuals over time allows description of the natural history of the illness and factors related to the recurrence of symptoms.

An early classic example is the psychiatric case register in Monroe County, New York, which included inpatient and outpatient child, adolescent, and adult contacts with facilities and private practitioners in the city of Rochester and the surrounding suburban and rural areas (Gardner et al., 1963). The Camberwell Cumulative Psychiatric Case Register includes information on adults and children making contact with inpatient, day-patient, and outpatient psychiatric services in Camberwell, London (Wing et al., 1968). More recently, the Kingston Psychiatric Record Linkage System was set up in Kingston, Ontario, a medium-sized city with relatively few private practitioners and three psychiatric inpatient facilities. The system links inpatient and outpatient contacts at the facilities, but not private practitioner contacts (Woogh, 1988).

Surveillance.   Surveillance is described by Last (1988) as "ongoing scrutiny, generally using methods distinguished by their practicality, uniformity, and frequently their rapidity, rather than by complete accuracy. Its main purpose is to detect changes in trend or distribution in order to initiate investigative or control measures." A surveillance system may be useful for the identification and description of psychiatric disorders that do not come to treatment, and may provide insight into the incidence trends of disorders that are rapidly changing over time. Such knowledge could point the way toward control of a problem that is getting out of hand.

For example, the Drug Abuse Warning Network (DAWN) is a system of selected emergency rooms, medical examiners, and crisis centers that provide information on the types of drugs and characteristics of persons involved in overdoses in a sample of cities throughout the country (Ungerleider et al., 1980). An alcoholism social indicator system that tracks problems that occur with higher frequency among alcoholics, such as violent deaths and vehicular accidents, also has been described (Westermeyer and Bearman, 1974).

Primary care.   Primary care provides a middle ground for the study of the frequency and patterns of psychiatric disorders in the community. Primary care patients are not, in most cases, seeking psychiatric services, nor are they randomly selected residents of the community. Surveys of patients in primary care have several of the advantages of institutional surveys, on the one hand, and community surveys, on the other. First, it has become clear that most cases of psychiatric disorders reaching treatment are seen not by psychiatric specialists but by primary care physicians. Thus, the types of cases seen in primary care (mostly depression and anxiety) are more representative of the cases in the community, with a broader spectrum of symptoms, than those seen in the specialized psychiatric sector. Second, when there is relatively free access to primary medical care, the primary care population is more representative of the general population, so that rates of psychiatric disorders in the primary care population approximate rates of these disorders in the community. Third, because a threshold of distress and problematic behavior must be crossed before a patient presents with psychiatric symptoms to a physician, ascertained cases may better reflect the self-perceived need for care than those found in community surveys (Shepherd and Wilkinson, 1988).

Epidemiological Surveys

Community surveys.   Despite insights that can be gained from the quantification of psychiatric disorders in treated populations, estimation of the true prevalence and incidence of psychiatric disorders requires surveys of the general population. The assessment of psychiatric disorders in the entire community also is necessary to properly investigate correlates of these disorders and to plan and evaluate the effectiveness of interventions.

In rare instances, if the community is small and geographically isolated or sharply defined, it may be possible to examine virtually every inhabitant and thus conduct a complete survey of the entire population. For example, in the Lundby study, nearly 99 percent of the 2550 inhabitants of two adjacent parishes in southern Sweden were examined (Essen-Möller, 1947). Rutter (1989) surveyed the entire population of about 3,500 children 9–11 years old living on the Isle of Wight. Such studies are rarely possible today, and it is necessary to select a representative sample of the inhabitants of the community for assessment of psychiatric disorders. If the sample is rigorously drawn, then the rates of psychiatric disorders in the population can be estimated from the sample, with sampling errors attached to the estimated rates.

There have been several important surveys of psychiatric disorders in communities in North America, for example, the Stirling County Study (Hughes et al., 1960) and the Midtown Manhattan Study (Srole et al., 1962). The conduct of more recent surveys of psychiatric disorders in the community relied on three developments. First, an accepted nosology of psychiatric disorders (such as DSM-III and ICD-9) was required, so that diagnoses could be standardized. Second, operationalized diagnostic criteria (such as the RDC criteria) were necessary. Third, a standardized interview for psychiatric disorders, either for psychiatrists, such as the Present State Examination (PSE) (Wing et al., 1974) and Structured Clinical Interview for DSM-III-R (SCID) (Spitzer et al., 1992) or for lay interviewers, such as the Diagnostic Interview Survey (DIS) (Robins, 1990), had to be developed, so that information on psychiatric symptoms could be obtained reliably (Dohrenwend and Dohrenwend, 1982).

The largest and most rigorous of community surveys of psychiatric disorders in the United States was the Epidemiological Catchment Area (ECA) Program of the National Institute of Mental Health, conducted in the early 1980s in five U.S. cities: New Haven, Baltimore, St. Louis, Durham, and Los Angeles (Robins and Regier, 1991). The ECA represents a landmark in the quantification of psychiatric disorders, providing estimates of prevalence and incidence rates of specific psychiatric disorders in defined communities. To the extent that the population of the surveyed communities reflects that of another community of interest, these rates can be applied to that community, and the number of cases of specific psychiatric disorders can be estimated. Also, using age, sex, and gender-specific rates, the numbers of cases for different demographic groups can be estimated. These numbers are extremely useful for assessing the needs for and the rational planning of mental health services for a community, and serve as the baseline for evaluation of new mental health programs in an area. In addition, information about specific risk factors allows psychiatric epidemiologists to investigate their relationship to psychiatric disorders.

Table 6-1 shows estimated one-month prevalence rates of selected disorders in Baltimore, Maryland, in 1981. The diagnoses were based on administration of the NIMH Diagnostic Interview Schedule (DIS) by trained lay interviewers. For contrast, estimates based on psychiatric examinations of a subset of the subjects in the second

Table 6–1   One-month prevalence (percent) of selected DSM-III
conditions, Epidemiologic Catchment Area Study, Baltimore, 1981

	Method of Case Ascertainment	
	DIS[a]	Psychiatrist[b]
Schizophrenia	0.7	0.5
Major depressive episode	2.3	1.1
Manic episode	0.4	0.4
Panic disorder	1.0	0.1
Obsessive-compulsive disorder	1.3	0.3
Alcohol use disorders	3.6	6.9
Drug use disorders	2.2	3.1
Phobias	11.2	21.3

Source: Anthony et al. (1985).
[a]Diagnostic Interview Schedule, by lay interviewers, of 3,481 subjects.
[b]Clinical examination, by psychiatrists, of 810 subjects.

stage of the same study are presented. It is seen that the estimated prevalence of
several of these conditions is influenced by the method of case ascertainment used.

Table 6-2 presents the estimated one-year incidence rates of selected disorders
from four ECA sites. It is seen from these estimates that more than one percent of
the adult population develops new cases of several of these disorders every year, an
important consideration for planning community psychiatric services. Furthermore,
although the annual incidence of several of these disorders (most notably schizophrenia) is quite low, the current prevalence may be considerable because of the chronicity
of these conditions and their onset in young adulthood.

These estimates provide a basis for judging the adequacy and appropriateness of
available community services and are informative about the quantity and types of
necessary services. The prevalence of psychiatric disorders is useful for determining
service needs but, as Bebbington (1990) points out, impaired social functioning may
be more important than symptoms as the relevant clinical feature. For example, as
part of the ECA study, Shapiro et al. (1985) investigated the need for psychiatric
services in a representative sample of noninstitutionalized subjects in Baltimore. Using
a composite of psychopathology and disability, they estimated that 11–15 percent of
the population had a need for psychiatric services, and 5–9 percent had an unmet
need.

Surveys of special populations.   Community psychiatrists may be interested in the
prevalence of psychiatric disorders in special segments of the population, for example,
those thought to be at high risk of disorders and those underserved by existing mental
health services. These populations may not be adequately covered in general community surveys if their numbers are relatively small or if they live in geographically
isolated areas not covered by the survey.

Table 6–2   Annual incidence (per 100 person-years) of selected
DIS/DSM-III disorders, Epidemiologic Catchment Area Study*

	Incidence
Phobic disorders	4.0
Alcohol use disorders	1.8
Major depressive disorder	1.6
Drug use disorders	1.1
Obsessive-compulsive disorder	0.7
Panic disorder	0.6
Schizophrenia	0.001

Source: Eaton et al. (1989).
*Baltimore, St. Louis, Los Angeles, and Durham.

One approach is to over-sample special segments of the survey population in a community survey. For example, in the ECA surveys, the Baltimore, New Haven, and Durham sites over-sampled the elderly, the St. Louis site over-sampled African-Americans, and the Los Angeles site over-sampled Hispanics. Alternatively, special surveys of these segments of the population may be conducted. For instance, the Baltimore Homeless Study randomly selected homeless subjects in missions, shelters, and jails in Baltimore in 1986 and 1987 (Breakey et al., 1989). Similarly, Susser et al. surveyed men at first entry to New York City municipal men's shelters in 1985 (Susser et al., 1989). These studies demonstrate the high rates of psychiatric disorders, especially schizophrenia and alcohol and other substance use disorders in the homeless and their substantial need for medical and psychiatric treatment.

Some other examples of special populations include refugees and recent immigrants to the community (Beiser and Fleming, 1986) and the elderly (Bowling and Farquhar, 1991). Such surveys identify special psychiatric problems and needs in these segments of the population, provide baseline measures for the evaluation and planning of programs, and identify subjects for the investigation of relationships between specific factors and psychiatric disorders.

Summary

The various sources of information differ in the type of information provided about psychiatric disorders, the availability and ease of obtaining the information, and the generalizability of the information obtained. No one source of information is ideal. The information provided to the community psychiatrist from the different sources is complementary and, taken together, can provide insight into the frequency of psychiatric disorders in the community. In addition, by expanding assessment beyond the clinical horizon, this information helps elucidate the full spectrum of psychiatric disorders, including subclinical and mild cases, and may help identify new syndromes in the community.

Discerning Patterns and Trends

Patterns by Person and Place

Psychiatric disorders are not randomly distributed throughout the community. One of the major contributions of epidemiology is to describe patterns of disease occurrence. These patterns provide clues to the etiology and prevention of psychiatric disorders. Furthermore, knowledge of the distribution of disorders is crucial for rational planning and evaluation of community services.

The frequency of specific psychiatric disorders has been shown to vary by geographic area and socioeconomic class. For example, Faris and Dunham found a relationship between first admissions to mental hospitals and area of residence in Chicago in the 1930s: areas with the highest levels of social disorganization had the highest rates of hospitalization (Faris and Dunham, 1939). In the early 1950s, Hollingshead and Redlich surveyed mental health facilities and private-practice psychiatrists treating patients in New Haven, Connecticut. They found a strong inverse relationship between social class and the treated prevalence of mental disorders. Treated cases in lower social classes were found to have more severe disorders, of longer duration, and were more likely to be treated in long-stay public psychiatric hospitals, as compared to those in the upper social classes (Hollingshead and Redlich, 1958). More recently, rural/urban differences in the prevalence of specific psychiatric disorders have been investigated. For example, residents of contiguous rural and urban counties in North Carolina were surveyed as part of the ECA study. It was found that major depression and drug abuse/dependence were more common in urban areas, whereas alcohol abuse/dependence was more prevalent in rural areas (Blazer et al., 1985).

Psychiatric disorders may occur differently according to other personal characteristics such as gender, age, or racial/ethnic group. Table 6–3 shows the one-month prevalence of selected DIS/DSM-III disorders by demographic factors, for all ECA sites combined. Schizophrenia, major depression, and alcohol abuse/dependence are more prevalent in the younger age groups, whereas cognitive impairment increases with age. Alcohol use disorders are much more common in men, but major depression is more prevalent in women. Schizophrenia and cognitive impairment are more prevalent in African-Americans than other groups. Schizophrenia, alcohol use disorders, and major depression are notable in subjects who are separated or divorced, whereas cognitive impairment is much more frequent in the widowed. Schizophrenia, major depression, and cognitive impairment are more prevalent in lower socioeconomic groups.

The *stress hypothesis* proposes that higher rates of psychiatric disorders in socially disorganized inner city areas and in lower socioeconomic classes is due to increased exposure to social stresses and adversities. In contrast, the *selection hypothesis* maintains that persons with psychiatric disorders, or predispositions to them, drift to areas of urban poverty (Dohrenwend, 1990).

Table 6–3   One-month prevalence (percent) of selected DIS/DSM-III disorders, by demographic factors, all Epidemiologic Catchment Area sites combined, 1981/1982

	Schizophrenia	Alcohol use disorders	Major depression	Severe cognitive impairment
Age				
18–24	0.8	4.1	2.2	0.6
25–44	1.1	3.6	3.0	0.4
45–64	0.5	2.1	2.0	1.2
65+	0.1	0.9	0.7	4.9
Sex				
Male	0.7	5.0	1.6	1.4
Female	0.7	0.9	2.9	1.3
Race/ethnicity				
Black	1.2	3.4	2.5	3.3
Hispanic	0.4	3.6	2.6	1.3
Other	0.6	2.7	2.2	0.9
Marital status				
Married	0.5	2.0	1.7	0.7
Single	1.1	4.2	2.5	1.0
Separated or divorced	1.5	5.9	4.7	1.6
Widowed	0.4	1.3	2.0	5.4
SES				
1 (high)	0.3	2.3	1.3	0.2
2	0.6	3.0	2.2	0.3
3	0.9	3.0	2.9	0.9
4 (low)	1.2	3.0	2.2	5.1

Source: Regier et al. (1993).

Time Trends

Psychiatric disorders in communities may show trends over time. The rates of some psychiatric disorders, such as schizophrenia, appear to have changed little over time whereas other disorders, such as depression, appear to have increased over time. Other conditions may occur epidemically, for example heroin abuse, or even in focal outbreaks, for example post-disaster anxiety and adolescent suicide.

Under steady-state conditions, in which the population is stable and incidence and duration of a disorder are not changing, point prevalence is a function of incidence rate and duration. This relationship between prevalence, incidence, and duration of psychiatric disorders has important implications for interpreting temporal trends in community psychiatry. For example, if the prevalence of a psychiatric disorder has increased over time, it may be due to an increase in the incidence rate (i.e., new cases of the disorder), or to an increase in the duration of the episodes of the disorder, or both. In turn, the duration will be increased by forces, such as new treatments, that increase survival times of those with the disorder. Increasing the duration of a disorder by reducing mortality due to the disorder or related causes will paradoxically lead to an increase in the prevalence, even if the incidence rate remains constant (Gruenberg, 1977). Conversely, a decline in the prevalence of a disorder may be due to a decrease in the incidence rate, or a decrease in the duration of the disorder, or both. The decrease in the duration may be due to more effective treatments, or to less favorable outcomes producing earlier mortality. It should also be noted that the prevalence of a disorder may show no change over time, if the incidence is increasing to the same extent that the duration is decreasing, or vice versa.

Time-Related Effects

Three time-related effects may explain secular trends in the rates of psychiatric disorders in a population. First, the rate of disorder can vary by age, regardless of when the person was born. This is an *age effect*. For example, the incidence rate of Alzheimer's disease increases sharply after the age of 65 years; as the population ages, the prevalence of Alzheimer's disease increases. Second, the rate of disease can vary by the calendar time through which a person has lived, regardless of his age. This is a *period effect*. For example, the rate of measles encephalopathy declined following introduction of immunization programs. People growing up in the years since immunization was implemented are less likely to have the disease than people growing up in other eras. Third, the prevalence of disease can vary by the year in which the person was born, that is, by the person's birth cohort. This is a *cohort effect*. For example, babies conceived and born during famine may carry a relatively high or low risk of a psychiatric disorder throughout their lives (Susser and Lin, 1992). Because these three time effects are interrelated, it may often be difficult to disentangle them.

For example, Klerman and Weissman discuss the apparent increase in rates of major depression, particularly in younger cohorts born after World War II, and the concomitant younger age of first onset. When the age-specific rates of depression are plotted separately, by birth cohort, it is found that the risk of major depression at every age is successively higher in later birth cohorts (cohort effect). There also is evidence of a period effect, in that subjects from all birth cohorts show an increase in rates of depression between 1965 and 1975 (Klerman and Weissman, 1989).

Time trends in the prevalence of disorders can also be affected by changes in the population. Changes in birth rates, mortality rates, and migration can change the structure of the community, placing a greater proportion of the population in age groups with greater rates of disorder. For example, even if the incidence rate for Alzheimer's disease in the elderly did not change, the prevalence of the disorder in the entire population would increase, simply because a greater proportion of the population is living to older ages. Therefore, in order to more meaningfully compare rates of disorders between places and over time, epidemiologists often use rates that are *adjusted* statistically for demographic factors, such as age, gender, and ethnic group. Alternatively, *specific* rates (e.g., age-specific or gender-specific rates) can be compared across places or times. Those involved in planning and evaluating mental health services, as well as those investigating relationships between risk factors and psychiatric disorders in communities, need to be aware of alternative explanations for secular changes in rates of psychiatric disorders.

Investigating Relationships

Analytic Epidemiology

To this point, we have discussed the contribution of *descriptive* epidemiology, i.e., describing the frequency and patterns of occurrence of psychiatric disorders in the community. These patterns are clues, suggesting possible relationships between a variety of factors and the frequency and distribution of disorders. Clues can also arise from the astute observations of psychiatrists observing patients in clinical settings. The purpose of *analytic* epidemiology is to evaluate the relationships or associations between psychiatric disorders and specific factors that may be involved in the initiation and progression of these disorders. Because of uncertainty from epidemiological evidence alone about the etiologic role of factors that appear to increase the probability of an outcome, they are referred to as *risk factors* or *risk correlates* rather than causes.

Outbreak Investigation

Classical epidemiology deals with the investigation of disease outbreaks, a rapid rise in the number of cases of disease in a discrete geographic area. Such outbreaks continue to occur for a variety of diseases caused by microorganisms. However, outbreaks of psychiatric disorders also can occur, and epidemiologic principles and methods can help elucidate the factors involved.

A *common source outbreak* is caused by exposure of a group to a common, adverse influence. Such outbreaks have occurred for psychiatric disorders, often in conjunction with natural or man-made disasters. Some examples are the Coconut Grove fire in Boston in 1943 (Adler, 1943), the 1972 Buffalo Creek flood in West Virginia (Special Section, 1976), the Three Mile Island nuclear reactor accident (Bromet et al., 1982) and the eruption of Mount St. Helens in 1980 (Shore et al., 1986). In this last study, high and low stress exposures in the area severely affected by the eruption were defined on the basis of property loss or death of a family member or close relative; a nearby control community unaffected by the eruption also was surveyed. It was found that generalized anxiety, major depression, and post-traumatic stress disorder were significantly associated with disaster stress, being lowest in the control community and highest in the high exposure areas. A particularly susceptible subgroup was composed of older females who were concerned about finances and had a prior physical health problem.

A *propagated outbreak* results from transmission of a pathogenic agent from one susceptible host to another. Outbreaks of apparently psychogenic origin were frequent in the Middle Ages. The Salem witch hunt was an example of the same phenomenon in colonial America (Veith, 1965). De Alarcon investigated the spread of heroin abuse in an English town, finding two major transmission pathways spreading from an initiator outside the town (de Alarcon, 1969). Outbreaks of hysteria in classrooms (Benaim et al., 1973) and of suicide and suicide attempts in adolescents and young adults (Phillips and Carstensen, 1986) have also been investigated.

Observational Studies

Cohort studies.   In the cohort (prospective, follow-up) study, two or more study groups are selected from a population initially free of the disorder. One of the study groups has not been "exposed" to the factor of interest, whereas the other group has been exposed to the factor. These groups are then followed forward in time to identify new cases. The follow-up may be completely prospective, in that the researcher follows the study population from the onset of the study period, or it may be retrospective, in that the exposure and outcome have occurred prior to the initiation of the study. In the latter case, secondary data collected for other purposes, such as medical records, are employed. The incidence rate of the outcome of interest in the exposed group is compared to that in the unexposed group. Expressed as a ratio, this is called the *rate ratio* or *relative risk.*

The cohort design has several advantages for investigating relationships in the community. It conceptually approximates a classical experiment, although individuals in the two groups are not randomly assigned to exposure. It is useful for studying rare exposures, and it allows examination of a variety of outcomes post-exposure. Since exposure predates outcome, outcome status cannot influence selection of subjects into the two groups, a type of selection bias that could lead to invalid interpretations of results. Furthermore, the direction of the exposure-outcome relationship is clear, adding credibility to any estimated association.

Cohort studies have provided intriguing evidence about the relationship between selected factors and psychiatric disorders. For example, Mednick et al. (1988) investigated all psychiatric hospitalizations over a 26-year period, in persons whose gestations overlapped with a severe type-A2 influenza epidemic that occurred from October 8 to November 14, 1957, in Helsinki, Finland. Controls were children born in the 6 years preceding the influenza epidemic. It was found that the "exposed" group was significantly more likely to have subsequent hospital admission for schizophrenia, but only if exposed during the second trimester. This excess was not observed for any other psychiatric diagnosis. These findings suggest a specific schizophrenogenic effect of prenatal exposure to influenza infection during the second trimester of gestation.

Case-control studies.   In the case-control (case-referent, retrospective) study, a group of incident or prevalent cases of disorder or other outcome is selected, and a group of non-cases (controls) is also selected. The two groups are compared with respect to past exposure to a factor of interest. The odds of exposure in the cases is compared to the odds of exposure in the controls. The ratio of these two odds is called the *odds ratio* or *relative odds* (also, the *cross-product ratio*). It can be shown that, if the disorder or other outcome under investigation is rare, then the odds ratio approximates the risk ratio and can be similarly interpreted. Subjects in case and comparison groups can be "matched" on other factors that the investigator wants to control.

The case-control design has several advantages compared to the cohort design. The study period is relatively short, since a long follow-up period is not required. It is useful for studying rare disorders. In addition, case-control studies generally are less expensive than cohort studies (Kleinbaum et al., 1982).

Case-control studies are useful for investigating risk factors for psychiatric disorders in the community. For example, Petronis et al. (1990) used data collected in the ECA surveys to investigate risk factors for suicide attempts. Forty subjects who had attempted suicide in the 2-year period around the baseline interview were compared with 160 controls who were matched on age and census tract. Significant risk factors for attempted suicide were depression (relative odds = 41), alcoholism (relative odds = 18), cocaine use (relative odds = 62), and being separated or divorced (relative odds = 11).

Summary

The etiology of psychiatric disorders appears to be very complex. Most conditions probably have a multifactorial etiology, and it is impossible to identify a single causal factor which, acting alone, invariably produces disorder. Rather, it is probable that many factors must act together, either sequentially or simultaneously, before a psychiatric disorder can occur. Causation cannot be proven on the basis of an observational epidemiological study. Ultimate proof of causation requires the experimental method, via randomized trials. Operationally, if it is demonstrated longitudinally that removing the putative cause—holding other factors constant—leads to reduction in the incidence of the disorder, then there is stronger evidence of a causal relationship. Therefore, rigorous evaluation of prevention programs may provide evidence of causal factors in psychiatric disorders.

Conclusion

This chapter has focused on epidemiologic methods useful for interpreting information about the distribution of psychiatric disorders in the community and for investigating the relationship of these disorders to sociodemographic and other factors. The techniques of psychiatric epidemiology also are applicable to assessing the need for mental health services in the community (Chapter 8) and for evaluating the efficacy of prevention programs (Chapter 24).

Community psychiatry focuses on the problems and needs of individuals as well as on the problems and needs of communities. These two roles are interdependent. Noxious and protective influences in the community impact on the mental health of the individual. Conversely, the ill individual places economic and social burdens on the community. Psychiatric epidemiology is fundamental in quantifying these problems, elucidating their patterns in the community, and evaluating the effectiveness of psychiatric responses to them.

References

Adler, A. (1943) Neuropsychiatric complication in victims of Boston's Coconut Grove disaster. *JAMA,* 123:1098–1101.

Anthony, J.C., Folstein, M., Romanoski, A.J., Nestadt, G., and Von Korff, M. (1985) Comparison of the Lay Diagnostic Interview Schedule and a standardized Psychiatric Diagnosis. *Archives of General Psychiatry,* 42:667–675.

Bebbington, P.E. (1990) Population surveys of psychiatric disorder and the need for treatment. *Social Psychiatry and Psychiatric Epidemiology,* 25:33–40.

Beiser, M., and Fleming, J. A. E. (1986) Measuring psychiatric disorder among Southeast Asian refugees. *Psychological Medicine,* 16:627–639.

Benaim, S., Horder, J., and Anderson, J. (1973) Hysterical epidemic in a classroom. *Psychological Medicine,* 3:366–373.

Blazer, D., George, L.K., Landerman, R., Pennybacker, M., Melville, M.L., Woodbury, M., Manton, K.G., Jordan, K., and Locke, B. (1985) Psychiatric disorders: a rural/urban comparison. *Archives of General Psychiatry,* 42:651–656.

Bowling, A., and Farquhar, M. (1991) Associations with social networks, social support, health status and psychiatric morbidity in three samples of elderly people. *Social Psychiatry and Psychiatric Epidemiology,* 26:115–126.

Breakey, W.R., Fischer, P.J., Kramer, M., Nestadt, G., Romanoski, A.J., Ross, A., Royall, R.M., and Stine, O.C. (1989) Health and mental health problems of homeless men and women in Baltimore. *JAMA,* 262:1352–1357.

Bromet, E., Parkinson, D., Schulberg, H., Dunn, L.O., and Gondek, P.C. (1982) Mental health of residents near the Three Mile Island reactor: a comparative study of selected groups. *Journal of Preventive Psychiatry,* 1:225–276.

de Alarcon, R. (1969) The spread of heroin abuse in a community. *World Health Organization Bulletin on Narcotics,* 21:17–22.

Dohrenwend, B.P. (1990) Socioeconomic status (SES) and psychiatric disorders: are the issues still compelling? *Social Psychiatry and Psychiatric Epidemiology,* 25:41–47.

Dohrenwend, B.P., and Dohrenwend, B.S. (1982) Perspectives on the past and future of psychiatric epidemiology. *American Journal of Public Health,* 72:1271–1279.

Eaton, W.W., Kramer, M., Anthony, J.C., Dryman, A., Shapiro, S., and Locke, B.Z. (1989) The incidence of specific DIS/DSM-III mental disorders: data from the NIMH Epidemiologic Catchment Area Program. *Acta Psychiatrica Scandinavica,* 79:163–178.

Essen-Möller, E. (1947) Individual traits and morbidity in a Swedish rural population. *Acta Psychiatrica et Neurologica,* (suppl. 100).

Faris, R. E. L., and Dunham, H.W. (1939) *Mental Disorders in Urban Areas: An Ecological Study of Schizophrenia and Other Psychoses.* Chicago: University of Chicago Press.

Gardner, E.A., Miles, H.C., Iker, H.P., and Romano, J. (1963) A cumulative register of psychiatric services in a community. *American Journal of Public Health,* 53:1269–1277.

Grob, G.N. (1985) The origins of American psychiatric epidemiology. *American Journal of Public Health,* 75:229–236.

Gruenberg, E.M. (1977) The failures of success. *Milbank Memorial Fund Quarterly,* 55:3–24.

Hollingshead, A.B., and Redlich, F.C. (1958) *Social Class and Mental Illness: A Community Study.* New York: Wiley.

Hughes, C.C., Tremblay, M., Rapoport, R.N., and Leighton, A.H. (1960) People of cove and woodlot: Communities from the viewpoint of social psychiatry. *The Stirling County Study of Psychiatric Disorder and Sociocultural Environment, Vol. II.* New York: Basic Books.

Kleinbaum, D.G., Kupper, L.L., and Morgenstern, H. (1982) *Epidemiologic Research: Principles and Quantitative Methods.* Belmont, California: Wadsworth.

Klerman, G.L., and Weissman, M.M. (1989) Increasing rates of depression. *JAMA,* 261:229–235.

Last, J.M. (ed.) (1988) *A Dictionary of Epidemiology.* New York: Oxford University Press.

Manderscheid, R.W., and Sonnenschein, M.A. (1992) *Mental Health, United States, 1992.* DHHS Pub. No. (SMA) 92-1942. U.S. Government Printing Office.

Mednick, S.A., Machon, R.A., Huttunen, M.O., and Bonett, D. (1988) Adult schizophrenia following prenatal exposure to an influenza epidemic. *Archives of General Psychiatry,* 45:189–192.

Petronis, K.R., Samuels, J.F., Moscicki, E.K., and Anthony, J.C. (1990) An epidemiologic investigation of potential risk factorsfor suicide attempts. *Social Psychiatry and Psychiatric Epidemiology,* 25:193–199.

Phillips, D.P., and Carstensen, L.L. (1986) Clustering of teenage suicides after television news stories about suicide. *New England Journal of Medicine,* 315:685–689.

Regier, D.A., Farmer, M.E., Rae, D.S., Myers, J.K., Kramer, M., Robins, L.N., George, L.K., Karno, M., and Locke, B.Z. (1993) One-month prevalence of mental disorders in the United States and sociodemographic characteristics: the Epidemiologic Catchment Area study. *Acta Psychiatrica Scandinavica,* 88:35–47.

Regier, D.A., and Burke, J.D. (1989) Epidemiology. In Kaplan, H.Z., Sadock, B.J. (eds.), *Comprehensive Textbook of Psychiatry Fifth Edition, Vol. 1.* Baltimore: Williams & Wilkins.

Regier, D.A., Goldberg, I.D., and Taube, C.A. (1978) The de facto U.S. mental health services system. *Archives of General Psychiatry,* 35:685–693.

Robins, L.N. (1990) Psychiatric epidemiology—a historic review. *Social Psychiatry and Psychiatric Epidemiology* 25:16–26.

Robins, L.N., and Regier, D.A. (eds.) (1991) *Psychiatric Disorders in America: The Epidemiologic Catchment Area Study.* New York: The Free Press.

Rutter, M. (1989) Isle of Wight revisited: Twenty-five years of child psychiatric epidemiology. *Journal of the American Academy of Child and Adolescent Psychiatry,* 28:633–653.

Shapiro, S., Skinner, E.A., Kramer, M., German, P.S., and Romanoski, A.J. (1985) Need and demand for mental health services in an urban community: an exploration based on household interviews. In Barrett, J.E., Rose, R.M. (eds.), *Mental Disorders in the Community: Progress and Challenge.* New York: Guilford Press.

Shepherd, M., and Wilkinson, G. (1988) Editorial: Primary care as the middle ground for psychiatric epidemiology. *Psychological Medicine,* 18:261–267.

Shore, J.H., Tatum, E.L., and Vollmer, W.M. (1986) Evaluation of mental effects of disaster, Mount St. Helens eruption. *American Journal of Public Health,* 76(Suppl):76–83.

Special Section: Disaster at Buffalo Creek (1976) *American Journal of Psychiatry,* 133:295–316.

Spitzer, R.L., Williams, J.B.W., Gibbon, M., and First, M.B. (1992) The Structured Clinical Interview for DSM-III-R (SCID). I. History, rationale and description. *Archives of General Psychiatry*, 49:624–629.

Srole, L., Langner, T.S., Michael, S.T., Opler, M., and Rennie, T. (1962) *Mental health in the metropolis: The Midtown Manhattan Study*. New York: McGraw-Hill.

Susser, E.S., and Lin, S.P. (1992) Schizophrenia after prenatal exposure to the Dutch hunger Winter of 1944–1945. *Archives of General Psychiatry*, 49:983–988.

Susser, E., Struening, E.L., and Conover, S. (1989) Psychiatric problems in homeless men. *Archives of General Psychiatry*, 46:845–850.

Ungerleider, J., Lundberg, G., Sunshine, I., and Walberg, C.B. (1980) The Drug Abuse Warning Network (DAWN) Program. *Archives of General Psychiatry*, 37:106–109.

Veith, I. (1965) *Hysteria: The History of a Disease*. Chicago: University of Chicago Press.

Westermeyer, J., and Bearman, J. (1974) A proposed social indicator system for alcohol-related problems. *Preventive Medicine*, 2:438–444.

Wing, L., Bramley, C., Hailey, A., and Wing, J. K. (1968) Camberwell Cumulative Psychiatric Case Register. Part I: Aims and methods. *Social Psychiatry*, 3:116–123.

Wing, J.K., Cooper, J.E., and Sartorius, N. (1974) *The Measurement and Classification of Psychiatric Symptoms*. New York: Cambridge University Press.

Woogh, C.M. (1987a) The case for psychiatric record linkage. *Canadian Journal of Psychiatry*, 32:470–475.

Woogh, C.M. (1988) An experience in psychiatric record linkage. *Canadian Journal of Psychiatry*, 33:134–139.

7

Administration:
The Psychiatrist as Manager

RONALD J. DIAMOND
LEONARD I. STEIN
KATHLEEN SCHNEIDER-BRAUS

Administration is a part of many professional activities. Administrative skills are required whenever resources need to be managed or allocated, or when a complex milieu needs to be developed or maintained. In organizations providing mental health services, psychiatrists play a critical role in these activities. Psychiatrists working in a public mental health system often have significant administrative influence and responsibility that goes beyond what is acknowledged in a formal job description. Many community mental health center psychiatrists do not appreciate the fact that they can significantly influence the mental health system to work more effectively for their clients. They often have great interest in improving patient care, but come away feeling frustrated and impotent when attempting interventions that might make the system work better.

This chapter will focus on the administrative skills and influence that can be developed by psychiatrists practicing in community mental health centers regardless of their assigned organizational role. Most clinical staff, including psychiatrists, ignore the informal power that influences all aspects of an organization. This influence is not limited to staff with formal administrative roles, but, as will be discussed below, is a daily part of how all staff interact with each other. The informal power of the psychiatrist will be examined in each of the following roles: as a clinician, as a team member, as a medical director, and, finally, as executive director. While most of the issues that will be discussed apply equally to both psychiatrists and non-medical staff, some have special salience for psychiatrists and can significantly increase the influence the psychiatrist can have in changing policy to improve patient care and psychiatrist job satisfaction. It is important to stress that we are not discussing influence and power for their own sake. Leadership requires an ethics of purpose (Blanchard and Peale,

1988); power and influence are legitimate tools when used to create a climate that promotes better care for persons with mental illness.

This chapter will not attempt to deal with the tasks a psychiatric administrator might face, such as personnel management, budgeting, new program development, etc. There are several excellent reviews available for readers interested in these topics (Talbott and Kaplan, 1983; Barton and Barton, 1983; Greenblatt, 1991).

Historical Overview: From Demedicalization to the Integration of Medicine in Community Mental Health

The role of the psychiatrist-administrator has changed dramatically over several dechades. During the 1950s, psychiatrists were the superintendents of almost all state mental hospitals and therefore were in direct control of the institutions that provided most publicly funded mental health care. The new community mental health centers established during the 1960s continued to have psychiatrists in firm administrative control. By the beginning of the 1990s, however, direct administrative control had largely passed from psychiatrists to other mental health professionals. Today, few mental health centers have psychiatrists as the chief executive officers or even team leaders of programs within centers. By the early 1990s, only three states had a psychiatrist as the commissioner of mental health. Even state hospitals are increasingly directed by professional administrators rather than psychiatrists. Several interrelated factors seem responsible for this decrease in the direct organizational power of the psychiatrist-administrator (Clark, 1986; Dewey and Astrachan, 1986).

First, psychiatrists now make up a smaller percentage of the clinicians in community programs (Winslow, 1979). This is not because psychiatrists are disappearing from these settings; the absolute number continues to increase, but the numbers of other non-medical staff have been increasing even faster. In the past decades it became clear that a multidisciplinary approach was required for effective treatment of persons with serious mental illness. Professionals from a number of different disciplines were trained with specific expertise in psychotherapy, case management, housing supports, and other aspects of psychosocial rehabilitation important to long-term community stability of persons with serious mental illness. Health care institutions, under scrutiny to justify expenses, had available a large pool of competent, yet lower paid, non-medical mental health clinicians to fill administrative posts. Second, exacerbating this trend, few psychiatrists seek out administrative positions or roles. Even though administration has become a bonafide specialty of its own with its own body of knowledge and advanced credentials, administrative expertise is often discounted by psychiatrists. This discounting occurs despite the painful awareness of the problems caused by clinicians who end up in high administrative posts without this expertise. Even those psychiatrists who have a job that includes significant management responsibility tend to see themselves primarily as clinicians or researchers rather than administrators.

Third, psychiatrists rarely receive training in administration during residency and rarely have faculty role models who see themselves as psychiatric administrators (Donovan, 1982). Even chief resident positions, which provide some exposure to faculty with administrative responsibility and some leadership experience, provide little training in managing an organization (Hagberg, 1984). This problem is not unique to psychiatry. Many professions requiring technical expertise, from medicine to engineering, tend to devalue management as requiring less skill and less training. In many professions such as teaching, nursing, and social work, becoming an administrator is considered a career advancement; in medicine, however, becoming an administrator may yield relatively little increase in pay and often a decrease in status. One psychiatrist-administrator lamented that administrators viewed him as a second-class manager because he was trained as a physician, and his peer physicians viewed him as a second-class doctor because he became an administrator (Schneider-Braus, 1992).

Finally, few community mental health programs have sufficient psychiatric consultation time to "waste it" on administrative tasks. Psychiatric time is expensive, and well-trained psychiatrists willing to work in community settings are sometimes difficult to find even when money is available. The limited psychiatric time that is available is often preserved for much-needed direct patient care. While this is a valid strategy, it can also reflect a more covert purpose on the part of the leadership of the organization. It is sometimes felt that a psychiatrist as an administrator would impose a "medical model" on the staff, although it is rarely specified what "medical model" means (Adler, 1981; Ribner, 1980). Non-MDs often use the term "medical model" pejoratively to mean a number of different things that they feel would be at odds with the overall treatment philosophy of their institution. At times, "medical model" is used to imply a narrow biological focus that minimizes the role of psychological factors in both etiology and treatment. At other times, it is used to imply a focus on pathology and illness rather than strengths and rehabilitation. Most often, it implies an authoritarian and hierarchical mode of administration that would place physicians at the top, giving orders to other staff. Physicians, of course, have a more favorable view of a "medical model" as a holistic, bio-psycho-social approach to treatment.

The Special Role of the Psychiatrist

Although the factors mentioned above have tended to both marginalize psychiatrists in community mental health programs and decrease their administrative power, other competing factors have tended to underscore the importance of psychiatrists (Beigel, 1984).

First, as community mental health centers have increasingly focused on providing treatment of persons with serious mental illness, the specific medical expertise of the psychiatrist has become more important (Windle et al., 1988). Areas that have traditionally been in the psychiatric sphere—such as psychopharmacology, decisions regarding hospitalization, and basic medical assessment—are now recognized by psychiatrist and non-medical staff alike as vital and central tasks. Careful psychiatric assessment is increasingly accepted as an important part of the overall assessment process. The old polarity between non-medical psychotherapists and psychiatrists has diminished as medical and non-medical clinicians are forced to work together toward a common purpose.

Second, state agencies and third-party payers have increasingly mandated psychiatrists to supervise treatment provided by non-medical staff. State certification programs and both public and private third-party payers now require high levels of psychiatric involvement. In many situations, psychiatrists are required to "prescribe" the treatment delivered by the non-medical provider and to supervise that treatment.

Finally, more psychiatrists are being trained now to work in multidisciplinary, community-oriented treatment settings. As a result of this training, these psychiatrists have a better conceptual understanding of the full range of interventions required for stabilizing and rehabilitating persons with serious and persistent mental illness (Stein et al., 1987). They have more respect for alternative points of view, are more comfortable with diversity of treatment models, and develop skills at being a system consultant that can assist the team to function more effectively. Psychiatrists with these skills and attitudes become a central part of the treatment process, rather than just limiting their involvement to providing medication management in a narrowly defined and limited role.

Definition and Dynamics of Power

From a political vantage, the previous discussion would not be complete without a discussion of the psychiatric profession's alarm over the loss of direct organizational power in mental health institutions. With power comes money, prestige, and the latitude to be creative in one's field. This loss has discouraged some professionals, and others have felt "called to arms" to take back their previous and "rightful" authority. Much time and effort has gone into political battles among professionals and professional organizations; it is unlikely that these battles have truly served the needs of the country's mentally ill.

Modern theories of administration stress that power cannot be attained or maintained by force or intimidation. The traditional, authoritarian, often patriarchal model of leadership has been replaced by a far more egalitarian model based on teamwork (Peters and Waterman, 1982). Modern organizations, from manufacturing plants to health providers, now have flatter hierarchies than in the past, and shared problem solving involving all of the participants is more important to getting the job done than traditional top-down control of the organization. An administrative philosophy of "quality improvement" (Deming, 1986; Juran, 1988) prescribes sharing the vision of the organization with all the employees regardless of their job within the administrative hierarchy. This shared vision facilitates teamwork and ultimately leads to sharing of power. This management philosophy is based on the premise that power is not a limited or finite quantity, and giving power to others increases one's own power rather than diminishing it (Burwick et al., 1990).

Power in traditional organizations is often simplistically defined by one's place on an organizational chart. Power in modern organizations is much more complicated. Mechanic (1964) defines power "as any force that results in behavior that would not have occurred if the force had not been present." Thus, the measure of an individual's power is the degree to which he or she can make things happen or prevent things from happening. Utilizing this conceptual framework, it becomes apparent that power is not *necessarily* related to the position one holds in the organizational structure of an institution. Persons low in a hierarchy can be very influential in shaping what actually happens within an organization. As already discussed, it is now rare for psychiatrists to be the chief executive officers in community mental health centers or state mental hospitals. In a very real sense, in these organizations, psychiatrists are now "lower participants" in terms of directly controlling resources or establishing policy. It is important, then, to understand the basic techniques that will allow any individual to gain influence within an organization.

The staff of a mental health program forms an interdependent group, in which the psychiatrist is only one member. Members of this group want to feel competent in their work and have some degree of recognition of their efforts and abilities (Covey, 1989). Thus the resources that are managed in an institution are not exclusively money, time-off, and benefits, which are the prerogative of the direct supervisors. Other resources relating to a sense of professional effectiveness and interpersonal support are frequently strong influences within collegial relationships. All staff function as part of a complex homeostasis, subject in many ways to the same forces that apply to families and other interactive units (Minuchin, 1974). The more a psychiatrist takes the time and effort to see the organization from the vantage point of fellow workers, the more he or she will be effective and influential in the organization. The resulting empathy increases the likelihood of a synergistic solution as a result of individuals working toward a common solution (Covey, 1989).

Organizational Structure of Community Mental Health Centers

There are important differences in how community mental health programs are organized and how decisions are made. They can have specialized teams or be organized as one integrated unit. Decision making can be highly centralized or decentralized, can be more hierarchical or more egalitarian. Most mental health centers have layers of management between the top administrator and the front-line clinicians who provide direct clinical service. The number of layers usually depends on the size and complexity of the organization; in large organizations there are senior administrators, assistant administrators, down to the team leaders or middle managers who directly supervise clinicians.

Along with these organizational variations, there are significant variations in the expected role of the psychiatrist. These expectations may be formal and overt, or informal and never acknowledged. For example, if the psychiatrist's offices are in a different part of the building from other staff, and if policies actively discourage non-medical staff from interacting with psychiatrists even over medication assessments, the development of collaborative relationships becomes almost impossible. Similarly, an expectation that psychiatrists will spend almost all of their time in direct face-to-face contact with clients will severely decrease the potential for psychiatrists to carve out a broader role for themselves.

Many such factors affect the role of the psychiatrist and the influence the psychiatrist will have in the organization. We will examine four different levels of hierarchical roles for the psychiatrist: clinician, team member, medical director, and, finally, executive director. Each has its own role and paradigm of administrative influence. As previously discussed, the influence to initiate or change some action is power, and it is important to keep in mind the purpose of seeking power with one's team and collegial co-workers. The kind of power being discussed will not help one obtain the biggest office, the most benefits, or the preferred parking spot. It will allow one to use one's special training and expertise to influence treatment decisions, treatment philosophy, and organizational policy.

Psychiatrist in the Role of Clinician: Influence without Authority

Even without direct supervisory authority, community psychiatrists have control over information and resources that are important to both their clients and the other team members. Psychiatrists, like other members of an organization, gain influence when they are perceived as useful and helpful. The more a psychiatrist helps to increase the effectiveness of other members of the team, the more the psychiatrist will come to have influence within the team. There are a number of ways that psychiatrists can increase or decrease this influence with their colleagues.

The most obvious source of influence comes from the psychiatrist's expertise. Psychiatrists are well aware that their expertise about medical topics is important to the organization. Often, other clinicians are forced to involve psychiatrists in a particular clinical situation because of needed information about medication. Expertise about medication and medical illness is essential, but if expertise is limited to medical issues it reinforces a narrow role for the psychiatrist. The more the psychiatrist can put medication issues into the larger context of the patient's life, the more useful he or she will be to both patients and other staff (Diamond, 1985). Equally important, the psychiatrist must be willing to communicate this information to his or her non-medical colleagues. Sharing expertise establishes one's legitimacy as an expert and extends one's influence. Psychiatrists increase both their effectiveness and influence if they see teaching non-medical colleagues about prescribed medication as an important part of their job.

There are a number of other ways that psychiatrists can increase their influence within an organization. Staff psychiatrists, because of their status, often have access to upper-level managers. They can, therefore, act as an interface between front-line staff and management and can help make management aware of policies that interfere with clinical work. This can be helpful to both front-line staff and administration.

This kind of intervention can improve the overall work environment and satisfaction of other mental health professionals. The psychiatrist's status also means that praise or criticism of another clinician may carry special weight in annual reviews, promotions, or the clinician's general professional reputation. It is wise for a psychiatrist to be aware of the importance accorded to his or her assessments of other clinicians. The rule of thumb for any successful administrator is to confront colleagues in private and praise them in public.

Availability and longevity within an organization also increase one's influence. A psychiatrist who is readily available is more likely to increase a non-medical colleague's own sense of effectiveness. This, in turn, increases the likelihood that the psychiatrist will be sought out in the future, listened to and included as part of the solution to a problem. Availability requires both physical and psychological accessibility—being physically present or easily reachable, and being collegial and helpful rather than dictatorial and demeaning.

As a person works in an organization longer, he or she will tend to be connected to more people within the organization, have more information about how things work, and will know more about how to get things done. From this, it follows that people tend to accumulate influence and informal power as their tenure in an organization increases. However, it is not absolute tenure that is important, but relative seniority. The extraordinary power of the secretary or nurse who has "been there forever" is well known, as is the relative impotency of the supervisor who has just arrived. Centers that have a stable work-force of non-medical staff but a rapid turnover of psychiatrists will thus have psychiatrists who do not have much power. This is a circular process because there is likely to be more psychiatrist turnover where psychiatrists feel they have little power to influence decisions, and this turnover will lead to psychiatrists who have little real power because of short tenure.

A number of other factors, apart from expertise and instrumental utility, also affect a person's role within an organization. A person will tend to have increased influence if he or she is perceived by other staff as having a commitment to the organization. In general, part-time workers are perceived as less committed than full-time staff, and temporary staff will have less influence than staff who are permanent.

Just as a large number of factors can increase one's usefulness and influence within an organization, there are factors that can decrease one's influence. If one alienates other mental health professionals or is perceived as interfering with their effectiveness, one's role will be sabotaged in subtle but powerful ways. Staff psychiatrists who withhold information from their colleagues, who are not reliably available, or who consistently seek praise and attention for themselves will tend to be excluded from their team. They will miss being given important information about a client, suggestions they make will be ignored or misinterpreted, they will tend to be excluded from important discussions about program planning, and they will see both their influence and their effectiveness diminish.

Psychiatrists are particularly vulnerable to factors that tend to diminish their influence within the mental health center. They are often part-time in the midst of other staff who are full-time; they are often perceived as less committed to the ideology of the agency; and the structure of their job often decreases their availability to other staff. While some of these potentially damaging factors are beyond the control of the psychiatrist, others are directly related to his or her behavior within the organization. The relative shortage of psychiatrists can encourage both them and the organization to feel that they are indispensable and irreplaceable. When this factor is perceived positively the influence of the psychiatrist is enhanced. At times, however, the other staff of the CMHC can feel "blackmailed," especially if the psychiatrist uses this as license to behave in ways that would not be tolerated from other staff. Blatant use of intimidation may yield a sense of short-term power, but it seriously undermines the psychiatrist's long-term effectiveness and place within the organization.

Psychiatrist in the Role of Team Member

Providing effective treatment to persons with serious mental illness requires organizing a system that can bring an array of services to the target population. Most mental health services focused on persons with serious mental illness have found that individual clinicians operating in relative isolation are less effective than teams of clinicians operating in close coordination with each other. There is no one way to organize these teams, and the design of services varies enormously from place to place. While some mental health agencies have just one service component or an all-inclusive clinic, most have developed a number of distinct programs or specialized teams, each with a specific focus or mandate. At the Mental Health Center of Dane County and in most of the mental health centers in the United States known to the authors, the teams are specialized to provide specific services such as crisis intervention, community support services, outpatient psychotherapy, or services for children. In Great Britain, Australia, and some places in the United States, generalist teams are set up that are responsible for all of the services needed for a limited geographical area. In either type of organization, staff from one team may have relatively little contact with staff from other teams, and staff may identify as much with their team as with the center as a whole. The development of a team approach has distinct implications for the psychiatrist (Gaitz, 1987). Psychiatrists who are not clearly identified as a member of a team are likely to be left out of the informal information networking that teams typically develop. Treatment planning often occurs in the team setting, and psychiatrists who are not part of the team will tend to be excluded from the treatment-planning process. Teams develop policies and practices, formally or informally, that influence how they will work with clients. For example, teams develop both written policies and informal norms about whether they will work with a patient who comes in intoxicated or whether a patient will be terminated if there is a threat of harm to a staff person. While some of these issues can be influenced by central administration, how the team will actually respond to a particular patient is a decision made in the team setting itself. If psychiatrists are not part of the team, they are not part of the process that makes the decisions.

It is often difficult to decide how to include psychiatrists within the team. Most of the non-medical staff are full-time in one team. Psychiatrists are more likely than other staff to work part-time, or to be assigned part-time to several teams. Thus the psychiatrist is not always present when team members come together to share information or make decisions. Since the psychiatrist is frequently not present and, thus, does not hear all of the information firsthand, the other team staff members are constantly making decisions about what information to pass on to the psychiatrist and what issues the psychiatrist should be involved with. How well the psychiatrist can function as an integrated member of the team depends on the skills of the psychiatrist as well as the attitudes of the other team members.

This is often complicated by the psychiatrist's difficulty in finding a comfortable place in the team hierarchy. Most psychiatrists are uncomfortable with the idea of having a non-physician as their "boss" (Leong, 1982). This is as much a cultural and political problem as a clinical one, but many psychiatrists feel that only another M.D. can truly understand and supervise their medical decisions. What happens if a psychiatrist who is medically responsible for a clinical decision disagrees with his or her team leader? In a well-functioning team with a skilled team leader and skilled psychiatrist, unresolvable disagreement does not occur. When important disagreements do occur, additional information is collected, the pros and cons of each solution are considered, and new options are pursued until a treatment plan can be developed that everyone can support. Teams do not always function ideally, however, and even psychiatrists who are comfortable with a non-medical team leader generally prefer some way of structuring their role so that they are formally supervised by another physician with whom they can legally share responsibility.

One alternative is for the psychiatrists to be neither above nor below the team leader, but to have their own supervisory structure outside the one for non-medical staff. The Mental Health Center of Dane County operates with this kind of parallel hierarchy. Each clinical program has a team leader who is responsible for running the team and supervising the clinical staff, and a team medical director who is administratively co-equal to the team leader but who has no formal administrative authority except over the other physicians on the team. This system functions extremely well, in large part because the medical directors of each team and the team leaders have been able to negotiate their inherently ambiguous relationship with each other.

There is a direct relationship between the amount of effort the psychiatrist is willing to exert in helping the team function and the amount of influence that psychiatrist will be given as a result of that effort. For example, a psychiatrist who clearly indicates that staff can call him or her after hours will have more influence than one who is perceived as less available. The help a psychiatrist offers may take many forms. Serving on committees or being involved in decisions outside those perceived as strictly medical indicates more widespread interest in the team. Occasionally coming in over an evening or weekend to see how those shifts operate, being available for emergencies, having lunch with staff rather than off on one's own, and attending social affairs will all give the psychiatrist information on how the team operates. In addition, these kinds of activities will be perceived by other staff as showing interest and will be responded to by invitations for involvement in a wider variety of ways. The most important issue is whether other staff in the team see the psychiatrist as being willing to help out, to "be there" when needed, or whether the psychiatrist is perceived as being more distant and less personally involved with the team. This is as much an issue of perception as one of actual time. A psychiatrist can spend large amounts of time and actually be willing to be helpful, but because of an aloof attitude or other subtle cues, may be perceived by staff as less involved or expending less effort, therefore being a less valuable or important member of the team.

The Psychiatrist in the Role of Medical Director

The American Association of Community Psychiatrists and the American Psychiatric Association have developed practice guidelines and a model job description for a medical director within a community mental health center (American Psychiatric Association, 1988). The suggested role of the medical director includes authority and supervision for all medical/psychiatric services; involvement in policy development; having a relationship to the Board of Directors or governing body; providing liaison to outside physicians, hospitals, and medical services; involvement in educational programs for both staff and students; involvement in quality assurance; and the provision of direct psychiatric service.

A psychiatrist named as medical director faces new responsibilities and needs new skills to be successful as an administrator. Whereas a psychiatrist as clinician only has responsibility for managing his or her own work, a psychiatrist administrator accomplishes his or her job by getting it done through other people. Unfortunately, physicians are not inclined to delegate. They tend to be action oriented and often feel guilty if they assign clinical work to their colleagues while they spend time doing "management work." Clinicians generally view administrative meetings to be, at best, a break from direct patient contact and, at worst, a boring waste of time. The medical director needs to be involved in planning, communicating, and managing the system; this requires not only the investment of time, but a mental shift in the evaluation of one's value to the organization.

The medical director must keep his or her goals in focus. The higher his or her position in the hierarchy of the organization, the more difficult it is to have direct control over what the front-line clinicians are actually doing. A top administrator has more power to develop policy, but less actual control over what happens between the clinician and the patient. The goal is that staff should do the job effectively even when the director is absent (Covey, 1989). This requires that staff understand and accept the mission of the institution and use it as a compass, making correct decisions that keep the team and the individuals within the team "on track." To be successful in this, the medical director and other members of the administration must spend a considerable amount of time communicating with staff, not only "taking the temperature" of the culture and morale of the teams, but also communicating consistently the mission and values of the institution. This is often done effectively by MBWA—"management by wandering around" (Peters and Waterman, 1982)—a style not unlike "rounding" in medical terminology.

Although some of a medical director's time will be spent in management tasks, it is important to perform some clinical work as well. This is the best way to see what front-line system problems need addressing and to keep current. Being a clinician with good repute is helpful in recruiting other psychiatrists and helps to maintain the medical director's legitimacy with the staff. As with the other roles discussed above, the qualities of commitment, hard work, and loyalty are important to ensure that the real power of the medical director does not shrivel in an organization, leaving only a hollow administrative post.

The second major change of focus for a psychiatrist who becomes a medical director is changing one's job description to include the staff's job satisfaction, success, and professional development. Physicians are trained to care for the health, satisfaction, and well-being of patients. If a staff member is unhappy, disgruntled, or unprofessional, a physician usually is displeased but not inspired to intervene. When one takes on the role of administrator, any staff problems that can affect the running of the system become, on some level, one's concern. Staff turnover, union contracts, budgetary restrictions, and recruiting all become part of the medical director's concern, if not directly his or her responsibility in the organizational structure.

Because few physicians have administrative training, most mental health centers have professional administrators managing a majority of these issues. The roles of medical directors range from being strictly a consultant to being an administrator who has direct budgetary control and functioning as an online supervisor on the organizational chart. Before accepting a medical director position, it is important to understand what responsibilities are included as part of the job. If the medical director is responsible for budgeting, personnel management, marketing, or public relations, it is important to have expertise in these areas. In large part, establishing and maintaining a healthy working relationship with the executive director and other members of the executive group is the key to success as medical director. These relationships will thrive on open communication about mission and goals. It is important that both the executive director and the psychiatrist move past a competitive mode to one of mutual respect for the other's talents and acceptance of the other's weaknesses. An executive director may be in awe of the psychiatrist who is able to manage a medical emergency, "talk down" an angry patient, or handle an explosive paranoid patient. Similarly, a psychiatrist may admire an executive director who is skilled in developing a complicated budget, is able to fire an ineffective and disgruntled employee gracefully, or can effectively negotiate union contracts. Each has taken years of training to develop these skills. Appreciating the other's abilities helps keep a functional relationship between the medical director and other members of the administration, which ultimately is the key to a successful leadership of the organization.

The effectiveness of the medical director is also dependent on his or her relationship with other staff, from middle management to front-line clinicians. No matter how the formal job description is worded, a large number of policy decisions can be considered to be either within or outside of the purview of the medical director. Arrangements will be made to make sure that the medical director is involved in making a decision or developing a policy if other clinical and administrative staff feel that the medical director's expertise would be useful. If the medical director is felt to be an impediment, the meeting to discuss the issue will be set up at an inconvenient time, or the medical director will hear about a decision in passing after the fact.

One further key responsibility of the medical director is recruiting, managing, and maintaining a competent psychiatric staff. One psychiatrist can hire another psychiatrist much more easily than can a non-medical administrator. Psychiatrists within a community often know each other, and a medical director can often encourage a colleague to work more effectively than can a non-medical administrator. Connections—through the state psychiatric association or the American Association of Community Psychiatrists (AACP), in addition to other pursuits such as research and publications—help enhance the institution's reputation and makes recruiting easier. A psychiatrist as medical director can often help to develop a job description that is attractive to potential psychiatric job candidates, yet also meets the service needs of the agency by helping to balance the needs for direct service with the staff psychiatrist's desire to spend some time consulting with staff, teaching, or pursuing other professional interests. A medical director can often describe a job in ways that encourages potential job applicants. Once hired, the personal supervision and relationship with the medical director can decrease the stress and isolation of the staff psychiatrist and provide supports that prevent burnout and job dissatisfaction.

It is useful to make a special note here regarding the task of terminating an employee. Taking away a person's livelihood, however justified, is never a pleasant task, and it never gets easy. Physicians, in particular, often choose medicine as a career in hopes of easing people's pain and suffering. Firing an employee causes unanesthetized pain for both the employee and the supervisor. With the experience of firing an employee comes a new appreciation for the care that goes into hiring of new staff. Putting effort into proper orientation and clearly communicating all responsibilities of the position are important to ensure the employee will be successful in the job.

While most community mental health programs have a medical director, some operate without one. The absence of a psychiatrist in a senior administrative position can cause a variety of difficulties. The lack of a medical director can make relationships with the rest of the medical community more difficult: A medical director, as a medical spokesperson for the community program, can establish connections with other psychiatric and non-psychiatric physicians in the community; the medical director can often help facilitate working relationships with hospital emergency departments and inpatient units and can help legitimize the role of the non-medical clinicians who work at the center. The lack of a medical director can make hiring and supervising staff psychiatrists difficult since feedback on performance is often more effective from one physician to another. Finally, a mental health program without a medical director has no physician responsible for the development of medically related policies, such as agency guidelines for assessing clients for medical illness, monitoring medication, informing clients and staff about medication side effects, as well as getting involved in public health issues such as TB screening.

Centers without a clear role for a medical director often lack a tradition of effective and collaborative medical leadership. Psychiatrists coming into such a situation may be assigned a restricted role of prescribing medication, with little opportunity for involvement with the non-medical staff or input into how clinical services can be improved. Psychiatrists with an interest in being part of the shaping and development of such a program will need to carve out a leadership role for themselves, whether or not they are formally designated as a "Medical Director." This can only be done by using the influence already discussed to demonstrate over time how a wider role for the psychiatrist will facilitate the clinical mission of the center.

As the following examples demonstrate, psychiatrists can attempt to assert themselves in ways that, paradoxically, decrease their influence with other staff, or alternatively, can behave in ways that will increase both their influence and authority:

1. A community mental health agency employed a psychiatrist who had a long history of trying to exert control through edicts that instructed non-medical staff when they should involve a psychiatrist. The psychiatrist sent other staff memos informing them that a psychiatrist should be the ultimate authority on all decisions about hospitalizing clients, and that a psychiatrist should be involved whenever a patient was at risk for harm to self or others. Other non-medical staff resisted allowing this psychiatrist to have control over their clinical decision making and strongly resisted creating the role of medical director because of concern that this would increase his power and control.

2. A new psychiatrist was initially treated with suspicion and limited to a narrow clinical role. She behaved quite differently from the senior psychiatrist, avoided edicts or suggestions of how other staff should do their job, but was willing to be useful when other staff were stuck with difficult clinical decisions. She was able to interact with staff regarding their decisions and helped them reconsider how they had arrived at those decisions. She helped develop non-hospital alternatives whenever possible. Within two years she was appointed as the center's first medical director, largely in acknowledgment of the role that she had already carved out for herself as an influential and sought-after clinician who helped the center do a better job with patients.

The Psychiatrist as Executive Director

As previously discussed, in the 1990s it has become rare to have a psychiatrist as executive director of a community mental health center. Those psychiatrists who assume this position need to acquire the skills needed to formally manage an organization. These range from the skills needed to develop budgets and salary schedules to understanding state laws governing clinics to being knowledgeable about personnel issues and OSHA requirements. The executive director is ultimately responsible for all of these areas, even if other staff have responsibility for specific areas. At the same time, the most important job for a CEO is not managing budgets, but effectively managing people. All the principles of influence discussed for the psychiatrist as clinician and team member, and the discussion of administrative tasks and training for the medical director, apply to the psychiatrist as executive director.

The increase in formal organizational power increases the need to work with other staff and to understand how one can influence as well as legislate. Moving to the role of executive director is a dramatic career change that takes a psychiatrist one step farther away from direct patient care. Many clinicians abandon practice entirely at this point because of competing demands and time constraints. In addition to providing leadership for the staff, the executive director represents the organization to the outside world: Contact with elected officials or benefactors may be necessary to establish and maintain funding sources; providing input into public mental health policy may be important to maintain community support; establishing connections with other institutions such as academic institutions or other nearby agencies may help keep different providers working as part of an integrated system; and finally, tact with the media becomes an important skill.

Advanced training can help develop the skills needed to be an effective administrator. Administrative Psychiatry is now a subspecialty recognized by board certification. Alternatively, clinicians interested in enhancing their administrative skills can get an advanced degree in business administration or public health. There are programs where one can obtain a medical MBA, including one available through the University of Wisconsin, that allows an applicant living anywhere in the country to obtain an advanced degree while holding an administrative post. Many physician-administrators join an organization such as the American College of Physician Executives, which offers a wide variety of excellent seminars ranging from beginning administration to high-level leadership.

Conclusion

Psychiatrists working in community mental health centers sometimes assume that they should have power and authority based on their years of training or their status as a physician. Often, there is an assumption that the psychiatrist is ultimately responsible for all aspects of a patient's treatment, and the psychiatrist should therefore have ultimate authority. These assumptions are not necessarily shared by most non-medical staff. Psychiatrists can be influential, but their influence must be earned. Psychiatrists can make a large impact, both on the organization and on the treatment of individual patients, but they must learn how to empower themselves so that such an impact is possible. Working in community psychiatry can be professionally rewarding, but it requires psychiatrists to learn a wide range of administrative skills. The most important of these skills is knowing how to exercise informal power and thus have a positive impact on policy and clinical practice.

References

Adler (1981) The Medical Model and Psychiatry's Tasks. *Hospital and Community Psychiatry,* 32:387–392.

American Psychiatric Association (1988) *Guidelines for Psychiatric Practice in Community Mental Health Centers.* Washington, D.C.: APA Press.

Barton, W.E., and Barton, G.M. (1983) *Mental Health Administration, Vol. 1.* Human Sciences Press: New York.

Beigel (1984) The remedicalization of community mental health. *Hospital and Community Psychiatry,* 35:1114–1117.

Blanchard, K., and Peale, N.V. (1988) *The Power of Ethical Management.* New York: William Morrow and Company, Inc.

Burwick, D.M., Godfrey, A.B., and Roessner, J. (1990) *Curing Health Care.* San Francisco: Jossey-Bass.

Clark, G.H. (1986) CMHCs and Psychiatrists: A Necessarily Polemical Review. In Clark, G.H. (ed.), *Community Psychiatry: Problems and Possibilities.* Spring House, PA: McNeill Pharmaceuticals.

Covey, S.R. (1989) *The 7 Habits of Highly Effective People.* New York: Simon and Schuster.

Deming, W.E. (1986) *Out of Crisis.* Cambridge: Massachussetts Institute of Technology, Center for Advanced Engineering Study.

Dewey, L., and Astrachan, B.M. (1986) Organizational Issues in Recruitment and Retention of Psychiatrists in CMHCS. In *Community Mental Health Centers and Psychiatrists.* Washington, D.C.: The American Psychiatric Association and The National Council of Community Mental Health Centers.

Diamond, R.J. (1985) Antipsychotic drugs and the quality of life: The patient's point of view. *Journal of Clinical Psychiatry,* 46(5):29–35.

Donovan, C.M. (1982) Problems of psychiatric practice in community mental health centers. *American Journal of Psychiatry,* 139:4.

Gaitz, C.M. (1987) Multidisciplinary team care of the elderly: the role of the psychiatrist. *The Gerontologist,* 27:553–556.

Greenblatt, M. (1991) Administrative Psychiatry. In Keill, S.L. (ed.), *Administrative Issues in Public Mental Health.* San Francisco: Jossey-Bass.

Hagberg, J.O. (1984) *Real Power: Stages of Personal Power in Organizations.* Minneapolis: Winston Press.

Juran, J.M. (ed.) (1988) *Juran's Quality Control Handbook.* New York: McGraw-Hill.

Leong, G.B. (1982) Psychiatrists and community mental health centers: Can their relationship be salvaged? *Hospital and Community Psychiatry,* 11:309–310.

Mechanic, D. (1964) Sources of Power of Lower Participants in Complex Organizations. In: Porter, D.E., Applewhite, P.B. (eds.), *Studies in Organizational Behavior and Management.* Scranton, PA: International Textbook.

Minuchin, S. (1974) *Families and Family Therapy.* Cambridge: Harvard University Press.

Peters, T.J., and Waterman, R.H. (1982) *In Search of Excellence: Lessons from America's Best-Run Companies.* New York: Harper & Row.

Ribner (1980) Psychiatrists and community mental health: Current issues and trends. *Hospital and Community Psychiatry,* 31(5):338–341.

Schneider-Braus, K. (1992) Managing a Mental Health Department in a Staff Model HMO. In Felman, J.L., Fitzpatrick, R.J. (eds.), *Managed Mental Health Care.* Washington, D.C.: American Psychiatric Press.

Stein, L.I., Factor, R.M., and Diamond, R.J. (1987) Training Psychiatrists in the Treatment of Chronically Disabled Patients. In Meyerson and Fine (eds.), *Psychiatric Disabilities.* Washington, D.C.: APA Press.

Talbott, J.A., and Kaplan, S.R. (eds.) (1983) *Psychiatric Administration: A Comprehensive Text for the Clinician Executive.* New York: Grune and Stratton.

Windle, C., Poppen, P.J., Thompson, J.W., Marvelle, K. et al. (1988) Types of patients served by various providers of outpatient care in CMHCs. *American Journal of Psychiatry,* 145:457–463.

Winslow, W.W. (1979) The changing role of psychiatrists in community mental health centers. *American Journal of Psychiatry,* 136:24–27.

8

Mental Health Services Research

MARK OLFSON
HOWARD H. GOLDMAN

Mental health services research uses a variety of epidemiological, experimental, and quasi-experimental methods to study the organization, financing, and performance of mental health services. Researchers study the need for and accessibility of services, the financial costs and clinical efficacy of services, and a host of other issues related to the delivery of care. The findings from mental health services research play an important role in the practice of modern community psychiatry. Community psychiatrists increasingly look to mental health services research to inform their decisions of who should receive which services and what benefits can reasonably be expected from these services.

This chapter describes the scope of mental health services research and highlights some of its major contributions. The chapter is divided into four sections: (1) an overview of the historic origins of mental health services research, (2) a description of methods commonly used by mental health service researchers, (3) a summary of the major components of the U.S. mental health services system, and (4) a selective review of studies on the efficacy of innovative community-based services for the severely mentally ill.

Historic Origins

Mental health services research began as an area of research within epidemiology. Medical superintendents of the asylums kept detailed records of admissions and discharges. Much of the early research in mental hospitals focused on the treated prevalence of mental disorders and the delivery of services. In the first half of the nineteenth century, Edward Jarvis investigated the patterns of admissions to and discharges from state-operated asylums. He discovered that the likelihood of admission was directly related to the proximity of the patient's residence to the hospital. Other studies focused on hospital design and costs of care.

During the second half of the nineteenth century, superintendents began to study the probability of recovery and relapse. By counting as a cure the "recovered" discharge of readmitted patients, some studies demonstrated better than 100 percent "cure rates"! Almost from the beginning, hospital planners and politicians concerned with state mental health policies used and at times misused the results of mental health services research.

The seventh United States decennial census (1850) institutionalized the study of the treated prevalence of mental disorder. This census surveyed the number of mentally ill and mentally retarded persons in specialized facilities. To the present day, and especially since the establishment of the National Institute of Mental Health (NIMH) in 1947, the enumeration of treatment provided to mentally ill Americans has been an important responsibility of the federal government, currently assumed by the Substance Abuse and Mental Health Services Administration (SAMHSA). As state and federal agencies have extended their role in the delivery of mental health services, there has been increased interest in the evaluation of services. With the addition of evaluation studies, mental health services research has grown from an area within epidemiology into a highly complex interdisciplinary field.

Methods Used by Mental Health Service Researchers

Mental health service researchers employ a wide range of research methodologies. Four major research strategies include (1) epidemiologic investigations, (2) systems-level research, (3) program-level research, and (4) model program assessment. A brief description of each research strategy is provided.

Epidemiology of Mental Health Services

This strategy examines the patterns and distribution of mental health care service provision. Although the focus is often on the volume or frequency of utilization, epidemiologic methods are also used to assess the range, composition, staffing, and financing of mental health services. Epidemiologic mental health services research generally takes the form of provider-based surveys or population-based surveys.

In the United States, the most extensive provider-based mental health service surveys are those conducted by the SAMSHA National Reporting Program. This program includes reports on the total universe of admissions and discharges from state and county mental hospitals, as well as samples drawn from community mental health centers and various other types of facilities (Manderscheid et al., 1993). These surveys have been used to study the pattern and composition of care provided to patient groups of special interest (Burns, 1991; Rosenstein et al., 1989; Wolff et al., 1989) and to provide information for service planning.

The most comprehensive population-based source of information on the care of mental illness in the United States is the NIMH Epidemiologic Catchment Areas Program (ECA) (Regier et al., 1993). Between 1979 and 1982, this program intensively studied the mental health and services utilization characteristics of 18,571 adult community residents from five sites across the nation. Based on ECA findings, Regier and colleagues (1993) have reported that approximately 5.9 percent of the adult U.S. population make a mental health visit to mental health specialists, 6.4 percent make a mental health visit to general medical providers, 3.0 percent seek such care from other human service professionals, and 4.1 percent receive such mental health care from the voluntary support sector over a one-year period. Although the presence of a mental disorder substantially increases the likelihood of making a mental health–related visit, most individuals with mental disorders do not receive services. Even for severe mental disorders, the rate of treatment is remarkably low. For example, less than half (45.1 percent) of the adult population who meet criteria for obsessive-compulsive disorder make even a single mental health visit to any provider during a given one-year period (Regier et al., 1993).

Similar results have come recently from the National Comorbidity Study. In this nationally representative survey of adult Americans, over a quarter of the population (29.5 percent) met criteria for a CIDI/DSM-III-R disorder. However, only about one-fifth (20.9 percent) of those who met such criteria received professional treatment during the course of one year (Kessler et al., 1994).

Systems-Level Research

Mental health services researchers also study the provision of care from a regional or systems-level perspective. In contrast to traditional clinical research, which often involves assessment of specific new treatments, the focus of systems research is on higher order organizational function. Systems-level research studies how service providers interact to meet the needs of a given patient population.

A noteworthy example of systems-level research is the evaluation of the Robert Wood Johnson Foundation Program on Chronic Mental Illness (Goldman et al., 1990a). This project explored the assumption that strengthening local mental health authorities promotes the development of comprehensive mental health care and social welfare services, which in turn improves the quality of life for the severely mentally ill (Goldman et al., 1990b). Nine U.S. cities were selected for the demonstration project. The project succeeded in creating structural change in the mental health service systems and improving continuity of care. However, these changes were not sufficient to produce improvements in the quality of life for mentally ill patients. The researchers conclude that structural change without a complementary focus on clinical and social care may not be sufficient to achieve the desired changes in patient outcomes (Goldman et al., 1994).

Program-Level Research

The evaluation of mental health programs is now a well-established area of services research. This research examines the nature and consequences of care provided in existing mental health programs. Because program-level research addresses the routine operation of existing services, it has the potential to be of immediate relevance to program planning and policy development. However, because of the difficulties in employing experimental methodologies, this type of research often has less internal validity than more controlled research.

An example of program-level research is the work of Lehman and colleagues on the quality of life of chronic patients in supervised community residences. In this research, clients of supervised community residence programs were found to perceive their living situations more favorably across a range of measures than inpatients at a state mental hospital (Lehman et al., 1986). Although non-random patient assignment limits the internal validity of the findings, this study points to problems with state hospital living conditions and potential strengths of well-designed supervised community residences.

Evaluation of Model Programs

Assessment of model programs is currently the most developed area of mental health services research. A variety of strategies has been used to evaluate innovative mental health services. Random patient assignment, case control studies, pre- and post-design, and detailed descriptions of individual programs have all been used to assess the performance of model programs.

Randomized controlled trials provide the most internally valid results, from which causal inferences may be drawn. In the late 1970s, Stein and Test (1980) conducted a major randomized controlled trial of a model community-based program of care versus traditional hospital- and clinic-based care. In this study, a group of 130 public mental hospital patients for whom inpatient treatment seemed indicated were randomly assigned to a community-based treatment team or existing public care. Clinical symptoms, occupational and social functioning, social burden (Test and Stein, 1980), and cost of care (Weisbrod et al., 1980) were closely monitored for 12 months. Across several functional areas, the outcome of the experimental group was more favorable than the control group. These results support the increased use of community-based interdisciplinary treatment teams (Assertive Community Treatment) and provide an illustration of the value of model program assessment in mental health services research (Olfson, 1990a; Burns and Santos, 1995).

The U.S. Mental Health Services System

In the United States, a complex and highly differentiated array of services provides mental health care. Provision of mental health services occurs within three major sectors: the specialty mental health sector, the general medical sector, and the human services sector (Regier et al., 1978). The specialty mental health sector comprises all specialized mental health facilities and providers. This includes psychiatric hospitals, community-based mental health programs, and mental health specialists in office-based practice. The general medical sector includes mental health care delivered by general hospitals without psychiatric units, nursing homes, and primary care clinicians. The human services sector includes mental health services provided by the clergy, family service agencies, crisis centers, and other providers.

As previously mentioned, epidemiological surveys indicate that only a small fraction (24.7 percent) of mentally ill persons receive professional treatment (Regier et al., 1993). At present, very little is known about the clinical, sociologic, economic, and attitudinal factors that govern the selection of mentally ill individuals into treatment.

Outpatient Care in General Medical Settings

It is estimated that the general medical sector provides mental health care to a larger proportion of the U.S. adult population (6.4 percent) than the specialty mental health sector (5.9 percent) (Regier et al., 1993). This ratio arises in large measure from the substantial numbers of outpatients who receive mental health treatment in outpatient primary-care settings.

The prevalence of psychiatric disorder in general medical settings is reported to be between 19 percent and 35 percent (Kessler et al., 1987; Hoeper et al., 1979; Blacker and Clare, 1988; Barrett et al., 1988). Although depressive disorders are the most prevalent (6 percent to 22 percent) (Jones et al., 1987; Schulberg et al., 1985), anxiety disorders, adjustment disorders, and substance abuse disorders also commonly present to primary-care clinics.

Mentally ill patients seen by primary-care physicians tend to be less severely impaired than those seen by mental health specialists. Compared with visits to psychiatrists, mental health visits to non-psychiatrist physicians tend to be shorter in duration, less often include therapeutic listening, and more commonly result in the prescription of a medication (Schurman et al., 1985).

Primary-care physicians vary widely in their level of interest, skill, and motivation in identifying and treating psychiatric illnesses. As a result, primary-care patients with mental disorders often escape detection (Perez-Stable et al., 1990), and concern exists that care provided to recognized cases is sometimes seriously deficient (Johnson, 1973). This concern has motivated studies of various strategies, such as patient questionnaire feedback and interview training, to improve the diagnostic and treatment practices of primary-care physicians (Higgins, 1994).

Survey data suggest that primary-care physicians usually do not make referrals for the mental health problems that they most commonly encounter (Hull, 1979). Only 0.07 percent (Locke et al., 1966) to 2.5 percent (Shortell and Daniels, 1974) of patients seen in general practice are referred for specialized mental health care.

Noncompliance with referrals for outpatient mental health services is a common occurrence (Nicholson, 1994). Estimates of referral noncompliance range from 30 percent to 74 percent, depending on the study population (Blouin et al., 1985; Sweeney et al., 1984; Jellinek, 1978). Patient resistance, inadequate insurance coverage for specialized services, and a scarcity of readily available specialists have been identified by primary-care physicians as important obstacles to specialty referral (Orleans et al., 1985).

An evolving literature suggests that specialized outpatient care is somewhat more effective than mental health care provided by general medical clinicians (Balestrieri et al., 1988). Most of this research has been conducted in the United Kingdom with patients who suffer from mild to moderate anxiety or depressive symptoms. However, much remains to be learned about which mentally ill patients are most efficiently treated in which sector.

Inpatient Treatment in General Medical Settings

On the inpatient side, large numbers of psychiatrically ill patients are treated in general hospitals that do not have a psychiatric unit (i.e., scatter beds). These patients, who until recently outnumbered those treated in general hospital psychiatric units, are typically treated on medical or surgical floors under the care of a non-psychiatrist physician. As compared with unit-based care, treatment in scatter beds is relatively brief in duration and seldom includes an organized program of psychosocial rehabilitation (Olfson, 1990b). Where psychiatrists are available to provide consultation, treatment in general hospitals without psychiatric units more closely resembles that provided in psychiatric units. Patients with more severe psychiatric conditions, especially those with psychotic symptoms or dangerous behavior, are often transferred to specialized inpatient facilities.

Nursing homes have become a major locus of residential care for persons with severe mental illness (Goldman et al., 1986; Goldman and Sharfstein, 1987). In addition to the large numbers of nursing home residents who suffer from dementing illnesses, substantial numbers of nursing home residents suffer from depressive disorders, anxiety disorders, or schizophrenia (Rovner et al., 1986; Strahan, 1990). However, no standards exist for the treatment of psychiatric illness in nursing homes.

Nursing homes vary in size, location, ownership, certification status, and level of care. Because of the diversity of facilities, it is difficult to generalize about the quality of psychiatric services available in nursing homes. However, some are not adequately staffed for psychiatric rehabilitation (Stotsky and Stotsky, 1983), and concern exists that psychoactive drugs are widely prescribed without adequate medical supervision (Avorn et al., 1989) and treatable mental illness is often undetected.

A recent national survey revealed that while more than three-quarters of nursing home residents with a mental disorder reside at facilities where mental health services such as counseling or psychotherapy are available, these services are seldomly actually provided. According to the survey, approximately one-fifth (19 percent) of mentally ill nursing home residents receive mental health services within one year (Smyer et al., 1994). Interestingly, residents of government facilities were more than twice as likely to receive mental health services than those in for-profit nursing homes (Smyer et al., 1994).

Substandard treatment of mental illness in nursing homes has been associated with adverse health outcomes. In one study, 13 percent of new admissions to proprietary nursing homes were found to have major depressive disorder. Most of these cases went unrecognized and untreated. At one-year follow-up, major depression was found to be an independent risk factor for mortality. Depression increased the likelihood of death by 59 percent (Rovner et al., 1991).

Little is known about the comparative efficacy of inpatient treatment in the general medical sector in relation to specialized psychiatric hospitalization. At present, there are no experimental studies that directly compare the health outcomes of mentally ill patients treated in scatter versus unit beds or in nursing homes versus psychiatric hospitals. Given the radically different styles of treatment provided in the two sectors and the equally impressive differences in associated costs, cost/benefit research in this area remains a high priority (Goldman and Sharfstein, 1987).

Inpatient Psychiatric Services

The major classes of facilities that provide specialized inpatient psychiatric care include state and county mental hospitals (state mental hospitals), general hospitals with psychiatric units, private psychiatric hospitals, Veteran's Administration medical centers (VAMCs), and community mental health centers (CMHCs).

Although state mental hospitals have been downscaled in recent years, in 1986 they still accounted for greater than three times more inpatient treatment days than any other class of mental health organization (Witkin et al., 1990).

At the same time there has been a marked increase in the number and diversity of psychiatric inpatients treated in general hospitals, with a concomitent reduction in average length of stay. In 1986 there were more than twice as many psychiatric admissions to general hospitals with psychiatric units than to state mental hospitals (Rosenstein et al., 1990).

General hospitals with psychiatric units differ from one another in several key characteristics including size, location, university affiliation, ownership, and operating auspices. Compared with psychiatric patients treated in state hospitals, patients treated in general hospital units are more likely to be admitted voluntarily, to stay less than two weeks, and to suffer from an affective disorder or an adjustment disorder.

The number of patients treated in private psychiatric hospitals, especially those operated on a for-profit basis, increased in the 1970s and 1980s. The availability of insurance for inpatient psychiatric care, a growing recognition that mental illness reduces employee productivity, and a decrease in the extent to which mental illness is stigmatized, are thought to have contributed to this growth (Dorwart and Schlesinger, 1988). National concern about the cost of this increased utilization in the context of spiraling health care costs led payers to implement measures to reduce utilization. Significant reduction in admission rates has been achieved through a variety of managed care mechanisms including precertification, concurrent review, and second opinion programs; case managers who serve as gatekeepers for high-cost patients; and prepaid financing mechanisms that provide incentives to reduce dependence on relatively high-cost inpatient care (Hodgkin, 1992).

Children account for a substantially larger proportion of the admissions to private psychiatric hospitals than they do to other types of inpatient mental health organizations (Rosenstein et al., 1990). In relation to inpatient services for adults, much less is known about the organization, content, and efficacy of mental health services provided to children. The mental health care of children remains an important area for future research.

Outpatient Psychiatric Services

Specialized outpatient mental health care is provided by several professional groups. The major groups include psychiatrists, clinical psychologists, clinical social workers, and clinical nurse specialists. Care is provided in group or solo office-based private practice or in institutional settings such as CMHCs, freestanding outpatient clinics, and clinics at the various types of hospitals. Each year there are approximately 19 million visits to office-based psychiatrists. Almost all of these visits include psychotherapy (89.5 percent), approximately half include a medication prescription (50.2 percent), and more than one-third (38.6 percent) of psychiatric visits include some form of counseling or advice (Schappert, 1993). The most common diagnostic groups seen in office-based private psychiatric practice are depressive disorders (36.8 percent), anxiety disorders (13.4 percent), personality disorders (10.2 percent), and schizophrenia and related disorders (8.8 percent). In 1989–1990, fewer than 2 percent of visits to psychiatrists in private practice resulted in the diagnosis of an alcohol- or substance abuse–related disorder (Schappert, 1993).

In institution-based outpatient settings, the patient mix varies considerably by facility type. For example, the proportion of outpatient admissions with social conditions or adjustment disorders is relatively high in free-standing outpatient clinics (37.7 percent), CMHCs (33.2 percent), and general hospital psychiatric clinics (31.3 percent), but relatively low in state mental hospital outpatient clinics (19.5 percent) and VAMC clinics (13.0 percent) (Rosenstein et al., 1990). In contrast, the proportion of outpatient admissions with schizophrenia is relatively high in state mental hospital clinics (21.0 percent) and VAMC clinics (17.2 percent), but lower in the other types of clinics such as general hospital psychiatric clinics (9.4 percent), CMHCs (7.6 percent), and freestanding clinics (5.2 percent) (Rosenstein et al., 1990).

The mix of services provided to outpatients also varies by institutional setting. For example, individual therapy is more commonly provided to schizophrenic patients treated at private psychiatric hospital clinics and CMHCs than to those treated in freestanding clinics or psychiatric clinics in VAMCs and general hospitals (Rosenstein et al., 1989). Outpatient psychiatric clinics also differ from one another in their staffing composition and in their staff-to-patient ratio.

Partial-Care Programs (Day Hospitals)

Partial-care programs typically provide specialized psychiatric treatment during the work-day week. Some programs additionally provide back-up telephone coverage during nights and weekends. Other programs provide services during the evening and allow patients to stay at night and work or attend school during the day. Schizophrenia and affective disorders are the most common diagnostic groups treated in partial-care programs (Rosenstein et al., 1990). The length of stay at partial-care programs is commonly 4 to 6 months. During this time, patients may receive supervision, group and individual therapy, socialization, medication management, and various recreational therapies.

The number of partial-care programs in the United States has grown in recent years (American Hospitals Association, 1994). However, there are more than ten admissions each year to specialized inpatient facilities for each patient admitted to a partial-care program (Rosenstein et al., 1990). Poor third-party reimbursement, concerns about patient safety, and a general unfamiliarity of psychiatrists with this treatment modality have impeded the proliferation of partial-care programs (Parker and Knoll, 1990).

Innovative Community Treatment Research

Community psychiatrists face the challenging task of providing a stable treatment environment for severely ill psychiatric patients. Over the last three decades, research has been conducted on several strategies to improve and extend patient function outside the hospital. Early innovations focused on alternatives to acute hospitalization. More recently, mental health services researchers have concentrated on strategies to enhance the quality of patients' lives in the community. Newer treatment interventions have tended to provide continuous or ongoing care that helps patients meet a range of basic needs such as housing, nutrition, medical care, social structure, and daily living skills. What follows is a summary of selected research findings on three alternatives to psychiatric hospitalization (home care, day hospitalization, and alternative institutions) and five strategies for enriching outpatient care (day hospitals, residential treatment, assertive community treatment, service access strategies, and clubhouses).

Alternatives to Psychiatric Hospitalization

Home care.   The most ambitious strategy of community-based treatment intercepts patients at or near the time of planned inpatient admission and returns them home with the support of a home care clinician. Available evidence suggests that acutely ill psychiatric patients, who are not dangerous and have families willing to participate in treatment, can often be managed with home care rather than hospitalization. However, more work is needed to assess the impact of home care on functional outcome.

In the 1960s Pasamanick and co-workers (1964, 1967) studied home care for acutely ill chronic schizophrenic patients. Patients selected for the intervention were neither homicidal nor suicidal and lived with a family member willing to supervise them. A randomly selected group of patients were discharged within a few days of hospital admission to the care of a visiting public health nurse supervised by a psychiatrist. At 6-month follow-up, home care patients were functioning as well as patients assigned to customary care, and the home care patients averaged fewer inpatient days.

These general findings were subsequently replicated with a diagnostically mixed group of non-chronically ill psychiatric patients who were neither suicidal nor homicidal and had family support (Fenton et al., 1979). A third study, which did not measure symptom level, failed to find that home care reduced total hospital days below the level delivered to patients receiving routine hospital and clinic care (Smith et al., 1976).

Day hospitals.   Day hospitalization has also been studied as an alternative to full hospitalization. Experimental evidence suggests that a subgroup of hospital-bound acutely ill patients—particularly non-dangerous patients, females, and those with acute rather than chronic conditions—can be successfully treated in this less restrictive setting. For patients who can be treated in day hospitals, the outcomes are generally similar to patients treated in full hospital settings (Creed et al., 1991).

In the 1960s Zwerling and Wilder randomly assigned unselected new psychiatric hospital admissions to inpatient care or day treatment (Zwerling and Wilder, 1964; Wilder et al., 1966). One-third of the day patients were immediately referred back for hospitalization, and an additional one-quarter were hospitalized later during their day hospital stay. At 2-year follow-up, the schizophrenic women assigned to day hospitalization tended to have better outcomes than those assigned to full hospitalization, but the reverse was true for schizophrenic men.

Herz and co-workers (1971) randomly assigned a carefully selected group of patients after three inpatient days to day hospitalization or continued inpatient care. Exclusion criteria resulted in bypassing more than three-quarters of hospital admissions. The study group was predominantly white, female, and had two or fewer previous hospitalizations. Day patients were discharged more rapidly and had a lower rate of readmission than the patients assigned to inpatient care. During the first month following admission, day patients were also less symptomatic than controls.

Alternative institutions.   In addition to day hospitals, other institutional alternatives to full hospitalization have been explored. These facilities offer a treatment environment that is less rigidly structured than traditional hospitalization, and they often have a lower staff-to-patient ratio. Clinical results have been mixed.

Polak and Kirby (1976) studied the effects of randomly assigning consecutive newly accepted inpatient admissions to standard state hospital care or carefully se-lected volunteer private homes. The homes combined aggressive medication manage-ment, crisis intervention, 24-hour nursing availability, and support from volunteers. A substantial proportion of the experimental patients (40 percent) were either lost to follow-up or removed from the study because they required hospitalization. The re-maining experimental patients were more satisfied with their treatment than the controls and were not significantly different from the controls on follow-up symptom ratings.

Rappaport and co-workers (1987) assessed the clinical consequences of treating psychiatric patients on a general hospital inpatient unit or in a short-term non-hospital treatment setting with a relatively low staff-to-patient ratio. The two groups had similar severity-of-illness ratings at the time of admission. At discharge, the hospitalized group were less ill than the experimental group and had been treated for a shorter period of time. This evaluation suggests that reducing the intensity of inpatient care risks diminishing treatment efficacy.

Strategies for Enriching Outpatient Care

Day hospitals.   Day hospitals have also been studied as a means of stabilizing and enhancing the functioning of psychiatric outpatients. For more severely ill patients, day hospital aftercare may promote improved social adjustment. For less severely ill patients, day hospital treatment combined with occupational rehabilitation may pro-mote improved social and occupational functioning.

The VA conducted a 10-site cooperative study that randomly assigned male schiz-ophrenic patients at hospital discharge to day treatment or medication maintenance (Linn et al., 1979). At long-term follow-up, day treatment patients at all 10 sites exhibited significantly higher social functioning than the controls. Six of the programs successfully delayed relapse or reduced clinical symptoms. The successful programs were characterized by occupational rather than group therapy and by sustained non-threatening treatment environments rather than high patient turnover.

In a second VA study, general psychiatric patients were randomly assigned to a conventional inpatient unit or to an experimental inpatient unit with aftercare access to a day hospital, group community housing, and a sheltered work program (Kuldau and Dirks, 1977). The patients were typically married, high school educated, em-ployed, and without previous hospitalizations. At follow-up, the experimental patients achieved a more favorable employment status, social adjustment, and had been read-mitted to the hospital significantly fewer times than the control group. In a similar study of non-chronically ill patients discharged to a day program or weekly group therapy, Glick and co-workers (1986) found no difference between the groups across several clinical outcome measures. The added support provided by the sheltered work program and group community housing may help explain the more favorable clinical outcomes reported by Kuldau and Dirks.

Residential programs.   Various experimental residential programs have been studied as a means of providing patients an opportunity to achieve meaningful social roles while protecting them from some of the harsher elements of the broader community. Available data suggest that residential programs are more likely to promote occupational and social functioning than to reduce symptom level or prevent relapse.

Fairweather pioneered work with the living-working lodge concept in Palo Alto, California (Fairweather etal, 1968). Set in the community, the lodge is a dormitory where former psychiatric inpatients live and run a for-profit janitorial and gardening service. Patients are first encouraged and later expected to assume responsibility for all aspects of the daily operation of the lodge and business.

A mixed group of long-term VA psychiatric inpatients were randomly assigned to the lodge or continued traditional care. Over a 2.5-year period, the lodge patients consistently spent more time than the controls in the community and in full employment. Measures of psychosocial adjustment and symptom level failed to uncover differences between the two study groups, and patients who left the lodge fared little better than controls.

Lamb and Goertzel (1972) randomly assigned a diagnostically mixed group of long-term state hospital patients to regular outpatient care or to a program that combined halfway house residence, day treatment, and vocational training. Although a greater proportion of experimental than control patients were rehospitalized during the first 6 months, this trend did not persist. Throughout the 2-year follow-up, the experimental patients achieved higher vocational and social functioning than the controls. As with many of the multifaceted treatment innovations, it is not possible to tease apart which of the service elements promoted the functional improvement.

Assertive community treatment.   Assertive community treatment (ACT) is a set of interventions based on direct patient assistance, instruction in basic living skills, and social support. Interdisciplinary treatment teams meet with severely ill psychiatric patients in the community and teach patients basic daily living skills. More important, the treatment teams ensure that patients have their basic material needs met.

The assertive community treatment strategy was pioneered by Stein and Test with the Training in Community Living program in Madison, Wisconsin (Stein and Test, 1980). Modifications of the original model have been studied in various service settings with diverse patient populations (Burns and Santos, 1995; Olfson, 1990a).

As previously mentioned, early research demonstrated that ACT was more effective than conventional treatment in controlling symptoms and improving the functioning of severely ill psychiatric patients. More recently, researchers have been unable to replicate these findings. However, patients have consistently expressed a preference for ACT over traditional care, and several studies have shown that ACT leads to reductions in hospitalization.

Case management.   The recognition that severely mentally ill patients have enduring but ever-changing service needs has led to the development of programs designed to connect patients with services in a timely and orderly manner. Case managers are mental health professionals who assume responsibility for ensuring that patients receive appropriate care.

Franklin and associates (1987) randomly assigned a mixed group of public sector psychiatric patients with two or more previous hospitalizations to customary care or case management. Case managers were mainly engaged in administrative tasks such as brokering services and making referrals. At follow-up, the experimental patients consumed more outpatient and inpatient care than the control group and were not significantly improved on quality of life measures.

Goering and co-workers (1988) followed inpatients assigned to case management and an equal number of matched controls given usual care. This study was set in a mental health system with known discharge planning problems. Both study groups had chronic psychiatric illnesses, poor employment histories, housing difficulties, and were socially isolated. Case managers focused on arranging for rehabilitation services and making appropriate referrals.

At 6-month follow-up, case managed patients and matched controls did not significantly differ from one another in symptom level or social adjustment. By 2 years, however, case managed patients had achieved significantly greater occupational functioning, housing status, and social adjustment than the controls.

Clubhouses.   Clubhouses are community-based day programs that provide a range of supportive and rehabilitative services. Clubhouses commonly encourage patients to assume a role in the daily operation of the institution (i.e., cooking meals, cleaning, clerical work) and provide patients with membership in a supportive social organization.

The only rigorous studies of clubhouse rehabilitation services have been performed at Fountain House in New York City (Beard et al., 1963; Beard et al., 1978). Recently discharged psychiatric inpatients, most of whom suffered from schizophrenia, were randomly assigned to clubhouse treatment or an outside referral. Clubhouse treatment significantly delayed but did not prevent hospital readmission and tended to increase employment.

Summary

There is much yet to be learned from the old but relatively undeveloped field of mental health services research. We still view much of the system of services as a "black box" and have difficulty defining the critical elements of service interventions. However, experimental and quasi-experimental research has helped to provide a rational basis for improving programs and systems of care.

An important finding to emerge from mental health services research is that for many seriously ill patients a variety of model community-based programs are capable of providing care that is at least as effective and often more effective than traditional hospital- and clinic-based care. Empirical data support the broader use of home care, day hospitals, residential programs, assertive community treatment, and clubhouses. Mental health services research has also increased our appreciation of the critical role of continuous and uninterrupted care rather than episode-based treatment.

Services research has broadened our view of the service needs of persons with severe mental illness. In addition to medically oriented psychiatric services, these patients often require assistance with housing, social support, training in daily living skills, vocational rehabilitation, and other basic social services.

Community psychiatrists face the formidable challenge of translating the findings of mental health services research into daily practice. Beyond their vital role as service providers, community psychiatrists are well positioned to conduct research to improve our understanding of how best to organize and provide care.

References

American Hospital Association (1994) *Hospital Statistics, 1994–95.* Chicago: American Hospital Association.

Balestrieri M., Williams, P., and Wilkinson, G. (1988) Specialist mental health treatment in general practice: a meta-analysis. *Psychological Medicine,* 18:711–717.

Barrett, J.E., Barrett, B.A., Oxman, T.E., and Gerber, P.D. (1988) The prevalence of psychiatric disorders in primary care practice. *Archives of General Psychiatry,* 45:1100–1106.

Beard, J.H., Malamud, T.J., and Rossman, E. (1978) Psychiatric rehabilitation and long-term rehospitalization rates: the findings of two research studies. *Schizophrenia Bulletin,* 4:622–635.

Beard, J.H., Pitt, R.B., Risher, S.H., and Goertzel, V. (1963) Evaluation of the effectiveness of a psychiatric rehabilitation program. *American Journal of Orthomolecular Psychiatry,* 33:701–712.

Blacker, C.V.R., and Clare, A.W. (1988) The prevalence and treatment of depression in general practice. *Psychopharmacology,* 95:S14–S17.

Blouin, A., Perez, E., and Minoletti, A. (1985) Compliance to referrals from the psychiatric emergency room. *Canadian Journal of Psychiatry,* 30:103–106.

Burns, B.J. (1991) Mental health service use by adolescents in the 1970s and 1980s. *Journal of the American Academy of Child and Adolescent Psychiatry,* 30:144–150.

Creed, F., Black, D., Anthony, P., Osborn, M., et al. (1991) Randomised controlled trial of day and inpatient psychiatric treatment: II. Comparison of two hospitals. *British Journal of Psychiatry,* 158:183–189.

Dorwart, R.A., and Schlesinger, M. (1988) Privatization of psychiatric services. *American Journal of Psychiatry,* 145:543–553.

Burns, B.J. and Santos, A.B. (1995) Assertive community treatment: An update of randomized controlled trials. *Psychiatric Services,* 46:669–675.

Fairweather, G.W., Sanders D.H., Maynard, H. (1968) *Community life for the mentally ill.* Chicago: Aldine Publishing.

Fenton, F.R., Tessier, L., and Struening, E.L. (1979) A comparative trial of home and hospital psychiatric care: One year follow-up. *Archives of General Psychiatry,* 36:1073–1079.

Franklin, J.L., Solovitz, B., Mason, M., and Clemons, J.R. (1987) An evaluation of case management. *American Journal of Public Health,* 77:674–678.

Glick, I.D., Flemming, L., DeChillo, N., Meyerkopft N., et al. (1986) A controlled study of transitional day care for non-chronically-ill patients. *American Journal of Psychiatry,* 143:1551–1556.

Goering, P.N., Wasylenki, D.A., Farkas, M., Lancee, W.J., et al. (1988) What difference does case management make? *Hospital and Community Psychiatry,* 39:272–276.

Goldman, H.H., Morrissey, J.P., Ridgely, M.S. (1994) Evaluating the Robert Wood Johnson Foundation Program on Chronic Mental Illness. *Milbank Quarterly,* 72:37–47.

Goldman, H.H., Lehman, A.F., Morrissey, J.P., Newman, S.J., Frank, R.G., and Steinwachs, D.M. (1990a) Design for the national evaluation of the Robert Wood Johnson Foundation Program on Chronic Mental Illness. *Hospital and Community Psychiatry,* 41: 1217–1221.

Goldman, H.H., Morrissey, J.P., and Ridgely, M.S. (1990b) Form and function of mental health authorities at RWJ Foundation program sites: Preliminary observations. *Hospital and Community Psychiatry,* 41:1222–1229.

Goldman, H.H., and Sharfstein, S.S. (1987) Are specialized services worth the higher cost? *American Journal of Psychiatry,* 144:626–628.

Goldman, H.H., Feder, J., and Scanlon, W. (1986) Chronic mental patients in nursing homes: Reexamining data from the National Nursing Home Survey. *Hospital and Community Psychiatry,* 37:269–272.

Herz, M.M., Endicott, J., Spitzer, R.L., and Mesnikoff, A. (1971) Day versus inpatient hospitalization: a controlled study. *American Journal of Psychiatry,* 127:1371–1382.

Higgins, E.S. (1994) A review of unrecognized mental illness in primary care: prevalence, natural history, and efforts to change the course. *Archives of Family Medicine,* 3:908–917.

Hodgkin, D. (1992) The impact of private utilization management on psychiatric care: a review of the literature. *The Journal of Mental Health Administration,* 19:143–157.

Hoeper, E.W., Nycz, G.R., Cleary, P.D., Regier, D.A., and Goldberg, I.D. (1979) Estimated prevalence of RDC mental disorder in primary medical care. *International Journal of Mental Health,* 8:6–15.

Hull, J. (1979) Psychiatric referrals in general practice. *Archives of General Psychiatry,* 36: 406–408.

Jellinek, M. (1978) Referrals from a psychiatric emergency room: relationship of compliance to demographic interview variables. *American Journal of Psychiatry,* 135:209–213.

Johnson, D.A.W. (1973) Treatment of depression in general practice. *British Journal of Medicine,* 2:18–20.

Jones, L.R., Badger, L.W., Ficken, R.P., Leeper, J.D., et al. (1987) Inside the hidden mental health network: examining mental health care delivery of primary care physicians. *General Hospital Psychiatry,* 9:287–293.

Kessler, L.G., Burns, B.J., Shapiro, S., Tischler, G.L., et al. (1987) Psychiatric diagnoses of medical service users: evidence from the Epidemiologic Catchment Area Program. *American Journal of Public Health,* 77:18–24.

Kessler, R.C., McGonagle, K.A., Zhao, S., Nelson, C.R., Hughes, M., Eshelman, S., Wittchen, H.U., and Kendler, L. (1994) Lifetime and 12-month prevalence of DSM-III-R psychiatric disorders in the United States: results from the National Comorbidity Study. *Archives of General Psychiatry,* 51:8–19.

Kuldau, J.M., and Dirks, S.J. (1977) Controlled evaluation of a hospital-originated community transitional system. *Archives of General Psychiatry,* 34:1331–1340.

Lamb, H.R., and Goertzel, V. (1972) High expectations of long-term ex-state hospital patients. *American Journal of Psychiatry,* 129:471–475.

Lehman, A.F., Possidente, S., and Hawker, F. (1986) The quality of life of chronic patients in a state hospital and in community residences. *Hospital and Community Psychiatry, 37*: 901–907.

Linn, M.W., Caffey, E.M., Klett, J., Hogarty, G.E., et al. (1979) Day treatment and psychotropic drugs in the aftercare of schizophrenic patients. *Archives of General Psychiatry, 36*: 1055–1066.

Locke, B.Z., Krantz, G., and Kramer, M. (1966) Psychiatric need and demand in a prepaid group practice program. *American Journal of Public Health,* 56:895–890.

Manderscheid, R.W., Rae, D.S., Narrow, W.E., Locke, B.Z., and Regier, D.A. (1993) Congruence of service utilization estimates from the epidemiologic catchment area project and other sources. *Archives of General Psychiatry, 50*:108–114.

Nicholson, I.R. (1994) Factors involved in failure to keep initial appointments with mental health professionals. *Hospital and Community Psychiatry,* 45:276–278.

Olfson, M. (1990a) Assertive community treatment: an evaluation of the evidence. *Hospital and Community Psychiatry,* 41:634–641.

Olfson, M. (1990b) Treatment of depressed patients in general hospitals with scatter beds, cluster beds, and psychiatric units. *Hospital and Community Psychiatry,* 41:1106–1111.

Orleans, C.T., George, L.K., Houpt, J.L., and Brodie, H.K.H. (1985) How primary care physicians treat psychiatric disorders: a national survey of family practitioners. *American Journal of Psychiatry,* 142:52–57.

Parker S., and Knoll, J.L. (1990) Partial hospitalization: an update. *American Journal of Psychiatry,* 147:156–160.

Pasamanick, B., Scarpitti, F.R., and Dinitz, S. (1967) *Schizophrenics in the Community.* New York: Appleton-Century-Crofts.

Pasamanick, B., Scarpitti, F.R., Lefton, M., Dinitz, S., et al. (1964) Home versus hospital care for schizophrenics. *Journal of the American Medical Association,* 187:89–93.

Perez-Stable, E., Miranda, J., and Munoz, R.F. (1990) Depression in medical outpatients: underrecognition and misdiagnosis. *Archives of Internal Medicine,* 150:1083–1088.

Polak, P.R., and Kirby, M.W. (1976) A model to replace psychiatric hospitals. *Journal of Nervous and Mental Disease,* 162:13–22.

Rappaport, M., Goldman, H.H., Thornton, P., Stegner, B., et al. (1987) A method for comparing two systems of acute 24 hour psychiatric care. *Hospital and Community Psychiatry, 38*: 1091–1095.

Regier, D.A., Goldberg, I.D., and Taube, C.A. (1978) The de facto U.S. mental health services system: a public health perspective. *Archives of General Psychiatry,* 35:685–693.

Regier, D.A., Narrow, W.E., Rae, D.S., Manderscheid, R.W., Locke, B.Z., and Goodwin, F.K. (1993) The de facto U.S. mental and addictive disorders services system: epidemiologic catchment area prospective 1-year prevalence rates of disorders and services. *Archives of General Psychiatry,* 50:85–94.

Rosenstein, M.R., Milazzo-Sayre, L.J., and Manderscheid, R. W. (1990) Characteristics of persons using specialty inpatient, outpatient, and partial care programs in 1986. In Manderscheid, R.W., Sonnenschein, M.A. (eds.), *Mental Health, United States, 1990,* pp. 139–172. Washington, D.C.: National Institute of Mental Health.

Rosenstein, M.R., Milazzo-Sayre, L.J., and Manderscheid, R.W. (1989) Care of persons with schizophrenia: a statistical profile. *Schizophrenia Bulletin,* 15:45–58.

Rovner, B.W., German, P.S., Brant, L.J., Clark, R., Burton, L., and Folstein, M.F. (1991) Depression and mortality in nursing homes. *JAMA,* 265:993–996.

Rovner, B.W., Kafonel, S., Flipp, L., Lucas, M.J., and Folstein, M.F. (1986) Prevalence of mental illness in a community nursing home. *American Journal of Psychiatry,* 143: 1446–1449.

Schappert, S.M. (1993) Office visits to psychiatrists: United States, 1989–90. *Advance Data,* 237:1–16.

Schulberg, H.C., Saul, M., McClelland, M., Ganguli, M., et al. (1985) Assessing depression in primary medical and psychiatric practices. *Archives of General Psychiatry,* 42:1164–1170.

Schurman, R.A., Kramer, P.D., and Mitchell, J.B. (1985) The hidden mental health network. *Archives of General Psychiatry,* 42:89–94.

Shortell, S.M., and Daniels, R.S. (1974) Referral relationships between internists and psychiatrists in fee-for-service practice: an empirical examination. *Medical Care,* 12:229–240.

Smith, F.A., Fenton, F.R., Benoit, C., and Barzell, R.N. (1976) Home-care treatment of acutely ill psychiatric patients. *Canadian Psychiatric Association Journal,* 20:7–13.

Smyer, M.A., Shea, D.G., and Streit, A. (1994) The provision and use of mental health services in nursing homes: results from the National Medical Expenditure Survey. *American Journal of Public Health,* 84:284–287.

Stein, L.I., and Test, M.A. (1980) Alternative to mental hospital treatment. I. Conceptual model, treatment program, and clinical evaluation. *Archives of General Psychiatry,* 37:392–397.

Stotsky, B.A., and Stotsky, E.S. (1983) Nursing homes: improving a flawed community facility. *Hospital and Community Psychiatry,* 34:238–242.

Strahan, G.W. (1990) Prevalence of selected mental disorders in nursing and related care homes. In Manderscheid, R.W., Sonnenschein, M.A. (eds.), *Mental health, United States, 1990,* pp. 227–240. Washington, D.C.: National Institute of Mental Health.

Sweeney, J.A., Von Bulow, B., Shear, M.K., Friedman, R., and Plowe, C. (1984) Compliance and outcome of patients accompanied by relatives to evaluations. *Hospital and Community Psychiatry,* 35:1037–1038.

Test, M.A., and Stein, L.I. (1980) An alternative to mental hospital treatment: III. Social cost. *Archives of General Psychiatry,* 37:409–412.

Weisbrod, B.A., Test, M.A., and Stein, L.I. (1980) Alternative to mental hospital treatment. II. Economic benefit-cost analysis. *Archives of General Psychiatry,* 37:400–405.

Wilder, J.F., Levin, G., and Zwerling, I. (1966) A two-year follow-up evaluation of acute psychotic patients treated in a day hospital. *American Journal of Psychiatry,* 122:1095–1101.

Witkin, M.J., Atay, J.A., Fell, A.S., and Manderschied, R.W. (1990) Specialty mental health system characteristics. In Manderscheid, R.W., Sonnenschein, M.A. (eds.), *Mental Health, United States, 1990,* pp. 1–139. Washington, D.C.: National Institute of Mental Health.

Wolff, N., Henderson, P.R., MacAskill, R.L., Rosenstein, M.J., Millazo-Sayre, L.J., Larson, D., and Manderscheid, R.W. (1989) Treatment patterns for schizophrenia in psychiatric hospitals. *Social Science and Medicine,* 4:323–331.

Zwerling, I., and Wilder, J.F. (1964) An evaluation of the applicability of the day hospital in treatment of acutely disturbed patients. *Israel Annals of Psychiatry and Related Disciplines,* 2:162–185.

9

Quantitative Methods in the Evaluation of Community Mental Health Services

GRAHAM THORNICROFT
PAUL BEBBINGTON

A new challenge for clinicians and researchers at the end of the twentieth century is to measure accurately the effects of patient interventions and mental health care in order to decide the best and most cost-effective means of delivery. This chapter first summarizes the characteristics of adequate measures in the field of community mental health and then gives an overview of the most commonly used scales. The intention is to act as a guide to clinicians who wish to evaluate the outcomes of their work, and to provide researchers with an initial entry into the vast array of measures that are available. The emphasis is on scales used for evaluating adult psychiatric services in the community; other important specialist areas, such as assessment of cognitive impairment and abnormal movements, are covered elsewhere in more detailed texts (Wetzler, 1989; Thompson, 1989; Parry and Watts, 1989; Freeman and Tyrer, 1989; Israel et al., 1990). Two examples are provided of how evaluation instruments were used in studies of the effects of community-based psychiatric services.

Establishing the psychometric qualities of new scales is detailed and time consuming. Although we would never use uncalibrated measures for height, weight, or temperature, many scales used for mental health service evaluation are unfortunately of unknown validity and reliability (Hall, 1979; Hall, 1980). It is important, therefore, to adopt a critical attitude toward this field of measurement, which in many key areas is in its infancy. In many domains of psychiatric measurement no gold standard exists against which to validate particular measures, and scales must therefore rely on lesser tests of adequacy.

The Psychometric Properties of Standardised Instruments

Research instruments are generally judged on the basis of their validity and reliability. A scale may be reliable and invalid or may be valid and unreliable, but a methodological goal in research is to devise scales with demonstrated strengths in both areas.

Validity

An instrument should first of all actually measure what it is intended to measure—it should be valid (in Latin *validus* meaning "strong"). Validity poses special difficulties in the area of psychological and psychiatric assessment, as the criteria against which to rate validity may themselves be indirect or imprecise. The range of validity estimates are characterized in the following ways. *Face validity* is the subjective judgment made by the user of the instrument about whether the individual items cover the appropriate range of problems relevant to the measure as a whole. This is not a statistical yardstick of validity so much as an initial impression about the degree to which the scale correctly includes relevant items. *Content validity* describes whether a test samples from the entire domain of that which is to be measured. Again, this is more an issue of personal judgment than a statistical measure of validity. More widely, the opinions of experts in the field may be taken about a new measure to provide an estimate of *consensual validity. Criterion-related validity* is acceptable when a new measure produces the same result as another instrument whose validity has already been established, where the latter is called the criterion measure. There are two types of criterion-related validity: *Concurrent* validity is used when the results of the two tests being compared are available simultaneously, while *predictive* validity is applicable where scores on the new test are used to predict subsequent scores on a proven test. Finally, *construct validity* addresses the psychological meaning of the test scores. It has been clearly described by Aiken (1985): "The construct validity of a test is not established by one successful prediction: It consists of the slow, laborious process of gathering evidence from many experiments and observations on how the test is functioning." Among these observations will be correlations with other measures of the construct under consideration, and the successful prediction of functional outcomes where these are known to be associated with the construct (Streiner and Norman, 1989).

Where a test is used for screening purposes, to identify probable cases of a condition, its validity is demonstrated in its ability to distinguish those with the condition from those without the condition (Table 9–1). Two validity indices are commonly used. *Sensitivity* is the probability of producing a positive test result if the disease is present; it is calculated as $a/(a+c)$. *Specificity* is the probability of producing a negative test result if the disease is absent; it is calculated as $d/(b+d)$.

Table 9–1   Screening test performance

Screen test result	Disease status		
	Positive	Negative	Total
Positive	a	b	a + b
Negative	c	d	c + d
Total	a + c	b + d	

Reliability

A rating scale must give repeatable results for the same subject when used under different conditions. This is referred to as *reliability*. There are two widely used methods to gauge reliability. *Inter-rater reliability* is a measure of the extent to which the instrument yields the same result when applied by two or more independent raters with the same subject. It is therefore applicable only to interviewer-rated scales and is best measured by the raters being present at the same live interview or, in a weaker form, separately rating the same recorded interview. The degree of agreement between raters may be calculated either for a total scale score, or for the ratings on individual items. A widely used measure of agreement is Cohen's kappa, which takes into account the likelihood of the raters agreeing by chance alone (Cohen, 1960). Usually kappa values of less than 40 percent indicate a poor level of agreement, and over 75 percent show very good agreement. *Test-retest reliability* describes how far the score of a rating scale remains constant when used by the same rater with the same subject at two or more points in time. If the scores are identical from the two rating occasions, the correlation is 1.0, but this does not occur in practice. Test-retest reliability is more applicable to stable variables, such as personality, than to symptoms that rapidly fluctuate, such as anxiety. It needs to be emphasized that a reliable measure is not necessarily valid.

In practice, when selecting a measure for a study of community psychiatry, a number of issues must be addressed. Does the scale being considered have published validity and reliability scores available, and how strong are these results? Do the age, sex, ethnic, diagnostic, and functional characteristics of the test population resemble the study population? If any doubt remains after addressing these questions, then a pilot study may be required to establish the psychometric properties of the selected measures under local conditions.

Key Domains in Mental Health Outcome Evaluation

Most outcomes of psychiatric treatment and management are measured at the level of the individual patient in terms of improvement in some area. These data may be aggregated later into indices of the performance of a specific program or of the whole service delivery system. In other situations, information may be collected at the system level alone, for example in determining the proportion of all admissions that are voluntary. The emphasis in this chapter is on the former, rating important mental health characteristics of individuals. Measures have been developed with a high degree of psychometric adequacy in three domains—the mental state, social behavior, and quality of life. These areas will therefore be described in most detail.

Mental State

There are several reasons to compare the mental states of psychiatric patients. We may wish to compare the phenomena exhibited by different groups of individuals in detail as a way of determining how similar they are. We may want to compare patients with themselves at a different point in time, that is, to evaluate change. We may require to relate specific phenomena, for example, hallucinations, to a range of social, psychological, and biological variables as a way of generating causal hypotheses. It may be necessary to identify and describe particular treatment targets. Many instruments have been developed to measure mental states, using different methods and concepts (Table 9–2). Some of the most important and widely used are reviewed here.

Phenomenology and diagnosis.   It is crucial to our understanding of the concept of mental symptoms that they have always been defined in terms of experiences. Although they are elicited through verbal report, they are not themselves verbal reports. In the formal process of diagnosis, verbal reports must be evaluated before they are accepted as representing an experience corresponding to a mental symptom. This has relevance for many of the instruments that are used to evaluate psychiatric status and can be illustrated by consideration of an instrument that has set the standard for measurement of mental states, the Present State Examination (PSE). The PSE has been developed over a period of 30 years. A ninth edition (PSE-9) (Wing et al., 1974; Wing et al., 1977), and a tenth (PSE-10), which forms part of a larger instrument, SCAN, developed under the auspices of the WHO/ADAMHA Project on Diagnosis and Classification of Mental Disorders are currently in use. The PSE is a *semi-structured* clinical interview, that is, it can be conducted in a flexible way in terms of the order of questioning, although the purpose is ultimately to cover a defined field of mental phenomena. The instrument's primary aim is to obtain a clear description of the phenomena of mental disorder. Only when this primary aim has been achieved is consideration given to the requirements for diagnostic classification. The argument for this is that although classifications change, the basic phenomena remain the same.

The PSE represents an attempt to reproduce, in a standardized form, the clinical judgments of psychiatrists that given symptoms are present. To ensure standardization, definitions are provided in a glossary and are then clarified and amplified in training courses. The PSE-9 covers 140 items, most of which are either symptoms or signs of psychiatric disorder and cover a very broad field of psychopathology. The instrument clearly is designed for administration by people of some clinical sophistication; al-

Table 9–2   Diagnostic and mental state instruments

Instrument	Authors	Comments
Brief Psychiatric Rating Scale (BPRS)	Overall and Gorham, 1962	Rating from patient interview, mainly for psychotic symptoms
Manchester Scale	Krawiecka, Goldberg, and Vaughan, 1977	Rating of symptoms of chronic psychosis
Present State Examination 9th version (PSE)	Wing, Cooper, and Sartorius, 1974	Detailed rating of 140 items from structured mental state interview. ICD output.
Schedule for Affective Disorders and Schizophrenia (SADS)	Endicott and Spitzer, 1978	Interview to allow Research Diagnostic Criteria (RDC) diagnosis
Diagnostic Interview Schedule (DIS)	Robins et al., 1985a	Structured operationalized patient interview by non-clinicians
Schedules for Clinical Assessment in Neuropsychiatry (SCAN)	Wing et al., 1990	Development of PSE 9. Structured interview with ICD and DSM IIIR outputs
Structured Clinical Interview for DSM IIIR (SCID)	Spitzer, Williams, and Gibbons, 1985	For use by trained clinicians to produce DSM-III-R diagnoses on axes 1 and 2.
Comprehensive Psychopathological Rating Scale (CPRS)	Asberg et al., 1978	65-item interview schedule designed to be sensitive to symptom change
Schedule for the Assessment of Positive Symptoms (SAPS)	Andreasen, 1984	Assesses hallucinations, delusions, bizarre behavior and thought disorder
Composite International Diagnostic Instrument (CIDI)	Robins 1985	Structure lay administered interview using some PSE items with DSM-III-R output
Schedule for the Assessment of Negative Symptoms (SANS)	Andreasen, 1983	Rates 5 subgroups of negative features from patient interview

though the rules for its administration are laid down, the examiner may always overrule them if clinical intuition demands it. It has also been used as a screening device by lay interviewers (Bebbington et al., 1981; Wing et al., 1977; Sturt, 1981). PSE-10 covers problems associated with appetite, alcohol and other substance use, and cognitive disorders, in addition to the disorders covered in PSE-9. Data from the schedules can be entered directly into a lap-top computer file.

SCAN (Schedules for Clinical Assessment in Neuropsychiatry) is a set of instruments aimed at assessing, measuring, and classifying the psychopathology and behavior associated with the major psychiatric disorders of adult life. It has four components, the Present State Examination, tenth edition (PSE-10), a Glossary of differential definitions, an Item Group Checklist (IGC), and a Clinical History Schedule (CHS) (Wing et al., 1990). A set of computer algorithms (CATEGO5) is used to process data entered from SCAN schedules. The output can include an Index of Definition, ICD-10, DSM-III-R and DSM-IV categories, and a printout of items meeting the various criteria. In its complete form, SCAN is intended for use only by clinicians with an adequate knowledge of psychopathology who have taken a course at a WHO-designated training center. There is a shortened version for use by lay interviewers trained in these centers (World Health Organization, 1992, 1994).

Using lay interviewers has been a long tradition in the United States, so that researchers have been concerned not to rely upon clinical skills but to eliminate the need for them. The Diagnostic Interview Schedule (DIS) (Robins et al., 1979, 1985a) deliberately incorporates a rigid structure of questions whose form is exactly pre-scribed. Interviewers are trained not to deviate from the printed format, so that the scope for clinical judgment is reduced to a minimum. This strategy is understandable in the context of the instrument's development, but many psychiatrists feel that it purchases reliability and comparability at the expense of validity.

The Composite International Diagnostic Instrument (CIDI) (Robins et al., 1988) represents an attempt to combine aspects of the DIS and the PSE. It does this by including neurotic and some psychotic items from PSE-9, but the resulting interview is highly structured in the same way as the DIS, being designed for use by lay inter-viewers. It provides classification according to the same three sets of criteria as the DIS. Because of the additional items, it also caters for some classes in the International Classification of Diseases (ICD9). This instrument is of interest because it is intended to pick up items equivalent to PSE items, but in a different way. Comparisons can thus be made between the two instruments (Farmer et al., 1987). The DIS has a role in field surveys, although it is incapable of matching the detailed symptom picture available with the PSE.

General psychiatric rating scales.   The General Health Questionnaire (GHQ) (Gold-berg, 1972) is self-administered and was originally designed as a screening instrument to identify people with a high likelihood of having non-psychotic disorders, both in general practice settings and in the community at large. It is a good screening instru-ment, with sensitivity and specificity between 70 percent and 90 percent. Although ideally the case status of subjects scoring above the threshold should be confirmed by a psychiatric interview, the instrument is often used as a measure of the severity of non-specific neurotic disturbance. The GHQ-28 yields four separate scales—somatic symptoms, anxiety/insomnia, social dysfunction, and depression—thus revealing a clear intention that it should be used to provide a stand-alone assessment. The tradi-tional thresholds identify a very high percentage of the population as significantly symptomatic, far more than the PSE-ID-CATEGO system or the DIS.

The Brief Psychiatric Rating Scale (BPRS) (Overall and Gorham, 1962) comprises 18 items that cover symptoms typical of affective disorders (e.g., anxiety, depressive mood, hostility) and of psychosis (e.g., hallucinations, unusual though content). It is one of the most widely used general rating scales and is often chosen to assess the effects of pharmacological treatment. It is probably best suited to severe disorders;

the quantification of relatively mild anxiety or depressive states is better served by more specific instruments.

The Schedule of Affective Disorders and Schizophrenia (SADS) is a semi-structured interview intended to be used by clinicians (Endicott and Spitzer, 1978). It is based on the diagnostic definitions contained in the Research Diagnostic Criteria (Spitzer et al., 1978). The first section of the instrument contains items to rate severity of current condition; the second part assesses lifetime history of mental illness. More recent variations of SADS assess lifetime morbidity, anxiety disorders, clinical change, and bipolar disorders.

The Structured Clinical Interview for DSM-III-R (SCID), is an interviewer-administered assessment of mental disorders, also designed to be used by people with clinical training, and produces diagnostic outputs consistent with the DSM-III-R classification (Spitzer, 1983). It was designed to supplement the DIS. A further version SCID-P has been developed to assess personality disorders. The advantages of SCID, compared with SADS, are that it is less time consuming and requires less intensive training (Riskind et al., 1987).

Scales for specific conditions.   One of the oldest and most frequently used scales for affective disorder is the Hamilton Depression Scale (Hamilton, 1967). Psychometrically, it is fairly crude, but this has not affected its popularity. Several authors (e.g., Bech et al., 1981) have modified the original format, which nevertheless retains the allegiance of most users. The ratings refer to the symptoms experienced over the last few days, and no distinction appears to have been made between intensity and frequency. It has quite good inter-rater reliability (Hamilton, 1967; Bech et al., 1979).

Two self-rating scales are widely used in the evaluation of depression. The Beck Depression Inventory (BDI) covers 21 categories of symptoms and attitudes (Beck et al., 1961). Each item is rated by asking patients to select which one of a graded series of statements corresponds most closely with their clinical condition. Like any self-rating scale it depends on the diligence and compliance of patients and can easily be falsified, should they wish. The Zung Self-Rating Depression Scale (Zung, 1965) and its shorter derivative, the Wakefield Inventory (Snaith et al., 1971) are other widely used measures of change in depressive states.

Like the Hamilton Depression Scale, the Hamilton Anxiety Scale (Hamilton, 1959) was designed for use in subjects diagnosed as having some form of an anxiety state. It comprises ratings of 13 symptoms, plus an overall rating of observed anxiety. It makes no distinction between generalized anxiety and panic attacks, which reduces its utility, although Bech and his colleagues have published amendments that circumvent this problem to some extent (Bech et al., 1981).

Scales for assessing mania are less common. The Biegel Mania Scale was one of the first (Biegel et al., 1971), but suffers from being over-long and over-complicated. It is completed by trained research nurses. It comprises 26 items rated on 5-point scales for both frequency and intensity. Modified versions have been published by Blackburn, Loudon, and Ashworth (1977) and by Young et al. (1978). The Bech-

Table 9–3   Social functioning instruments

Instrument	Authors	Comments
Social Behaviour Scales	Wykes and Sturt, 1986	Key information interview. 21 key areas of observed behavior rated on 5-point scale. Brief.
Disability Assessment Schedule (WHO/DAS)	WHO, 1988	Key informant interview. Includes behavior, role performance and modifying factors. A generic instrument.
Social Behaviour Assessment Schedule	Platt et al., 1980	Key informant interview. Includes section on family burden. Quite lengthy.
REHAB	Hall and Baker, 1983	Key-informant ratings of general and deviant behavior. For more disabled patients.
Basic Everyday Living Schedule	TAPS, 1990	Key information interview. 26 key areas, rating opportunity and performance. Lengthy.
Social Role Performance Schedule	Hurry and Sturt, 1981	Key informant interview. Patient rated in 8 areas of role performance. Brief.
Global Assessment Scale (GAS)/Global Assessment of Functioning Scale (GAF)	Endicott and Spitzer, 1978; APA, 1987	GAS modified to GAF for DSM IIIR. Both use 0–100 single scale for combined social and clinical functioning. Very brief. Easily learned.
Social Adjustment Scale	Weissman and Bothwell, 1976	Self-report questionnaire
Index of Activities of Everyday Living	Katz and Lawyerly, 1963	Early rating made from interview with key-informant

Rafaelsen Mania Scale (Bech et al., 1978) is an attractive alternative. Eleven items characteristic of manic states are rated for severity on 5-point scales, giving a score range of 0 to 44. The instrument has adequate reliability despite the difficulties inherent in rating manic behavior.

Social Functioning

For many purposes, the assessment of social functioning skills and impairments is of greater importance in community mental health evaluation than is symptomatology (Phelan et al., 1994; Jones et al., 1995). The degree of dependence or autonomy of each patient will be highly associated with the range and intensity (and hence cost) of treatment and care required. While a consensus has emerged about the headings under which mental state phenomena may be described, a much broader variety of items is included under the rubric of social functioning. As Table 9–3 shows, scales in this area include reference to abnormal observed behavior, impaired social role

Table 9–4   Quality of life instruments

Instrument	Authors	Comments
Quality of Life Index	Spitzer, Dobson, and Hall, 1981	5 self-rated visual analogue scales. Designed for use by cancer patients
Quality of Life Interview	Lehman, 1982	Strucured interview by lay interviewers
Quality of Life Profile	Oliver, 1992	Short version derived from a factor analysis of the Quality of Life Interview
Quality of Life Questionnaire	Bagel, et al., 1982	Structured patient interview
Quality of Life Scale	Heinrichs, Hanlon, and Carpenter, 1984	Semi-structured interview by clinician
Quality of Life Checklist	Malm, May, and Dencker, 1981	Rating scale for semi-structured interview

performance, overall global disability, and everyday living skills. There is relatively little published academic work that addresses the comparability of such scales (Sturt and Wykes, 1987), and researchers are best advised to conduct their own scrutiny, giving consideration to the time expenditure needed for administration of each scale, the target area measured, and the adequacy of its construction.

Quality of Life

The concept of quality of life (QOL) is one of the most intuitively appealing and least well operationally defined areas of mental health service evaluation (Lehman, 1995). This global concept combines freedom from symptoms, adequate social performance, and the ability to engage in activities that are rewarding. Most approaches to the measurement of this concept have failed to place the instrument within a clearly defined model (Lehman and Burns, 1990), so that any attempt to establish construct validity across schedules is fraught with dangers. Further, patients' satisfaction with life has been shown to closely correlate with the presence of anxiety and depression, so QOL measures need to be accompanied by mental state scores. The most thoroughly established scales are those devised by Lehman (1982), which take about 45 minutes to administer. A number of quality of life measuring instruments are listed in Table 9–4.

Family Care-Giving

The concept of care-giving shares characteristics with that of social performance, for one person's poor social performance is another person's care-giving (Schene et al., 1994). Both concepts are relative to social expectations that are likely to be very variable. Thus, as Platt and colleagues (1980) have emphasized with regard to social performance, measurement can never be entirely satisfactory. The existence of a burden indicates the breakdown of the reciprocal arrangements that people arrive at in their relationships, such that one person is doing "more than their fair share." This may merely result in their taking on an overlarge proportion or number of shared tasks, but it may also restrict their activities outside the relationship. This change in pattern can be assessed against approximate norms but is often accompanied by subjective dissatisfaction. Such dissatisfaction occasionally arises from judgments of the situation that may not be entirely justified, but it is an integral part of care-giving in that it is there to be dealt with.

The dissection of care-giving through the effects on the performance of various roles by the patient's relatives was an approach first used by Mills (1962). Grad and Sainsbury (1963a,b) advanced the measurement of care-giving by using a 3-point scale rather than the descriptive sketches given by their predecessors. Hoenig and Hamilton (1966, 1969) made the important distinction between "objective" care-giving (e.g., effects on health, financial loss) and "subjective" care-giving (the extent to which relatives felt they carried a burden). These techniques were applied by Creer and Wing (1974) in their study of the relatives of patients with schizophrenia. Despite the qualifications that surround this measurement, the methods used in the study of care-giving have now reached a reasonable level of sophistication, although no instrument has yet achieved wide circulation. There is a gradually emerging consensus that care-giving should be assessed in relation to the effect on the carers' subjective and objective role performance. (Creer, Sturt, and Wykes, 1982; Fadden 1984).

Service Utilization

The evaluation of mental health service interventions and innovations will often need to address changes in the patterns of service contacts of individuals and of patient groups. To establish and monitor locally based mental health services, clear, systematic, and continuing methods of collecting clinical and social-need data (Brewin et al., 1987) and service-utilization data are required. National data on service utilization are collected in many industrialized countries. Often, however, there is very little attempt at quality control, and the data are subject to weak diagnostic practices. The use of such data is often limited because they are published by central authorities with little appreciation of the local needs for information. A much more comprehensive method for eliciting, coding, and storing these data is the case register, defined as a local information system that records the contacts with designated social and medical services of patients or clients from a defined geographic area (Wing, 1989). Although such systems were formerly labor intensive, the recent availability of on-site micro and mini computers has made their more widespread use a practical option in many places.

The routine collection of clinical contact data can reveal patterns of service with respect to diagnoses (Der and Bebbington, 1987; Tansella and Williams, 1989), social class (Wiersma et al., 1983), and geographical mobility (Lesage and Tansella, 1989). Further, the use of standardized coding and diagnostic systems allows comparisons of service use within local areas (Giel and ten Horn, 1982), within regions (Torre and Marinoni, 1985), and between countries (ten Horn et al, 1986; Sytema et al., 1989). Such data can therefore indicate how treated morbidity varies with local socio-demographic characteristics, with the nature and extent of local service provision, and with the service trends at the national level. While one of the primary aims of developing local mental health services is to deliver services to identified priority groups of patients, the type of detailed information produced by case registers is required to ensure that the outcome is consistent with the declared aims of the service.

As mental health services research becomes more sophisticated, other domains for measurement are defined and instruments are developed. Examples include social support and social networks (Brugha et al., 1987), patient satisfaction (Bowling, 1991), need for care (Brewin et al., 1987) and residential environment (Garety and Morris, 1984).

Applications

Two illustrations will provide a fuller understanding of the issues that arise in practice when selecting instruments for mental health service research. The first study followed up long-term patients served by the COSTAR outreach program in Baltimore; the second study, conducted by the Team for the Assessment of Psychiatric Services (TAPS), assessed the effects of discharging long-stay inpatients from Friern and Claybury Hospitals into the community as a part of the closure program of psychiatric hospitals in Britain.

COSTAR Study

The COSTAR (Community Support Treatment and Rehabilitation) program is a mobile treatment and case-management service for the long-term mentally ill in inner-city Baltimore which is described in detail in Chapter 16.

The aims of the study described here were to establish the sociodemographic, psychiatric, and social network characteristics of the study population, to describe their social, cognitive, and mental states, and to relate these variables to duration of contact with the COSTAR program. Three hypotheses are tested: that a long contact group (more than 12 months in COSTAR), when compared with the newer group (12 months or less in COSTAR), will show (1) lower levels of psychiatric symptomatology, (2) improved social function, and (3) enhanced social networks.

Six assessment instruments were chosen for this study, guided by the following considerations: (1) they should have been widely used and at least their reliability characteristics were available; (2) they were fairly brief; and (3) they were relevant to important areas of clinical and social functioning for long-term adult patients with psychotic disorders. The scales used were sociodemographic data and psychiatric history at entry to the program, Brief Psychiatric Rating Scale (BPRS) (Overall and Gorham, 1962), Social Behavior Schedule (SBS) (Wykes and Sturt, 1986), Mini Mental State Examination (MMSE) (Folstein et al., 1975), Social Network Schedule (SNS), and the Global Assessment Scale (GAS) (Endicott et al., 1976).

The 18 items from the Brief Psychiatric Rating Scale (BPRS) were rated on a five point scale (0 to 4), and the total score lay in the range 0 to 72. The overall mean BPRS score was 10.5 (95 percent CI 9.1–11.9). The most frequently rated items were suspiciousness (48 percent), emotional withdrawal (44 percent), hallucinations (35 percent), motor retardation (34 percent), posturing (26 percent), and disorganized thoughts (25 percent), indicating that many of the patients continued to manifest both the positive and negative symptoms of psychosis. There was no difference in the total BPRS scores between the long- (mean 10.0, CI 7.9–11.9) and short-contact (mean 11.3, CI 9.5–13.4) groups.

The most frequently occurring social behavior problems, in terms of SBS items, were passive leisure interests (47 percent), underactivity (42 percent), poor hygiene (36 percent), and slowness (19 percent). Of the first 20 items of the SBS, 2 showed no difference between the two groups, 5 items showed less severe social behavior problems among the short-contact group, and 13 items showed better social functioning in the long-contact group, most marked for slowness (p = 0.03), poor personal hygiene (p = 0.07), and depressed mood (p = 0.09). With a cut-off of 2 or more for each item, the total number of social behavior problems was lower in the long- (mean 2.3, 95% CI 1.7–2.9), than in the short-contact group (mean 3.1, 95% CI 2.5–3.7, Student's t p = 0.06).

The most striking differences between the long- and short-contact groups were in the quantity and quality of their social networks. The long-contact group had more primary group members, more contact with relatives, and more weekly and infrequent contacts. However, the mean measure of network density (the extent to which network members know each other) was no different between groups (Thornicroft and Breakey, 1991; Thornicroft et al., 1995).

This study illustrates that useful evaluative research can be conducted using limited resources: In this case one research worker conducted all the baseline and follow-up interviews. Without an external comparison or control group, the study can be seen as generating hypotheses that more stringent research designs may test with greater analytical rigor.

Friern and Claybury Hospitals Study

In 1985, North East Thames Regional Health Authority set up the Team for the Assessment of Psychiatric Services (TAPS) to study the clinical and social outcomes of long-term patients discharged into the community from two large psychiatric hospitals in the region (TAPS, 1990; Leff, 1993). This study, unique in its scale and detail, is following up patients discharged from Friern and Claybury Hospitals in North London, both of which were scheduled to close in 1993. The main questions that

TAPS addresses are: How is the move from hospital to community being managed? Has the move proved better for long-term patients? How does the expense of community care compare with that of looking after people in long-term hospitals? How does transfer from hospital affect psychogeriatric patients? What are the effects of moving acute services into local districts?

This summary is of the main outcome results for the 278 long-stay patients discharged from both hospitals during the first 3 years of this reprovision program. The long-stay patients are defined as those adults having continuous residence in hospital for one year or more who, if over 65 years of age, do not have a primary diagnosis of dementia.

The research used a prospective matched design to compare outcomes for discharged patients with patients remaining in hospital. On discharge from hospital each leaver was matched with another patient who was likely to remain in hospital for a further year. Matching variables were age, sex, hospital, total time in hospital, total number of social behavior problems, and case note diagnosis (categorized as psychotic illness, neurotic illness and personality disorder, and organic illness). These matching variables were chosen on the basis of past research and created a matched control group of "stayers" with similar expected natural histories for their illnesses compared with their counterparts who were leaving hospital. In addition to the main study, research is being carried out with three other groups: new long stay patients, who have remained in hospital over one year; psychogeriatric patients, who have a primary diagnosis of dementia; and acute patients, whose supporting services will also leave the psychiatric institutions as they close.

TAPS uses eight rating scales in assessing patients. These were extensively piloted before use in the main study and are summarised in Table 9–5. They include several measures of quality of life of long-term patients, including psychiatric symptoms, social behavior, physical disorders, quality of the treatment setting, and social networks. Of the 278 patients leaving hospital for whom data are reported here, in their first year after discharge 39 (14 percent) were readmitted to hospital and six discharged patients died, of whom one committed suicide. In the comparison group of similar patients remaining in hospital, five died—a difference that was not statistically significant. Only one patient was imprisoned. Two percent probably became vagrant in the follow-up year, half of whom had been homeless on admission to hospital. Placement in a "bed and breakfast with care" scheme was associated with losing contact with services, and it seemed that some patients were being placed inappropriately in this form of accommodation. Finally, after the first four years of the reprovision process, a small group of patients (6 percent) has been identified whose needs cannot be met by locally based facilities as they currently exist. We compared the results for leavers and stayers in several areas of social and clinical functioning (mental state, social behavior, social network, and basic everyday living skills), and there were no overall changes either for leavers or stayers over this first follow-up year.

At each stage of the research, patients' own opinions about their move away from hospital were recorded. About half (43 percent) of the stayers said they wanted to leave hospital when first interviewed, and about as many (34 percent) gave the same

Table 9–5   Assessment instruments used in TAPS study

Basic Everyday Living Skills

A rating of the opportunity given to patients to undertake everyday tasks such as cooking, shopping, and cleaning, and their actual performance of these tasks.

Environmental Index

A method of ranking environmental "restrictiveness," which is a measure of patients' opportunities for independent activity.

Patient Attitude Questionnaire

A set of questions on patients' subjective attitudes about their current accommodation and treatment (Thornicroft et al., 1992).

Personal Data and Psychiatric History

A checklist of data derived from case records providing basic demographic information.

Physical Health Index

A rating of physical health problems and the degree of medical care required, extracted from case records and career interviews.

Present State Examination

A structured diagnostic interview conducted with patients. It generates data relating to the previous month concerning a range of psychiatric symptoms, diagnostic information, and the likelihood of being identified as a diagnostic "case" (Wing, Cooper, and Sartorius, 1974).

Social Behaviour Schedule

A set of questions answered by an informant allowing patients to be rated on a range of problematic social behaviors. A total social behavior problem count is calculated (Wykes and Sturt, 1986).

Social Network Schedule

A measure of the quality and quantity of patients' social contacts during the previous month.

reply when interviewed later. Among leavers, however, two-thirds (65 percent) initially wanted to leave hospital, and when followed up one year after discharge only 15 percent wanted to leave their new homes. Before discharge, 75 percent of patients mentioned some positive aspect of their current setting; this rose to 96 percent after discharge. In particular, patients preferred the greater degree of autonomy and permissiveness offered by their community homes. In the community, patients were also asked which staff were most helpful. Residential care staff were seen as most helpful (mentioned by 83 percent of patients), followed by GPs (61 percent), social workers (34 percent), psychiatrists (33 percent), and community psychiatric nurses (23 percent). Although a small group (14 percent) did continue to express a preference for living in hospital, the majority wanted either to remain in their current setting indefinitely (50 percent) or to move to more independent accommodation (21 percent).

Issues for Future Community Mental Health Service Evaluation

This chapter has outlined functional areas in which individual patient measures of outcome are well developed. However, many important areas remain woefully undeveloped in terms of the available assessment instruments, most notably consumer and care provider satisfaction and acceptability. We have tried to stress, especially for physicians who may have had no training in the psychometric properties of assessment schedules, that these issues are of central importance. Indeed, we would go further and say that there is very limited value in using questionnaires and rating scales that have not undergone rigorous testing to establish their characteristics (Ruggeri, 1994).

Until relatively recently the use of uniform outcome assessment across the Atlantic was rare. This situation is now rapidly changing. Increasingly, collaborative U.S.-U.K. studies are using common instruments, of which the BPRS and GAS/GASF are notable examples. A second relatively recent development is the use of standardized measures in routine clinical practice. In England, the government strongly encourages measurement of the outcomes of care in everyday clinical work and stipulates that care providers must be prepared to defend their practices in terms of effectiveness and improved health outcome. In this case the boundaries between community mental health service evaluation and routine clinical performance measurement are becoming increasingly indistinct.

References

Aiken, L. (1985) *Psychological Testing and Assessment.* Boston: Allyn & Bacon.

American Psychiatric Association. (1987) *Diagnostic and Statistical Manual of Mental Disorders* (DSM-III-R, third edition, revised). Washington, DC: American Psychiatric Association.

Andreasen, N. (1983) *Scale for the Assessment of Negative Symptoms* (SANS). Iowa City: University of Iowa.

Andreasen, N. (1984) *Scale for the Assessment of Positive Symptoms* (SAPS). Iowa City: University Iowa.

Asberg, M., Montgomery, S., Perris, C., Shalling, D., and Sedvall, G. (1978) The comprehensive psychopathological rating scale. *Acta Psychiatrica Scandanavica,* Supplement 271: 5–27.

Bagel, D., Brodsky, G., Steward, L., and Olson, M. (1982) The concept and measurement of quality of life as a dependent variable in evaluation of mental health services. In Stahlar, G., Tash, W. (eds.) *Innovative Approaches to Mental Health Evaluation.* New York: Academic Press.

Bebbington, P., Hurry, J., Tennant, C., Sturt, E., and Wing, J. (1981) Epidemiology of mental disorders in Camberwell. *Psychological Medicine,* 11:561–579.

Bech, P., Rafaelsen, O.J., Kramp, P., and Bolwig, T.G. (1978) The mania rating scale: Scale construction and inter-observer agreement. *Neuropharmacology,* 17:430–431.

Bech, P., Bolwig, T.G., Kramp, P., and Rafaelsen, O.J. (1979) The Bech-Rafaelsen Mania Scale and the Hamilton Depression Scale. *Acta Psychiatrica Scandinavica,* 59:420–430.

Bech, P., Allerup, P., Gram, L.F., Reisby, N., Rosenberg, R. Jacobsen, O., and Nagy, A. (1981) The Hamilton Depression Scale. Evaluation of objectivity using logistic models. *Acta Psychiatrica Scandinavica,* 63:290–299.

Beck, A., Ward, C., Mendelson, M., Mock, J., and Earbaugh, J. (1961) An inventory for measuring depression. *Archives of General Psychiatry,* 4:561–571.

Biegel, A., Murphy, D., and Bunney, W.E. (1971) The manic-state rating scale. *Archives of General Psychiatry,* 25:256–262.

Blackburn, I.M., Loudon, J.B., and Ashworth, C.M. (1977) A new scale for measuring mania. *Psychological Medicine,* 7:453–458.

Bowling, A. (1991) *Measuring Health: A Review of Quality of Life Measurement Scales,* Milton Keynes: Open University Press.

Brewin, C., Wing, J.K., Mangen, S., et al. (1987) Principles and practice of measuring needs in the long term mentally ill: the MRC needs for care assessment. *Psychological Medicine,* 17:971–981.

Brugha, T.S., Sturt, E., MacCarthy, B., Potter, J., Wykes, T., and Bebbington, P.E. (1987) The Interview Measure of Social Relationships: the description and evaluation of a survey instrument for assessing personal social resources. *Social Psychiatry,* 22(2):123–128.

Cohen, J. (1960) A coefficient of agreement for nominal scales. *Educational and Psychological Measurement,* 20:37–46.

Creer, C., and Wing, J. K. (1974) *Schizophrenia at Home.* Surbiton, Surrey: National Schizophrenia Fellowship.

Creer, C., Sturt, E., and Wykes, T. (1982) The role of relatives. In Wing, J.K. (ed.), Long term community care: experience in a London borough. *Psychological Medicine,* Monograph, Supplement 2:29–39.

Der, G., and Bebbington, P. E. (1987) Depression in inner London: a register study. *Social Psychiatry,* 22:73–84.

Endicott, I., Spitzer, R., Fleiss, J., and Cohen, J. (1976) The global assessment scale. *Archives of General Psychiatry,* 33:766–771.

Endicott, J., and Spitzer, R. (1978) A diagnostic interview: the schedule for affective disorders and schizophrenia. *Archives of General Psychiatry,* 35:837–844.

Fadden, G.B. (1984) The relatives of patients with depressive disorders: A typology of burden and strategies for coping. Institute of Psychiatry, London University, M.Phil. thesis.

Farmer, A., Katz, R., McGuffin, P., and Bebbington, P.E. (1987) A comparison between the Present State Examination (PSE) and the Composite Diagnostic interview (CIDI). *Archives of General Psychiatry,* 44:1064–1068.

Folstein, M., Folstein, S., and McHugh, P. (1975) Mini Mental State, a practical method for grading the cognitive state of patients for the clinician. *Journal of Psychiatric Research,* 12:189–198.

Freeman, C., and Tyrer, P. (1989) *Research Methods in Psychiatry.* London: Royal College of Psychiatrists, Gaskell.

Garety, P.J. and Morris, I. (1984) A new unit for long-stay psychiatric patients: Organisation, attitudes and quality of care. *Psychological Medicine,* 14, 183–192.

Giel, R., and ten Horn, G. (1982) Patterns of mental health care in a Dutch register area. *Social Psychiatry,* 17:117–123.

Goldberg, D. P. (1972) *The Detection of Psychiatric Illness by Questionnaire.* Maudsley Monograph no. 21. Oxford University Press: London.

Grad, J., and Sainsbury, P. (1963a) Evaluating a community care service. In Freeman, H., Farndale, J. (eds.), *Trends in Mental Health Services,* pp. 303–317. New York: MacMillan Company.

Grad, J., and Sainsbury, P. (1963b) Mental illness and the family. *Lancet,* i:544–547.

Hall, J. (1979) Assessment procedures used in studies on long-stay patients. *British Journal of Psychiatry,* 135:330–335.

Hall, J.N. (1980) Ward rating scales for long-stay patients: a review. *Psychological Medicine,* 10:277–288.

Hall, J., and Baker, R. (1983) REHAB: a user's manual. Aberdeen: Vine Publishing.

Hamilton, M. (1959) The assessment of anxiety states by rating. *British Journal of Medical Psychology,* 32:50–55.

Hamilton, M. (1967) Development of a rating scale for primary depressive illness. *British Journal of Social and Clinical Psychology,* 6:278–296.

Heinrichs, D., Hanlon, T., and Carpenter, W. (1984) The quality of life scale: an instrument for rating the schizophrenic deficit syndrome. *Schizophrenia Bulletin,* 10:388–398.

Hoenig, J., and Hamilton, M.W. (1966) The schizophrenic patient in the community and his effect on the household. *International Journal of Social Psychiatry,* 12:165–176.

Hoenig, J., and Hamilton, M.W. (1969) *The Desegregation of the Mentally Ill.* London: Routledge and Kegan Paul.

Hurry, J., and Sturt, E. (1981) Social performance in a population sample: relation to psychiatric symptoms. In Wing, J.K., Bebbington, P.E., Robins, L. (eds.), *What is a Case? The Problem of Definition in Psychiatric Community Surveys,* pp. 202–213. London: Grant MacIntyre.

Jones, S., Thornicroft, G., Coffey, M., and Dunn, G. (1995) Report of a six month study of the reliability and validity of the Global Assessment of Functioning. *British Journal of Psychiatry* (in press).

Katz, S., and Lawyerly, S., (1963) Methods for measuring adjustment and social behaviour in the community. 1: rationale, description, discriminative validity and scale development. *Psychological Reports,* 13:503–535.

Krawiecka, M., Goldberg, D., and Vaughan, M. (1977) A standardized psychiatric instrument for rating chronic psychotic patients. *Acta Psychiatrica Scandanavica,* 55:299–308.

Leff, J. (1993) The TAPS Project. *British Journal of Psychiatry,* Supplement 19, vol. 162.

Lehman, A. (1982) The well-being of chronic mental patients—assessing their quality of life. *Archives of General Psychiatry,* 40:369–374.

Lehman, A. (1995) Measures of quality of life among persons with severe and persistent mental disorders. *Social Psychiatry and Psychiatric Epidemiology* (in press).

Lehman, A., and Burns, B. (1990) Severe Mental Illness in the Community. In Spiker, B. (ed.), *Quality of Life Assessment in Clinical Trials.* New York: Raven.

Lesage, A., and Tansella, M. (1989) Mobility of schizophrenic patients, non-psychotic patients and the general population in a case register area. *Social Psychiatry and Psychiatric Epidemiology,* 24:271–274.

Malm, U., May, P., and Dencker, S. (1981) Evaluation of the quality of life of the schizophrenic outpatient: a checklist. *Schizophrenia Bulletin,* 7:477–487.

Mills, E. (1962) *Living with Mental Illness: A Study in East London.* London: Routledge and Kegan Paul.

Oliver, J.P.J. (1992) The social care directive: development of a quality of life profile for use in community services for the mentally ill. *Social Work & Social Sciences Review,* 3(1): 5–45.

Overall, J., and Gorham, D. (1962) Brief psychiatric rating scale. *Psychological Reports,* 10: 799–812.

Parry, G., and Watts, F. (1989) *Behavioural and Mental Health Research: a Handbook of Skills and Methods.* London: Lawrence Erlbaum.

Phelan, M., Wykes, T., and Goldman, H. (1994) Global Function Scales. In Thornicroft, G., Tansella, M. (eds.), Designing Instruments for Mental Health Service Research. *Social Psychiatry and Psychiatric Epidemiology,* 29:5.

Platt, S., Weyman, A., Hirsch, S., and Hewett, S. (1980) The social behaviour assessment schedule (SBAS): rationale, contents, scoring and reliability of a new interview schedule. *Social Psychiatry,* 15:455–460.

Riskind, J., Beck, A., Berchick, R., Brown, G., and Steer, R. (1987) Reliability of DSM-III Diagnoses for major depression and generalised anxiety disorder using the structured Clinical Interview for DSM-III. *Archives of General Psychiatry,* 44:817–820.

Robins, L.N. (1985) The Composite International Diagnostic Interview. *DIS Newsletter,* Spring, 1–2. St. Louis, MO: Washington University School of Medicine.

Robins, L.N., Helzer, J.E., and Croughlan, J. (1979) *The National Institute of Mental Health Diagnostic Interview Schedule.* Rockville, Maryland: National Institute of Mental Health.

Robins, L.N., Helzer, J.E., Orvaschel, H., Anthony, J.C., Blazer, D.G., Burnham, A., and Burke, J.D. (1985a) The Diagnostic Interview Schedule. In Eaton, W.W., Kessler, L.G. (eds.), *Epidemiologic Field Methods in Psychiatry: The NIMH Epidemiologic Catchment Area Program.* Orlando, Fla.: Academic Press.

Robins, L.N., Wing, J.K., Wittchen, H.U., Helzer, J.E., Babor, T.F., Burke, J.D., Farmer, A., Jablensky, A., Pickens, R., Ruggeri, D.A., Sartorius, N., and Towle, L.H. (1988). The Composite International Diagnostic Interview. *Archives of General Psychiatry,* 45:1069–1077.

Ruggeri, M. (1994) Patients' and relatives' satisfaction with psychiatric services. In Thornicroft, G., Tansella, M. (eds.), Designing Instruments for Mental Health Service Research. *Social Psychiatry and Psychiatric Epidemiology,* 29:5.

Schene, A., Tessler, P., and Gamoche, G. (1994) Instruments for measuring family or caregiver burden in severe mental illness. In Thornicroft, G., Tansella, M. (eds.), Designing Instruments for Mental Health Service Research. *Social Psychiatry and Psychiatric Epidemiology,* 29:5.

Snaith, R.P., Ahmed, S.N., Mehta, S., and Hamilton, M. (1971) Assessment of the severity of primary depressive illness. Wakefield self assessment depression inventory. *Psychological Medicine,* 1:143–149.

Spitzer, R. (1983) Psychiatric diagnoses—are clinicians still necessary? *Comprehensive Psychiatry,* 24:399–411.

Spitzer, R., Endicott, J., and Robins, E. (1978) Research Diagnostic Criteria: rationale and reliability. *Archives of General Psychiatry,* 35:773–782.

Spitzer, W., Dobson, A., and Hall, J. (1981) Measuring quality of life of cancer patients: a concise QL index for use by physicians. *Journal of Chronic Disease,* 34:585–597.

Spitzer, R., Williams, J., and Gibbons, M. (1985) *Instruction Manual for the Structured Clinical Interview for DSM-III-R* (SCID). New York: Biometrics Research Department, New York State Psychiatric Institute.

Streiner, D., and Norman, G. (1989) *Health Measurement Scales.* Oxford: Oxford University Press.

Sturt, E. (1981) Hierarchical patterns in the distribution of psychiatric symptoms. *Psychological Medicine,* 11:783–794.

Sturt, E., and Wykes, T. (1987) Assessment schedules for chronic psychiatric patients. *Psychological Medicine,* 17:485–493.

Sytema, S., Balestrieri, M., Giel, R., TenHorn, G., and Tansella, M. (1989) Use of mental health services in South-Verona and Groningen. *Acta Psychiatrica Scandinavica,* 79: 153–162.

Tansella, M., and Williams, P. (1989) The spectrum of psychiatric morbidity in a defined geographical area. *Psychological Medicine,* 19:765–770.

TAPS (Team for the Assessment of Psychiatric Services) (1990) *Better Out than In?* London: North East Thames Regional Health Authority.

TenHorn, G., Giel, R., Gulbinat, W., and Henderson, J. (eds.) (1986) *Psychiatric Case Registers in Public Health: A Worldwide Inventory, 1060–1985.* Elsevier: Amsterdam.

Thompson, C. (1989) *The Instruments of Psychiatric Research.* Chichester: Wiley.

Thornicroft, G., and Breakey, W.R. (1991) The COSTAR programme. 1: Improving social networks of the long-term mentally ill. *British Journal of Psychiatry,* 159:245–249.

Thornicroft, G., Breakey, W., and Primm, A. (1995) Case management and network enhancement of the long-term mentally ill. In Brugha, T. (ed.), *Social Support and Psychiatric Disorder.* Cambridge: Cambridge University Press.

Thornicroft, G., C. Gooch, C. O'Driscoll, and S. Reda. (1993) The TAPS project 7. The reliability of the Patient Attitude Questionnaire. *British Journal of Psychiatry,* 162 (Supplement 19):25–29.

Torre, E., and Marinoni, A. (1985) Register studies: data from four areas in Northern Italy. *Acta Psychiatrica Scandinavica,* 136:87–94.

Weissman, M., and Bothwell, S. (1976) Assessment of social adjustment by self-report. *Archives of General Psychiatry,* 33:1111–1115.

Wetzler, S. (1989) *Measuring Mental Illness.* Washington, D.C.: American Psychiatry Press.

Wiersma, D., Giel, R., de Jong, A., and Slooff, C. (1983) Social class and schizophrenia in a Dutch cohort. *Psychological Medicine,* 13:141–150.

Wing, J.K., Baber, T., Brugha, T., Burke, J., Cooper, E., Giel, R., Jablenski, A., Regier, D., and Sartorius, N. (1990) SCAN: Schedules for Clinical Assessment in Neuropsychiatry. *Archives of General Psychiatry,* 47:589–593.

Wing, J.K., Cooper, J.E., and Sartorius, N. (1974) *The Measurement and Classification of Psychiatric Symptoms.* Cambridge: Cambridge University Press.

Wing, J.K., Henderson, A.S., and Winckle, M. (1977) The rating of symptoms by a psychiatrist and non-psychiatrist: a study of patients referred from general practice. *Psychological Medicine,* 7:713–715.

Wing, J.K., Nixon, J.M., Mann, S.A., and Leff, J.P. (1977) Reliability of the PSE (ninth edition) used in a population survey. *Psychological Medicine,* 7:505–516.

Wing, J.K. (ed.) (1989) *Health Services Planning and Research. Contributions from Psychiatric Case Registers.* London: Gaskell.

World Health Organization (1988) *The WHO/DAS. Disability Assessment Schedule.* Geneva: WHO.

World Health Organization (1992). *SCAN—Schedules for Clinical Assessment in Neuropsychiatry.* Geneva: WHO.

World Health Organization (1994). *SCAN—Schedules for Clinical Assessment in Neuropsychiatry. Version 2.* Geneva: WHO.

Wykes, T., and Sturt, E. (1986) The measurement of social behaviour in psychiatric patients: an assessment of the reliability and validity of the SBS schedule. *British Journal of Psychiatry,* 148:1–11.

Young, R.C., Briggs, J.T., Ziegler, V.E., and Meyer, D.A. (1978) A Rating Scale for Mania: Reliability, Validity and Sensitivity. *British Journal of Psychiatry,* 133:429–435.

Zung, W.W.K. (1965) A Self-Rating Depression Scale. *Archives of General Psychiatry,* 12:63–70.

10

The Catchment Area

WILLIAM R. BREAKEY

Can you see the ward or district organization with a district center with reasonably accurate records of the facts needed for orderly work? . . . I long to get the means and the privilege of trying a few mental hygiene districts, no doubt best shaped, as things are now subdivided, so as to have the school of the district as the center of attention, with a specially trained physician and two or three helpers living in the district without any trumpets and without legislation; as far as possible inconspicuous, but charged to obtain the friendship and cooperation of the teachers, the district workers of various charity organizations and the physicians and ministers of the region. They would have to know their districts as a social fabric and they can do so if their districts are not too large.

(Adolf Meyer, 1915, p. 190)

Long before community-based service systems were established under state and federal policies, Adolf Meyer articulated the concept of mental health services closely identified with a particular community, staffed by professionals who are intimately familiar with the district and closely linked with its institutions. This principle was also strongly emphasized more recently as a basic premise of deinstitutionalization, that patients would be better when responsibility was transferred from large, impersonal state institutions to local community-based organizations that can be responsive to their communities and accountable for the provision of services. This concept is embodied in the term *catchment area.*

This term was borrowed from hydrology. It referred originally to the area or terrain from which rainfall or surface water drains into a river system, lake, or reservoir. The drainage of water is a passive process, and the usage of the term in mental health services has been justly criticized because participation in mental health services should certainly not be passive. The term can also be criticized because of its reference to terrain rather than population. For these reasons, other terms have been introduced, such as *service area,* or, in Europe, *sector.* Sectors for mental health service provision were set up in France in the 1960s; in Britain, health districts were established in the 1970s for public health services generally, including mental health services. Italy,

Sweden, and other countries followed the same pattern (Lindholm, 1983). More recently health districts in England and Wales have been further subdivided into smaller mental health service sectors to promote accessibility and accountability (Johnson and Thornicroft, 1993). However, catchment area continues to be the term most widely used in the United States, and it has come to embody ideas of accountability and responsibility to a specific area and the people who live there. It implies a population-oriented focus in the provision of services by a group of professionals who are well versed in the ethos of the people who live in the area, have a good understanding of their needs, and are determined to address those needs.

The concept of service units addressing the needs of defined geographic areas had been inherent in the state hospital system for more than a century, and health districts had been a tool of health administration, but the designation of mental health catchment areas came into its own as a central and essential principle for deinstitutionalization in *Action for Mental Health* (Joint Commission, 1961) and was incorporated in the Community Mental Health Centers legislation of the 1960s. Foley and Sharfstein (1983) describe the concept:

> The extent of a CMHC's program area (the "community" of a CMHC) was defined in demographic terms as one containing a population of 75,000 to 200,000 within specific geopolitical boundaries. The service area, for which the 1963 law holds the CMHC responsible, may be several countries of a rural state, an entire small city, a few contiguous suburbs in a metropolitan area, or one or two neighborhoods in a densely populated inner city. These population catchment areas not only would reflect the demographic and geographic diversity of the nation, but also the variations in age, race, language and culture, and socioeconomic status. CMHC responsiveness to the unique needs of its service area population was defined as one goal of the governing board, or advisory committee of each CMHC; moreover, a needs assessment phase was required as part of the funding process (p. 261).

The new policies required the division of the country into approximately 1,500 catchment areas, and the catchment area focus remained a key element of the federal program, although centers were established in fewer than half of the defined areas. After the demise of the federal program in 1981, the concept of catchment persisted under state plans, as a way of assigning responsibility and compelling accountability of service providers to specific populations.

Access

Catchment areas provide a framework for the allocation of resources by state or city mental health agencies, with the intent of ensuring that each section of the population has access to services within easy reach. As early as 1866, Edward Jarvis had demonstrated that utilization of mental hospital services decreased in proportion to distance from the hospital, what has been called "Jarvis' Law." This principle has since been found to apply even within the relatively confined area of a small urban area (Breakey and Kaminsky, 1982), so that service providers, to serve the population well, must be distributed in the various neighborhoods and districts.

In an urban area, where a population of 75,000 to 200,000 people may be contained in a reasonably small geographic area, the catchment area concept would appear to promise relatively easy access to everyone, as far as distance is concerned. This is less so in sparsely populated rural areas, where catchment areas are extremely large, in terms of terrain, if not in population. In 1982, for example, one catchment area in Arizona covered 65,000 square miles and one in Montana covered 50,000 square miles (Ozarin, 1982). Issues of access are clearly very different in these circumstances.

Accountability

In the absence of catchment areas, it is difficult to assign responsibility for the care of a particular person, or to hold any agency accountable for the provision of specific services. If a city, for example, is divided into areas and the responsible agency in a particular area is defined, a person can demand from that agency that services to which he or she is entitled be provided. Defining such responsibility on the basis of where a person resides has obvious practicality. Mental health authorities at city, county, or state level can develop contracts with agencies, defining their responsibilities to their specific target population and establishing performance criteria for continuing funding support.

Cultural Sensitivity

Catchmenting, or sectorization, enables community mental health programs to address another important principle, that of cultural relevance. Providers can develop familiarity with the culture of different groups in their circumscribed area, so that services can be planned to meet their needs in the most appropriate way, provided by professionals who are familiar with the culture of their patients. Lack of such cultural sensitivity can constitute a barrier to treatment or render treatment offered less than effective. It is axiomatic in community mental health services that staff should be sensitive to the particular cultural issues in the community and that the composition of the staff team should as closely as possible reflect the racial/ethnic makeup of the population served.

Planning

The catchment area provides a basic unit for planning. Although planning for mental health services occurs at state, city, or regional levels, and these plans, along with the political and fiscal realities of the state, will generally dictate local policies, the most relevant detailed planning occurs at the catchment area level. Community mental health service providers should be able to advocate on behalf of their own catchments where local conditions will determine the best mix of services to be provided.

Advocacy of this sort usually addresses issues of service needs, but the concept of need is complex. Needs may be perceived differently by government, by professionals, by mentally ill individuals themselves, or by other members of the community. Needs for services depend not only on prevalence rates for psychiatric disorders, but on the nature of the community, the strength of its social institutions, and the individual resources of its citizens. Needs can be estimated directly or indirectly. Direct estimates rely on data collection from the target population. Standardized methods exist for measuring needs for services at an individual level and have been effectively used in mental health services research, but applying these techniques to the population of a catchment area is generally impractical. Instead, indirect approaches must be used, using data from sources such as demographic profiles from local censuses, epidemiological data from published surveys, and case registers.

Censuses are conducted at 10-year intervals in the United States: Data are available through local planning offices. Enumerations are provided for the nation as a whole, by state, by region, or at the level of census tracts, which are small enumeration areas, each containing several hundred people. Census tract data can easily be used to compile a demographic profile of a catchment area, indicating the composition of the population as a whole, but also permitting pockets of special populations to be identified, such as specific ethnic groups, or concentrations of older people. Sociodemographic characteristics of a population can in themselves provide a general indication of level of need. A method has been developed in England to use socioeconomic indices to predict needs for general health services as a basis for health resource allocation. The same method has subsequently been shown also to predict utilization of mental health services (Jarman et al., 1992). If the demographic structure of the population is known, estimates of prevalence in a local area are derived by applying data from epidemiological surveys (Shapiro et al., 1985; Zautra and Simons, 1978). Age-, sex-, and race-specific prevalence data can be combined with other social and demographic indicators, such as poverty levels, to predict the levels of need and demand for services in a specific community. The NIMH Epidemiological Catchment Area Study, which provides prevalence estimates based on data gathered from five areas of the United States in the early 1980s (Regier et al., 1988), provides an excellent source of weighted prevalence rates which can be applied to a specific population (Breakey, 1982).

Case registers have been used in many places to gather data systematically about persons who have received services in the area (Miles et al., 1964; Wing 1989). Case registers collect data on treated prevalence, rather than true prevalence. They provide a measure of utilization, rather than of need. Nonetheless, utilization patterns can provide useful indications of where need exists and can point to where there is likely to be unmet need (Babigian, 1977; Roghmann et al., 1982). Although concerns about confidentiality have been a major impediment to the implementation of case registers, particularly in the United States, they have the advantage that the data can be accumulated by service providers in the course of delivering the services, at relatively low cost. The disadvantages include the fact that data collected in the course of service delivery are never as carefully collected as in a research study.

These methods may be combined in practice. For example, utilization data derived from a small area can be used to develop estimates for a larger area if the demographic data are available to permit adjustment of the rates (Goodman and Craig, 1982). Input can be obtained from local informants to identify specific areas within the catchment where needs are particularly great (Hull et al., 1979).

Administrative Decentralization

If decision-making authority is effectively delegated to the local level, catchmenting has the advantages, and disadvantages, of decentralization. On the one hand, decisions can be made with the needs of the specific population in mind, by those who are presumed to have the best local knowledge and who are advised by representatives of the catchment population. On the other hand, local areas can be inward-looking and satisfied with the status quo, not familiar with new ideas or concepts, and unwilling to try new approaches. In the competition for resources that inevitably occurs, a local area may be disadvantaged if its mental health service providers are less skillful or assertive in seeking new opportunities.

Continuity of Care

Continuity of care was a prime concern of the original CMHC movement. Where mental hospitals were remote from the population served and from "aftercare" agencies, care for patients easily became fragmented. The notion of a series of services within a circumscribed area, well-coordinated and responsive to its local population, promised marked advantages and was another rationale for the catchment area emphasis. Several methods have been developed to promote continuity of care. Tracking systems for catchment area patients permit the service providers to know when a patient is admitted to hospital or has dropped out of treatment, so that appropriate interventions can be made to ensure that the course of treatment is pursued in as coherent a way as possible. Case managers can stay in contact with individuals as they move through the system of services in the catchment area, again maximizing the consistency and continuity of the treatment approaches.

Allocation of Resources

The catchmenting of a city or county provides an opportunity for resources to be allocated in proportion to need. Poorer areas can be predicted to have higher morbidity and require more intensive services. Catchment area boundaries, for example under the original federal CMHC legislation, were in some cases altered so that neighborhoods with high poverty indices were not all assigned to the same catchment areas. Needless to say, such decisions can become highly politicized and can have the opposite effect if resources are steered away from those areas whose representatives may have less power or be less interested in advocating for mental health services.

Problems with the Catchment Area Concept

In general, the catchment area concept has been very successful in providing a structure for service provision and accountability in mental health service systems. It has become apparent, however, that this approach has certain limitations. As community mental health service systems have become more elaborate and the needs of patients have become better understood, it is clear that not all services can, or even should, be provided in every area. For instance, specialized programs addressing the needs of only a small segment of the population cannot generally be supported by a single catchment area, or would not be adequately utilized if they restricted their patients to one area. Examples might be programs for the visually or hearing impaired, or programs catering to the language and cultural needs of certain minority ethnic groups. Some services may be particularly costly, so that it is not feasible for the mental health funding agencies to provide them in every catchment area. Some programs serve populations that are not confined within a catchment area, notably homeless people, who will never be eligible for services where eligibility is defined by street address. Such programs may be provided with a state-wide or city-wide mandate, reaching across catchment area boundaries.

Another limitation of the catchment concept is that the boundaries in many cases do not coincide with the boundaries observed by other service agencies, such as police districts, school districts, or social service districts. This is particularly problematic in relation to children's services, where providers deal with a wide variety of other service providers, including schools, juvenile correctional services, child protective services, welfare departments, and other agencies whose service district boundaries may be very different from those of the mental health catchment area. The delineation of catchment area boundaries is an administrative act, performed for administrative reasons and influenced by political considerations. Boundaries may be gerrymandered to try to provide a certain mix of ethnic groups, to avoid segregation, or to meet demographic requirements for certain types of funding support. Ideally, boundaries should be cognizant of natural neighborhood boundaries and natural transportation patterns, but this may be difficult to achieve and does not necessarily occur (Huffine and Craig, 1973). Administrative lines are frequently drawn through, rather than around, neighborhoods, so that persons on one side of the street are served by one community mental health program, and their friends and relatives across the street are served by another.

Whatever their problems, however, catchment areas, service areas, or sectors provide many advantages for the administration and provision of public mental health services. Whatever new forms of health administration emerge, some form of catchment organization will continue to provide the basic units for planning and the assignment of responsibility.

References

Babigian, H.M. (1977) The impact of community mental health centers on the utilization of services. *Archives of General Psychiatry,* 34:385.

Breakey, W.R. (1982) A public health approach to schizophrenia. *The Johns Hopkins Medical Journal,* 150:188–195.

Breakey, W.R., and Kaminsky, M.J. (1982) An assessment of Jarvis' Law in an urban catchment area. *Hospital and Community Psychiatry,* 33:661–663.

Foley, H.A., and Sharfstein, S.S. (1983) *Madness and Government: Who Cares for the Mentally Ill?* Washington D.C.: American Psychiatric Press.

Goodman, A.B., and Craig, T.J. (1982) A needs assessment strategy for an era of limited resources. *American Journal of Epidemiology,* 115:624–632.

Huffine, C.L., and Craig, T.J. (1973) Catchment and community. *Archives of General Psychiatry,* 28:483–488.

Hull, J.W., Huebner, R.B., Small, K.H., and Pion, G. (1979) Map survey strategy for locating areas with mental health problems. *Community Mental Health Journal,* 15:219–228.

Jarvis, E. (1866) Influence of distance from and nearness to an insane hospital on its use by the people. *American Journal of Insanity,* 22:361–406.

Jarman, B., Hirsch, S., White, P., and Driscoll, R. (1992) Predicting psychiatric admission rates. *British Medical Journal,* 304:1146–1151.

Johnson, S., and Thornicroft, G. (1993) The sectorization of psychiatric services in England and Wales. *Social Psychiatry and Psychiatric Epidemiology,* 28:45–47.

Joint Commission on Mental Illness and Health (1961) *Action for Mental Health: Final Report of the Commission.* New York: Basic Books.

Lindholm, H. (1983) Sectorized psychiatry. A methodological study of the effects of reorganization on patients treated in a mental hospital. *Acta Psychiatrica Scandinavica,* Supplementum 304.

Meyer, A. (1915, 1952) Where should we attack the problem of the prevention of mental defect and mental disease? In Winters, E.E. (ed.), *Collected Papers of Adolf Meyer.* Baltimore: Johns Hopkins University Press.

Miles, H.C., Gardner, E.A., Bodian, C., and Romano, J. (1964) A cumulative survey of all psychiatric experience in Monroe County, NY. *Psychiatric Quarterly,* 38:458–487.

Ozarin, L.D. (1982) Federal perspectives: the activities of the National Institute of Mental Health in relation to rural mental health services. In Keller, P.A., Murray, J.C. (eds.), *Handbook of Rural Mental Health.* New York: Human Sciences Press.

Regier, D.A., Boyd, J.H., Burke, J.D. Jr., Ree, D.S., Myers, J.K., Kramer, M., Robins, L.N., George, L.K., Karno, M., and Locke, B.Z. (1988) One-month prevalence of mental disorders in the United States, based on five Epidemiologic Catchment Area sites. *Archives of General Psychiatry,* 45:977–986.

Roghmann, K.J., Babigian, H.M., Goldberg, I.D., and Zastowney, T.R. (1982) The increasing number of children using psychiatric services: analysis of a cumulative psychiatric case register. *Pediatrics,* 70:790–801.

Shapiro, S., Skinner, E.A., Steinwachs, D.M., and Regier, D.A. (1985) Measuring need for mental health services in a general population. *Medical Care,* 23:1033–1043.

Wing, J.K. (ed.) (1989) *Health Services Planning and Research: Contributions from Psychiatric Case Registers.* London: Gaskell.

Zautra, A., and Simons, L.S. (1978) An assessment of a community's mental health needs. *American Journal of Community Psychology,* 6:351–362.

Cultural and Ethnic Sensitivity

ANNELLE B. PRIMM
BRUNO R. LIMA
CYPRIAN L. ROWE

In the United States, the term *minority* is used in a non-pejorative sense to reflect the current numerical status of African Americans, Asian Americans, Hispanics, and native Americans with respect to whites. It is understood that inherent in this terminology is the marginalization of any grouping of individuals not considered white, regardless of actual numerical representation. The politics of minority status and the history of the four major groups encompass an experience of (1) slavery; (2) migration, both voluntary and involuntary, with varying degrees of assimilation and acculturation; (3) internment; (4) exploitation of land and labor; (5) segregation; (6) exclusion; and (7) outward experiences of racism, discrimination, and oppression. These experiences have an impact on the collective psyche of the groups and contribute to their social attitudes regarding mental illness and psychopathology.

The terms *culture* and *ethnicity* will be used interchangeably in this chapter in describing the mental health experience of the four major minority groups. There is considerable heterogeneity within each group with respect to socioeconomic status, national origin, and other variables. However, because of the overrepresentation of minority groups among those of low socioeconomic status, public sector services have a particular responsibility to respond to their needs.

African Americans constitute 12 percent of the U.S. population, roughly 30 million people, according to the 1990 U.S. Census (U.S. Bureau of the Census, 1994). The majority have a history of slavery common to their background, and many have mixed with native Americans and Caucasians. Many migrated from rural areas of southern states in the mid-twentieth century to inhabit northern industrial urban areas in large numbers. Currently, the largest group of African Americans live in the South. Roughly one-third of African Americans live below the federally defined poverty line.

In the United States, the term *Hispanic* refers to a person with cultural roots in any other country in the Americas except Canada, regardless of race. A Hispanic population of 22 million was reported by the 1990 Census, constituting 9 percent of the population. The country of origin was Mexico for 60 percent, followed by Puerto Rico at 14 percent, Cuba at 5 percent, and the remaining countries at 21 percent. It is predicted that Hispanics will experience a population increase of 65 percent between 1990 and 2010, making them the fastest growing population group in the United States. These figures serve as a forecast of an even greater need for mental health services in the future as prevalence rates increase with population growth (Kramer, 1983). According to the U.S. Bureau of the Census (1994), Hispanics are nearly three times more likely than white Americans to be poor.

Reports of population statistics combine into one category persons belonging to the American Indian, Eskimo, Aleut, Asian, or Pacific Islander, and other groups. They numbered approximately 19 million, constituting 3.8 percent of the total U.S. population in the 1990 Census. American Indians and Alaska natives comprised the smallest population among minority groups, numbering roughly 2.0 million in the 1990 Census. This group has special status due to federal government obligation. Approximately half live in urban metropolitan areas; however, the main focus is on their presence in rural areas and reservations. Poverty is widespread and the attendant problems of unemployment and low educational level abound. Alcohol figures prominently in morbidity and mortality among American Indians and Alaska natives (Manson et al., 1987).

In 1990, the population of Asians and Pacific Islanders totaled 7.5 million. This group encompasses a wide variety of origins. The Asian group includes the Chinese, Filipino, Asian Indian, Japanese, Korean, Southeast Asian (Cambodian, Hmong, Lao, Vietnamese), and others. The Guamanians, Hawaiians, Samoans, and current and former inhabitants of Trust Territory islands (Micronesia, Marshall Islands, etc.) constitute the major Pacific Islander groups. When compared with the other minority groups, Asian Americans are less likely to be poor. This group has been referred to as the "model minority," and their disproportionately low utilization of mental health services has contributed to this. It is known, however, that they have needs for mental health services at least to the same extent as other groups. Many members of the Asian American subgroups, like Hispanics, have recently migrated and have language barriers and assimilation to contend with as immediate stressors (Westermeyer, 1989).

Cultural bias can have an impact on how public mental health services are established, marketed, and operated, given that psychiatrists and other mental health professionals are invested with their own perspectives which derive from their own cultural membership, both personal and professional (Kleinman, 1993). Providing mental health services to populations requires an appreciation of the demographic composition of the community being served so that while universal quality of care is strived for, attention is paid to the characteristics of the population and how they affect the extent to which groups utilize services. In addition, particular regard must be given to the attitudes of ethnic groups toward psychopathology and mental illness.

This chapter will focus on the cultural factors influencing the mental health experience of people of color or ethnic minorities. A special emphasis will be placed on African Americans, who constitute the largest minority group in the United States.

Accessibility and Utilization of Mental Health Services

An important aim of the Community Mental Health Center legislation of the 1960s was to provide mental health services to members of racial and ethnic minority groups (Cheung and Snowden, 1990). Historically, these groups had been underserved, partly due to their overrepresentation among the poor, which placed psychiatric care financially out of reach for most (Cheung and Snowden, 1990). With the establishment of community mental health centers, mental health care could be provided to the public regardless of ability to pay.

Some reports have shown an overrepresentation of black consumers of mental health services compared to whites. These differences are largely explained by greater inpatient utilization by blacks and use of mental health specialists for economic and physical health needs (Cheung and Snowden, 1990; Broman, 1987). Eligibility for Medicaid has been shown to substantially increase the likelihood of outpatient mental health service use, but race still exerts an influence on utilization (Taube and Rupp, 1986). The National Survey of Black Americans found that less than 50 percent of African Americans with an emotional problem sought any type of help, and data from the NIMH Epidemiologic Catchment Area Survey (ECA) illustrate similarly that more than 50 percent of non-whites had unmet mental health care needs (Neighbors, 1985; Shapiro et al., 1985).

For Hispanic Americans also, low utilization of mental health services is the rule, extending far below the rates seen with whites. The ECA revealed that less than half of Mexican Americans with any DIS/DSM III disorder made health or mental health visits compared with nearly 71 percent of non-Hispanic whites (Hough et al., 1987). Mexican Americans who entered treatment also had half the number of visits per person than did the non-Hispanic white group.

Asian Americans and Pacific Islanders have the lowest utilization rates in proportion to their population size compared to all other ethnic groups. This does not appear to be a reflection of lower rates of mental illness in this group, as one study reveals prevalence rates of depression at least as high as that in whites (Kuo, 1984). The disparity between use of mental health services and prevalence may be accounted for by severe stigma of mental illness in Asian American groups and problems of access for new immigrants and refugees, as well as other factors (Cheung and Snowden, 1990). The use of outpatient care by native Americans and Alaskan natives equals that of their population proportion, but information on their help-seeking patterns is limited.

It is clear that use of mental health services by minority groups is also determined by factors other than socioeconomic status, including history, religion, language, migration, acculturation, and culture-bound belief. These influences modify the connection between need and utilization through two sets of factors: the use of alternative resources and the presence or perception of barriers to receiving mental health care. The tendency to seek help for mental health problems from alternative sources is borne out by the findings of The National Survey of Black Americans. In this study, the majority of subjects who were seeking help made contact with non–mental health specialty sources such as a physician's office, emergency room, or minister, while less than 10 percent sought services from a mental health practitioner directly (Neighbors, 1985). Another survey of an urban black population found that one-third of the sample would consult an informal source of help for a serious mental health problem (Hendricks et al., 1981). Clergy, traditional healers, and extended family networks are common examples of the sources of help that may be used either alone or in combination with medical care from a family doctor (Chunn et al., 1983; Larson et al., 1988). Hispanics use the family, a neighbor or friend, *compradazgo* (a term used to describe the relationships between godparents, godchildren, and the biological parents of the godchildren), and folk healers (Canino and Canino, 1993). Folk treatments used among Hispanics such as *espiritismo, curanderismo,* and *santeria* reveal the importance of spiritualism in understanding mental illness (Alonso and Jeffrey, 1988). In a study of help-seeking among Korean-Americans, the likelihood of referral of a mentally ill person to a mental health provider by a pastor was found to be dependent on whether the clergyman held a psychological versus a religious conceptualization of mental illness (Kim-Goh, 1993). Thus, seeking help from clergy could serve as either a barrier or a conduit to receiving specialty mental health care.

The stigma associated with psychiatric disorders and mental health services continues to be a major barrier to access. African Americans who have a history of slavery and the experience of racial discrimination are stigmatized by their racial identification and its association with inferior status. Seeking services directly from a mental health professional places the individual at risk for receiving another stigmatizing label, mentally ill. Thus, the double stigma—black and mentally ill—is understandably avoided by African Americans and presents a significant barrier to seeking mental health care. The double stigma of mental illness is felt among other ethnic groups as well. Among Asian Americans, mental illness in a family member is a mark of shame, a problem to be borne by the family and hidden if at all possible (Gaw, 1993). Recently immigrated Asian groups, particularly Southeast Asian refugees, who have entered the United States in large numbers in recent decades, encounter barriers of language difference as well as cultural unfamiliarity with mental health services and a taboo against receiving them at all.

Other major barriers are general lack of trust in dominant group mental health providers, fear of abuse based on past experiences of a segregated mental health system, the need to maintain the sanctity of family business, and concerns about confidentiality (Acosta et al., 1982). Among American Indians who reside on Indian reservations, fear of sharing secrets with others in a psychiatric treatment setting is compounded by a general mistrust of white doctors employed by the federal government. Thus, the historical association of American Indians and the federal government in a relationship of "forced control" has an negative impact on the perception of mental health services (Thompson et al., 1993).

In African Americans, denial presents an additional barrier to help-seeking. Often help is not sought until a crisis point is reached and family stability is threatened. Some blacks believe that mental illness is an affliction of whites and that mental health care is a luxury reserved for affluent whites. Often denial is buttressed by a tendency toward fatalistic acceptance of one's lot and religious belief exemplified by statements such as, "Put it in the Lord's hands." In a related fashion, religion, spirituality, prayer, and folk healing are commonly used by African Americans and American Indians as means of salvation from ill-health.

Language presents the most important barrier for Hispanics. A large percentage of both first- and second-generation Hispanics consider Spanish their dominant tongue. Some speak dialects that are combinations of Spanish and English. For those who are illegal aliens and refugees, the language barriers to seeking formalized mental health care are compounded by fears of being discovered and apprehended by immigration authorities.

Cultural Issues in Patient Evaluation and Diagnosis

Stereotypes easily enter into the evaluation and diagnostic process. Often, referral information precedes face-to-face contact with a patient. Clinician bias, based on past experience, sets the stage for inappropriate conclusions and misinterpretations, as well as outright misdiagnosis. For instance, the opening statement that traditionally introduces identifying data on a patient—such as, "This is a 25-year-old African American woman mother of three, unemployed"—conjures a visual image that shapes an impression of the individual before she is actually seen. It is important that the clinician be cognizant of unconscious biases so that the patient will not be prejudged or misdiagnosed.

Language presents another possibility for bias to enter into the diagnostic process. Since verbal communication is the main vehicle for psychiatric evaluation, comprehension between patient and practitioner is key. Individuals speaking non-standard dialects such as black English are at a disadvantage and may be subject to being misunderstood or even being assumed to be unintelligent, lazy, or antisocial (Russell, 1988). If the patient perceives pressure to speak standard English and is not proficient in it, an awkward effort or inappropriate use of language may be misinterpreted as evidence of formal thought disorder or other psychopathology, such as thought blocking, looseness of associations, perseveration, or neologisms. It is best to encourage the patient to speak in the native tongue on the assumption that the information shared in that language will be the most accurate reflection of the internal experience of the patient. Furthermore, the gathering of more accurate information will lead to more accurate diagnosis and appropriate treatment.

Nonverbal communication involves assessment of gesture, posture, eye contact, and interpersonal distance. Ethnic differences in interpersonal distance are most pronounced between whites, blacks, and Hispanics, from wider to narrower distance being preferred, progressively (Sue, 1981). When the therapist and patient are of different ethnic groups, there is potential for discomfort on the part of either party, misinterpretation of nonverbal communication and/or inappropriate assignment of pathology. Particularly when there is difficulty in establishing rapport or a therapeutic relationship, the space between therapist and patient as demarcated by office furniture arrangement takes on special meaning. A patient may feel estranged if the distance established by office furniture arrangement is out of the bounds within which people in his culture interact. Eye contact is also prone to misinterpretation. Sustained, direct eye contact is regarded as socially rude among members of some African American and Asian groups. Nonverbal communication through body contact is also culturally mediated. Those groups in which Christianity is commonly practiced, especially African Americans, attach special value to touch related to the "laying on of hands" in a religious sense. The belief exists, even in the context of the psychiatric encounter, that no healing can take place unless the practitioner has touched the patient. Rebuffing an innocuous tactile gesture from an African American patient may risk rapport by communicating a lack of empathy and rejection.

In screening for delusional beliefs in the mental status examination, great care must be taken not to automatically assume that suspicions or fearful notions of attack are delusional. Mental health professionals must learn that implausible events in their own social context may not be considered out of the ordinary in some ethnic minority communities. In many instances, patients who have been victims of or witnesses to violence may be understandably fearful, harboring persecutory beliefs. For groups that by virtue of their minority status have been discriminated against by dominant groups, paranoia emerges as the primary form of delusion in mood disorders and schizophrenia. It is important to remember, however, that allegations of racism must be taken seriously and explored carefully before being dismissed as delusional.

Using standardized diagnostic instruments, the ECA showed that blacks have higher one-month prevalence rates of schizophrenia than Hispanics or others (Table 6–3). In Britain, where comparatively higher rates of schizophrenia have been found among Afro-Caribbeans than in other groups, there has been controversy over whether this phenomenon is observed due to misdiagnosis, ethnic density, viral exposure in utero, cannabis use, or other environmental factor impinging on the genetically predisposed (Cochrane and Bal, 1988; Sugarman and Craufurd, 1994). Yet, outside of epidemiologic surveys, there has been wide documentation of overdiagnosis of schizophrenia in African Americans (Adebimpe, 1981; Bell and Mehta, 1980; Jones and Gray, 1986) and Hispanics (Mukherjee et al., 1983), among those patients who meet criteria for diagnoses of affective disorder with psychotic features.

Some of the misdiagnosis and false positive cases of schizophrenia can be attributed to lack of adherence to the basic cluster of symptoms that demarcate affective and psychotic disease categories and the lack of use of standardized diagnostic instruments. In addition, due to the pathoplasticity of illness, culture and individuality shape the appearance of disease, challenging the clinician to recognize the same diseases in different contexts (McHugh and Slavney, 1983). For example, hallucinations and other first-rank symptoms in affective disorders are more prominent in young blacks and Hispanics than in other groups (Mukherjee et al., 1983).

Clinicians must become adept at recognizing the general pattern, presentation, and course of an illness before learning to recognize the same disease with a cultural overlay, such as the increases in somatic symptoms with depression that may occur in African Americans. This approach involves the interweaving of an emic (from within the culture) and an etic (extra-cultural) approach to diagnosis (Westermeyer, 1985). Several culture-bound syndromes present commonly within certain societies and groups. Examples include bulimia, mainly in white females; "falling out" among African Americans, in which collapse is associated with paralysis and mutism or blindness with the restoration of hearing and comprehension; *susto* in Hispanics, a folk diagnosis describing a debilitating state that follows a severe fright or startle experience (Simons and Hughes, 1993); and *koro,* an affliction of Japanese men in which the penis is believed to have reverted into the abdomen (Westermeyer, 1985). *Nervios* ("nerves") is a condition in Hispanics which involves a sudden impact of emotion that leads to partial loss of consciousness, sometimes accompanied by pseudoseizures or by screaming, moaning, or tearing of clothing.

Ethnocultural beliefs in sorcery, voodoo, spirit intrusion, spirit possession, and soul loss should not be mistaken for strict psychopathology when they are endorsed as accepted belief by outside informants belonging to the patient's cultural group. The religious and spiritual beliefs of African Americans, especially those from the southern states and those who have migrated from the South to northern urban centers, may include preoccupation with the Holy Ghost, belief in spirit possession, and glossolalia (speaking in tongues in a religious-linked state of dissociation). It should be noted that these beliefs are not necessarily examples of delusional ideas or severe thought disorder. The therapist should consult with family members, religious leaders, or spiritual healers in order to assess whether or not beliefs in the supernatural are in keeping with the cultural context and accepted belief system of the patient's sociocultural sphere.

Cultural Issues in Treatment

Given the underutilization and high rates of treatment dropout for ethnic minority groups, it is important to consider treatment issues likely to increase tenure in treatment and to facilitate effective treatment. Mental health providers must become knowledgeable about the specific subculture to which the patient belongs, the values held by the group, and the particular social, economic, and medical problems the group encounters. In addition, the practitioner must incorporate these elements into planned intervention with members of the ethnic group. A clinical approach should integrate standard principles of practice with a working understanding of language use, culturally sanctioned patterns of behavior, and all other values held by the individual. In this way interventions will have cultural salience and a greater chance of acceptability by the patient.

It is also important to appreciate that different ethnic groups may respond differently to psychopharmacological agents. Racial variations in drug-metabolizing enzymes, plasma protein binding, conjugation, and cell membrane transport appear to play a role in the pharmacokinetics of antidepressants, neuroleptic medications, and mood stabilizers (Lin et al., 1993). Greater incidence of tardive dyskinesia has been reported in non-whites, specifically in African American and Asian American groups (Glazer et al., 1994; Pi et al., 1993). Sensitivity to medication side effects, such as extrapyramidal symptoms, and long-term adverse effects, such as tardive dyskinesia, have a potential impact on medication compliance, treatment dropout, iatrogenic morbidity, long-term course, and overall outcome.

Differences in the ethnicity of practitioner and patient should be acknowledged and aired openly, particularly when psychotherapy is the primary mode of treatment. Open discussion of difference helps to build a trusting therapeutic relationship so that the individual knows that it is safe to talk about racial issues in the context of therapy and that difference will not be artificially obscured. Patients' views about mental illness, treatment, and expectations should be explored. Treatment should be clarified as early as possible so that mismatch of expectation and actual service does not occur. Ethnic groups that do not have a history of use of mental health services may have concerns about confidentiality and privacy that prevent them from being disclosing in individual or group psychotherapy. For this reason, the establishment of trust is crucial. It may be necessary for the therapist to use self-disclosure to balance the personal information being exchanged between the patient and the therapist.

Therapists who use language as a gauge of intelligence may underestimate the ability of a patient to benefit from certain types of psychotherapy, particularly insight-oriented therapies. African Americans have been stereotyped as being lazy, paranoid, antisocial, lacking the ability to be psychologically minded, introspective, and self-disclosing (Block, 1981). Clinicians should maintain a low threshold for recognizing transference and countertransference that revolve around racial or ethnic difference. For instance, the fixed pattern of class and authority relationships between blacks and whites in America originating from slavery places blacks in a persistently lower caste position. Such fixed relationships have implications for how African Americans are perceived by whites regardless of their actual social station, creating tension if expectations of disadvantaged status are not met. This also has implications in that some African Americans defer to whites as unquestionable authority figures. Such fixed patterns in history have implications for how African Americans and other groups are treated in the context of psychotherapy and should be a basis for self-exploration and supervision of the therapist.

''Hallucinatory whitening,'' also referred to as the ''illusion of color-blindness,'' is an example of a reaction to countertransference (Jones et al., 1970; Bell et al., 1983). Well-meaning white therapists make statements to convince minority patients that they are seen just like white patients, or that when seeing a minority patient, they see no color at all. Such statements appear benign on the surface but represent a veiled example of racism. The attitude suggests that in order to see a person of color as equal, he or she must be imagined to be white. This denies the patient a specific identity, which should be acceptable to the therapist as is, without psychological adulteration. Therapists should use informed supervision and a high degree of self-exploration to avoid this pitfall, as it may have an impact on treatment progress and treatment tenure.

The results of some studies support the use of ethnic specific mental health programs or staffing as a mechanism for improving ethnic minority utilization of mental health services (Takeuchi et al., 1995; Wu and Windle, 1980). However, same-ethnicity patient-therapist pairings have not been demonstrated to be conclusively more effective than mixed pairings (Sue, 1977). Frequently, African American patients request a black therapist if at all possible as they feel more trusting of someone of their own ethnic background. Aside from the obvious benefits of feeling that one is more likely to be understood, some potential negative consequences are that the therapist overidentifies with the patient to the point that the therapy is ineffective, diagnostic issues are confused, or socioeconomic status or other variables emerge as significant points of difference or resentment—the "cultural blind spot syndrome" (Lin, 1984). Thus, a clinician of the same background as the patients being served should not be exempt from participating in cultural competence or sensitivity training.

In some cases, in order for treatment to proceed, mental health practitioners must be prepared to interweave their armamentarium of therapeutic approaches with traditional folk beliefs and practices, crafting a treatment plan the patient will agree to and become invested in. An example of this is seen in the psychiatric treatment of American Indians in which healing ceremonies such as "sweats" that provide cleansing and catharsis are used along with conventional modalities of Western treatment (Thompson et al., 1993).

Organization of Services

The first step to designing culturally relevant mental health services is to appreciate the demographic makeup of the population served and to strive to gear the services toward the characteristics of the groups that make up the population. Community mental health needs can then be appreciated and potential barriers to mental health service utilization can be determined. Barriers exist in many forms: language, financial hardship, lack of knowledge of existence of services, use of alternative resources, geographical distance and lack of transportation, stigma of mental illness, and fear. These barriers, taken singly, may not be considered universally problematic, but when compounded with the estrangement of minority group members from mental health services, they serve to make it even less likely that people of color will use mental health services at all.

It is not uncommon that members of minority groups seek help for emotional problems from sources other than mental health professionals, such as priests or pastors, traditional healers, or family physicians. Therefore, it is important that community psychiatry programs initiate and nurture relationships with a variety of practitioners and helpers in the community so that they are aware of the program as a resource for troubled help-seekers. Communications networks of cultural organizations, churches, ethnic newspapers and newsletters, and radio and television, offer vehicles for publicizing the services available at mental health centers while working to reduce stigma. Mental health practitioners should be visible in the community, providing teaching about mental health and mental illness in an array of different settings. Participation in health promotion events and other activities in minority communities helps to raise awareness of mental illness and treatment resources among those who are often the last to know, the last to receive, and the least able to afford health care. Culturally syntonic self-help resources, support groups, and advocacy groups can also serve as sources of education about mental health and avenues for help-seeking.

Recent and first-generation immigrants of Hispanic and Asian groups are likely to use their native language exclusively. Thus, services must be developed to accommodate their communication needs and overcome a potential major obstacle to receiving care. The use of bilingual mental health professionals is crucial so that evaluation and treatment can be conducted without the additional barrier presented by a translator. Registration documents, diagnostic instruments, and other written materials should be translated into the patient's native language.

Ideally, mental health services should be established in locations that facilitate engagement without undue inconvenience. This means that whenever possible, services should be located within or near general health centers or social services agencies near bus routes. Using a setting already accepted by the ethnic community helps to remove the barrier of unfamiliarity. Services can be made more accessible by accommodating the habits and daily activities of the community being served. Hours of operation should be tailored to work schedules and varied cultural roles. If child care services are not available on site, children should be accommodated along with the identified consumer parent or guardian. Depending on the beliefs of the minority group served, Hispanic families in particular may wish to be involved in the initial and perhaps subsequent contacts with the mental health provider.

The clinic receptionist, often the first person a new patient sees, should be welcoming and manage the milieu of the waiting area so as not to create unnecessary strife or anxiety among those present. It is helpful if the receptionist speaks the language of the minority group being served so that there are no communication barriers at the portal. The milieu is important and should be tailored to reflect an appreciation for the cultural group being served. Magazines, decoration, art work, and community information with direct links to the cultural group should be displayed to help make patients feel more at home and comfortable in the environment.

Outreach services should be well developed so that visits may take place at home, school, or any potential site in the community where members of the minority group congregate. This is one way to circumvent the "tip of the iceberg" phenomenon wherein it is assumed that the only persons who need help in a given community are those who are currently engaged in treatment. Mobile outreach services help establish connections by performing the first contact on neutral territory or on the patient's own turf, facilitating the formation of a trusting relationship with the individual and the family.

Community mental health programs must engage in assertive hiring of personnel, both professional and paraprofessional, who are members of the same ethnic or cultural groups served by the agency. It would be difficult and impractical to hire staff such that all mental health providers share a common ethnic background with patients they are serving. However, continuation of care of many ethnic patients can be facilitated by pairing them with therapists and service providers with whom they do not perceive a barrier of racial or ethnic difference. Sue (1981) asserts that race and ethnicity are distal rather than proximal factors in therapist-patient matching. However, regardless of empirical support of such claims, it is important to recognize that if the patient perceives that a barrier exists, it is difficult to dislodge the patient's belief.

Consideration of affinity for type of treatment is important for maintaining tenure for certain ethnic groups. For example, treatment of American Indians through group therapy and family-network approaches has been effective (Manson et al., 1987). Cultural sensitivity and cross-cultural competence of therapists and treatment personnel should be ensured through the institutionalization of culturally related didactic seminars, case conferences, grand rounds, and individual and group supervision. Administrators should be prepared to contract for experts to address these issues with staff, who should be encouraged to attend extramural educational activities as well. Cross-cultural training for mental health professionals has the potential for achieving maximization of minority use of services and minimizing treatment dropout (Lefley, 1984).

Given that members of minority groups are generally more likely than whites to be poor, the therapist has a vital role in resource coordination for low-income persons. An appreciation of the disproportionate impact of deinstitutionalization on African Americans and other people of color should be appreciated, given their higher rates of homelessness and incarceration (Deas-Nesmith and McLeod-Bryant, 1992). Therapists must take a stance of helping to improve lives and not watch inactively while patients stagnate in patterns reflecting the historical disenfranchisement of minority groups. Such efforts encompass assistance with jobs, education, housing, general medical care, substance abuse, violence, and safety.

Summary

Cultural sensitivity in the provision of mental health care must begin with the fact that the mental health needs of diverse ethnic or cultural groups exceed their utilization of mental health services. Among the reasons for the disparity between need and actual use are denial, concerns about stigma, lack of access due to socioeconomic status and geographical distance, distrust of mainstream practitioners, lack of knowledge of available services, language barriers, and reliance on alternative sources of help such as traditional healers, clergy, and informal support networks. In order to ensure that members of ethnic minority groups receive services, mental health program planners have a responsibility to know the culture of the population they are serving, fashion programs that eliminate the barriers through outreach and education, and establish partnerships with alternate help sources.

References

Acosta, F.X., Yamamoto, J., and Evans, L.A. (1982) *Effective Psychotherapy for Low-Income and Minority Patients.* New York: Plenum Press.

Adebimpe, V. (1981) Overview: white norms and psychiatric diagnosis of black patients. *American Journal of Psychiatry,* 38:279–285.

Alonso, L., and Jeffrey, W.D., (1988) Mental illness complicated by the Santeria belief in spirit possession. *Hospital and Community Psychiatry,* 39:1188–1191.

Bell, C.C., Bland, I.J., Houston, E., and Jones, B.E. (1983) Enhancement of knowledge and skills for the psychiatric treatment of black populations. In Chunn, J.C., Dunston, P.J., Ross-Sherrif, F. (eds.) *Mental Health and People of Color.* Washington, D.C.: Howard University Press.

Bell, C., and Mehta, H. (1980) The misdiagnosis of black patients with manic depressive illness. *Journal of the National Medical Association,* 72:141–145.

Block, C. (1981) Black Americans and the cross-cultural counseling and psychotherapy experience. In Marsella, J., Pedersen, P. (eds.), *Cross Cultural Counseling and Psychotherapy.* New York: Pergamon Press.

Broman, C.L. (1987) Race differences in professional help seeking. *American Journal of Community Psychology,* 15:473–489.

Canino, I.A., and Canino, G.J. (1993) Psychiatric care of Puerto Ricans. In Gaw, A.C. (ed.), *Culture, Ethnicity and Mental Illness.* Washington, D.C.: American Psychiatric Press.

Cheung, F.K., and Snowden, L.R. (1990) Community mental health and ethnic minority populations. *Community Mental Health Journal,* 26:277–291.

Chunn, J.C., Dunston, P.J., and Sheriff, F. (1983) *Mental Health and People of Color Curriculum Development and Change.* Washington, D.C.: Howard University Press.

Cochrane, R., and Bal, S. (1988) Ethnic density is unrelated to incidence of schizophrenia. *British Journal of Psychiatry,* 153:363–366.

Deas-Nesmith, D., and McLeod-Bryant, S. (1992) Psychiatric deinstitutionalization and its cultural insensitivity: consequences and recommendations for the future. *Journal of the National Medical Association,* 84:1036–1040.

Gaw, A.C. (1993) Psychiatric care of Chinese Americans. In Gaw, A.C. (ed.), *Culture, Ethnicity and Mental Illness.* Washington, D.C.: American Psychiatric Press.

Glazer, W.M., Morgenstern, H., and Doucette, J. (1994) Race and tardive dyskinesia among outpatients at a CMHC. *Hospital and Community Psychiatry,* 45:38–42.

Hendricks, L.E., Howard, C.S., and Gary, L.E. (1981) Help-seeking behavior among urban black adults. *Social Work,* 26:161–163.

Hough, R.L., Landsverk, J.A., Karno, M., Burnam, A., Timbers, D.M., Escobar, J.I., and Regier, D. (1987) Utilization of health and mental health services by Los Angeles Mexican Americans and non-Hispanic whites. *Archives of General Psychiatry,* 44:702–709.

Jones, B.E., Lightfoot, O.B., Palmer, D., Wilkerson, R.G., and Williams, D.H. (1970) Problems of black psychiatric residents in white training institutes. *American Journal of Psychiatry*, 127:798–803.

Jones, B.E., and Gray, B.A. (1986) Problems in diagnosing schizophrenia and affective disorders among blacks. *Hospital and Community Psychiatry*, 37:61–65.

Kim-Goh, M. (1993) Conceptualization of mental illness among Korean-American clergymen and implication for mental health service delivery. *Community Mental Health Journal*, 29:405–411.

Kleinman, A. (1993) How is culture important for DSM-IV? In *Cultural Proposals and Supporting Papers for the DSM-IV Task Force*. Submitted to the NIMH-Sponsored Group on Culture and Diagnosis, Third Revision, 13–33.

Kramer, M. (1983) The increasing prevalence of mental disorders: a pandemic threat. *Psychiatric Quarterly*, 55:115–143.

Kuo, W. (1984) Prevalence of depression among Asian-Americans. *Journal of Nervous and Mental Disease*, 172:449–457.

Larson, D., Hohmann, A.A., Kessler, L.G., Meador, K.G., Boyd, J.H., and McSherry, E. (1988) The couch and the cloth: the need for linkage. *Hospital and Community Psychiatry*, 39:1064–1069.

Lefley, H. (1984) Cross-cultural training for mental health professionals: effects on the delivery of services. *Hospital and Community Psychiatry*, 35:1227–1229.

Lin, E.H.B. (1984) Intraethnic characteristics and patient-physician interaction: cultural blind spot syndrome. *Journal of Family Practice*, 16:91–98.

Lin, K.M., Poland, R.E., and Silver, B. (1993) Overview: the interface between psychobiology and ethnicity. In Lin, K.M., Poland, R.E., Nakasaki, G. (eds.), *Psychopharmacology and Psychobiology of Ethnicity*. Washington, D.C.: American Psychiatric Press.

Manson, S.M., Walker, R.D., and Kivlahan, D.R. (1987) Psychiatric assessment and treatment of American Indians and Alaska natives. *Hospital and Community Psychiatry*, 38:165–173.

McHugh, P.R., and Slavney, P.R. (1983) *The Perspectives of Psychiatry*. Baltimore: Johns Hopkins University Press.

Mukherjee, M.D., Shukla, S., Woodle, J., Rosen, A.M., and Olarte, S. (1983) Misdiagnosis of schizophrenia in bipolar patients: a multiethnic comparison. *American Journal of Psychiatry*, 140:1571–1574.

Neighbors, H.W. (1985) Seeking professional help for personal problems: black Americans' use of health and mental health services. *Community Mental Health Journal*, 21:156–166.

Pi, E.H., Gutierrez, M., and Gray, G.E. (1993) Tardive dyskinesia: cross-cultural perspectives. In Lin, K.M., Poland, R.E., Nakasaki, G. (eds.), *Psychopharmacology and Psychobiology of Ethnicity*. Washington, D.C.: American Psychiatric Press.

Russell, D.M. (1988) Language and psychotherapy: the influence of non-standard English in clinical practice. In Comas-Diaz, L., Griffith, E.E.H. (eds.), *Clinical Guidelines in Cross-Cultural Mental Health*. New York: Wiley and Sons.

Shapiro, S., Skinner, E.A., Kramer, M., Steinwachs, D.M., and Regier, D.A. (1985) Measuring need for mental health services in a general population. *Medical Care*, 23:1033–1043.

Simons, R.C., and Hughes, C. (1993) Culture-bound syndromes. In Gaw, A.C. (ed.), *Culture, Ethnicity and Mental Illness*. Washington, D.C.: American Psychiatric Press.

Sue, S. (1977) Community mental health services to minority groups, some optimism, some pessimism. *American Psychologist*, 32:616–624.

Sue, D.W. (1981) *Counseling the Culturally Different: Theory and Practice.* New York: John Wiley and Sons.

Sugarman, P.A., and Craufurd, D. (1994) Schizophrenia in the Afro-Caribbean community. *British Journal of Psychiatry,* 164:474–480.

Takeuchi, D.T., Sue, S., Yeh, M. (1995) Return rates and outcomes from ethnic specific mental health programs in Los Angeles. *American Journal of Public Health,* 85:638–643.

Taube, C., and Rupp, A. (1986) The effect of Medicaid on access to ambulatory mental health care for the poor and near-poor under 65. *Medical Care,* 24:677–686.

Thompson, J.W., Walker, R.D., and Silk-Walker, P. (1993) Psychiatric care of American Indians and Alaska natives. In Gaw, A.C. (ed.), *Culture, Ethnicity and Mental Illness.* Washington, DC: American Psychiatric Press.

U.S. Bureau of the Census (1994) *Statistical Abstract of the United States (114th edition).* Lanham, MD: Bernham Press.

Westermeyer, J. (1989) *Mental Health for Refugees and Other Migrants.* Springfield, Illinois: Charles C. Thomas, Publisher.

Westermeyer, J.J. (1985) Psychiatric diagnosis across cultural boundaries. *American Journal of Psychiatry,* 142:798–805.

Wu, I.H., and Windle, C. (1980) Ethnic specificity in the relative minority use and staffing of community mental health centers. *Community Mental Health Journal,* 16:156–168.

12

Citizen and Consumer Participation

WILLIAM R. BREAKEY
LAURIE FLYNN
LAURA VAN TOSH

People who were not professionally trained in health or mental health have always played major roles in the development of improved mental health services. William Tuke, Dorothea Lynd Dix, Clifford Beers, the families of Gheel, and Bill W., the founder of Alcoholics Anonymous, for example, all made fundamental, lasting contributions. Countless other individuals and groups have contributed to the development of ideas and the progress of reforms. Yet, by and large, until relatively recently, official mental health service planning, policy making, and service provision has been dominated by professionals, and other major stake-holders have been largely excluded. The reasons for this exclusionary policy are complex but undoubtedly include the belief of physicians and other professionals that they are best able to understand the important issues in providing mental health services and also the stigma surrounding people with mental illnesses that exists within the helping professions just as it does in society at large (Fink and Tasman, 1992).

Gradual change has nonetheless been under way for a long time and much has changed already. It is now widely accepted that nobody understands the experience of mental illness better than the patients and their families, who have lived through it. Doctors are now expected to obtain patients' informed consent for whatever treatments they prescribe, and it is standard practice for patients to share in the development of a treatment plan. Consumers and their families are included in the formulation of federal, state, and local mental health policy. Influential approaches to psychiatric rehabilitation and case management are structured around consumer choice and the client's setting of the goals (Anthony et al., 1990). Self-help groups have major roles in the treatment of substance-use disorders and in other spheres also.

However, there is still a long way to go in perfecting the collaboration between those who experience mental illness, those who love and care for them, and the professionals whose job it is to help them. Psychiatrists must develop the skills and attitudes necessary to relate constructively to nonprofessionals who are active in the mental health service arena: patients, their families, advocates, and others. The psychiatrist's responsibility is to bring his or her own special expertise as teacher, physician, and researcher to the enterprise. At the same time, the psychiatrist must acknowledge the validity of the experience and expertise of nonprofessionals and must be willing to learn from others and to collaborate actively with them in bringing about improvements in the mental health service system.

A Note on Labels

There is no single completely satisfactory word in current use to describe a person with a major mental illness, active or in remission, who may or may not be currently in treatment, or who has at some time been diagnosed as such. At one time, people in institutions were referred to as *inmates,* and sometimes, after discharge as *ex-inmates.* This focus on the institutional status of people, likening them to prisoners, has fortunately passed into history, along with *lunatic* and *insane* (except as a legal term).

Patient is the term used by a physician or other health care professional to describe the particular relationship that exists within the healing professions between them and those they serve. They see this as a very special relationship, hallowed by centuries of noble tradition and signifying a special commitment on the part of the professional and certain obligations on the part of the patient, who then receives the benefits of the ''sick role.''

Some have felt this relationship to be infantilizing, and prefer to use *client* to describe the contract that exists between the provider and the recipient of services. They consider this term to convey a greater sense of equality in the relationship, with less sense that the person receiving the service is of inferior status.

Professionals in the field of rehabilitation emphasize that while ''patient'' or ''client'' may be appropriate in the clinical setting, those labels should not continue to attach to a person when he or she leaves the doctor's office and fulfills other roles in life. Clubhouse programs, for example, use *member* to describe the people who participate in their activities, and *resident* for those who occupy their housing programs.

With the increasing assertiveness of current or former recipients of mental health services, *consumer* has been adopted to imply that they can have an active and critical role in determining what is acceptable. Others object to this term as being too commercial in its implications and origins, implying an exploitative relationship between the supplier of goods and those who seek them. This terminology has been extended to include *primary consumers,* those who are or have been patients within the mental health service system, and *secondary consumers,* those, such as parents or close friends, who have also had a stake in the treatment and rehabilitation process.

Some former patients describe themselves as *survivors.* In this way they emphasize the suffering associated with mental illness. They have survived an ordeal; in some cases they have survived the legal processes for involuntary treatment, the humiliation of restraint or seclusion, the other vissicitudes of mental hospital life, and the unwanted effects of medications. Some do not believe in the concept of mental illness and use the term "survivor" to indicate that they have survived wrongful labeling, treatment within the mental health service system, and stigmatization. Many professionals view this term as excessively confrontational. Others agree that it aptly describes the experience. Sometimes the combination *consumer-survivor* is employed.

In the opinion of the authors of this chapter, each of these labels has its strengths and weaknesses. There is little evidence that any of the terms in current use is less stigmatizing than any other. Until better terminology evolves, we will use whichever seems to provide the most appropriate description of the many roles of a person who experiences mental illness or who is labeled as such.

The Need for Advocacy against Stigma

Public attitudes are all-important in the development of policy, the establishment of priorities, and the allocation of resources. Attitudes towards mental illness have long been influenced by misunderstanding, misinformation, fear, and shame. Old notions of demonic possession and other superstitions linger not far beneath the surface. Even within the medical professions, mental illness is not thought of as "real illness" and psychiatrists are sometimes not thought of as "real doctors." Psychiatry has at times contributed to the stigma surrounding mental illness, for example, by developing theories that relate the origins of disorders to failures of parenting, and by infantilizing patients through emphasizing their vulnerabilities rather than their strengths. Psychiatrists have devalued their field by uncritical acceptance of theories that are later shown to be of little value (McHugh, 1992). The victims themselves have often been blamed for their illnesses, which are attributed to a character flaw, or a lack of personal discipline. The stigma surrounding mental illness is real and persistent (Fink and Tasman, 1992). In one study, 71 percent of respondents said that mental illness was due to "emotional weakness," 65 percent said that "bad parenting" was at fault, 35 percent blamed "sinful behavior," 45 percent stated that people with mental illness "bring on their own illnesses," and 43 percent believed that such illnesses as schizophrenia and bipolar disorder are hopeless. Only 10 percent indicated a belief that mental disorders have a biological basis involving the brain (Utah AMI, 1989).

Stereotyping is as pernicious as stigma. The term "mental patient," often used by news media, for instance, to describe the perpetrator of some crime, conjures up negative images and is assumed to categorize a homogenous class of people. The demeaning assumption that they are all alike is one of the reasons that survivors of this process have found it necessary to protest loudly their own individuality and dignity. Prior to the development of advocacy organizations, mentally ill individuals and their families were generally intimidated from making a public stand on their own behalf. The first major organization to provide strength in numbers for this purpose was the National Committee for Mental Hygiene. This organization was founded in 1909, inspired by Clifford Beers's *A Mind That Found Itself* and encouraged by notable medical figures of the time, including Adolf Meyer. In 1950 it united with two other groups to form the National Mental Health Association. The national association and its local affiliates include in their membership a wide variety of people from various backgrounds, many of them professionals in the field, who volunteer their time and share a common interest in advocating on behalf of people with psychiatric disorders.

More recently those people directly affected by mental illness have formed organizations to support one another and advocate more forcefully on their own behalf. First, a movement developed among families of people affected by mental illness, who organized themselves to provide effective advocacy for improved services, research, and the reduction of stigma. Then, wanting to speak more forcefully from their unique perspective, mentally ill people themselves began to create powerful organizations for advocacy and mutual support. Such organizations emphasize empowerment; they took a lead in the development of Patients' Bills of Rights and in establishing the right to refuse treatment. Several legal advocacy organizations have focused on the issues affecting people with mental illness and their treatment. The Judge David L. Bazelon Center for Mental Health Law and the National Association of Rights Protection and Advocacy have had leading roles in this arena.

Additional important contributions to public understanding (both positive and negative) have been made by writers, film-makers, and journalists in various media. Many have had important roles in forming public consensus about mental health policy, exposing injustices, exploring ethical and legal issues, and in decreasing, or increasing, stigma.

In a variety of ways, therefore, the development of mental health services has been influenced by, and continues to depend on, the energetic involvement of individuals and groups not conventionally considered to be among the mental health professions.

Mandatory Citizen Participation

A basic tenet of community psychiatry has been that the community itself has a vital role in the establishment of mental health service priorities and the development of services. Thus, when the community mental health center movement developed in the 1960s, citizen participation was a central concept. This principle has been consistently reinforced and developed by the Community Support Program of the Center for Mental Health Services, formerly of the National Institute for Mental Health (Parrish, 1989). Under the federal CMHC program, community advisory boards and community-based governing boards were mandated to ensure that programs were as responsive as possible to the needs of their target populations. Stuggles occurred between professionals and local community boards in some places in the early years.

Now their role is collaborative, partly because providers have become more open to guidance, partly because the concept of consumerism is more widely accepted in contemporary culture, and partly because citizens have become better informed about health and mental health.

Citizen advisory structures are still mandated by law (P.L. 99–660, The State Mental Health Planning Act, and P.L. 99–319, The Protection and Advocacy Act for the Mentally Ill, have both supported consumer and family involvement) and are now standard in all jurisdictions. There are state advisory boards, made up of civic leaders, representatives of legal and medical professions, consumers and their families, and others. Similar boards are constituted at city and catchment area levels to ensure as far as possible that service providers are sensitive to community needs.

A program director must develop effective collaboration with the program's advisory or governing board. The board can contribute to the effectiveness of planning and operating a program in three ways. First, it can advocate with the program and its director on behalf of the community, reflecting the priorities and concerns of the community for mental health and mental health services, and ensuring that the program is responsive to these concerns. In so doing, it serves an evaluation and monitoring function, in support of quality in the provision of services. Second, the board can advocate for the program in the community, demystifying psychiatry, destigmatizing mental illness, and encouraging help-seeking when appropriate. Third, the community board or advisory group can, with the program and its director, advocate for greater resources to be made available to the community for mental health programs.

Citizen boards are set up in various ways, each of which has advantages and disadvantages. In some areas, elections have been organized within the catchment area. In others, boards are made up of persons representing key organizations within the area, such as social service departments, community organizations, consumer groups, police, schools, and ethnic organizations. In other places, the program director recruits individuals who are known to have an interest in mental health issues and the willingness to participate; the board itself, once established, elects its own new members through a nomination process. In all cases, it is now considered obligatory to include primary and secondary consumers.

The program director's job is to ensure that the board functions well. Like many organizations, boards wax and wane in their effectiveness. Members must see clearly that they are useful, that they are not merely providing rubber stamp approval for what the director would do anyway. Specific projects, such as consumer satisfaction surveys, public education programs, site visiting of specific program components, or confrontation of state or local mental health service administrators, when needed, help the board to keep its purpose in focus and to maintain its motivation to provide effective input.

Organized Advocacy

For many years the preeminent organization for public education and advocacy for the rights of psychiatric patients and for a more responsive service system was the

National Mental Health Association. Clifford Beers had suffered greatly with affective disorder and had suffered also at the hands of the staffs of the public and private psychiatric hospitals of his day (Beers, 1907). Beers inspired a group of people to form the Connecticut Committee for Mental Hygiene in 1908, and with enormous energy founded the National Committee for Mental Hygiene less than a year later. Since its origin, the organization has spread throughout the country and has been emulated worldwide. In 1953, it was renamed the National Mental Health Association. State mental health associations, operating under the umbrella of the national association, undertake advocacy at state levels, and local chapters provide advocacy, support, and public education in urban and rural communities. The Mental Health Association embraces a wide constituency of civic-minded people from all walks of life who are concerned with decreasing stigma and increasing understanding of mental illness and the needs of people with psychiatric disabilities. The membership includes psychiatrists and other professionals, in addition to former and current patients and members of their families. The association strives to maintain a balance between professionals and nonprofessionals. Psychiatrists are welcomed and have provided leadership locally and nationally. National and state organizations employ staffs who, among other responsibilities, organize lobbying efforts in legislatures when issues relevant to mental health services or the interests of the mentally ill are discussed. The national organization was influential in the development of the National Institute for Mental Health in 1948, the development of the Community Mental Health Centers in the 1960s and 1970s, and in the health care reform debates in the 1990s, always seeking to ensure that people with psychiatric disorders are treated fairly and with dignity. At local levels, mental health associations have been in the forefront of movements for reform of state hospitals, recognition of and respect for the rights of patients, and dissemination of public information about psychiatric disorders and legislation for parity for psychiatric patients in health insurance coverage. Throughout its history, the Mental Health Association has emphasized prevention and positive mental health, which has led it, among other things, to stress the importance of services for children and to engage in major efforts for public education about mental health issues. The National Committee for Mental Hygiene established Mental Health Week in 1949, which in 1960 was expanded to Mental Health Month, observed in May each year. Their public information service publishes material on a variety of mental health topics.

The Mental Health Association also emphasizes the importance of research. As the National Committee for Mental Hygiene, it made a major contribution to the fight to establish the National Institute for Mental Health in the 1940s, and the association continues to advocate each year for maintaining and increasing federal support for psychiatric research.

In some areas, local mental health associations have developed service programs in addition to their advocacy roles, funded through charitable donations or state mental health funds. In this way they have taken an active role in filling some of the gaps in the service system. The disadvantage for an advocacy organization, however, is that accepting public funds may compromise its advocacy.

Self-Help Groups

Self-help groups in the area of mental health, perhaps more aptly described as mutual help groups (Killilea, 1976), enable their members to help each other through support, problem-solving, and advocacy. Advocacy has two aspects, both of which are important in this context: advocacy on behalf of an individual who needs assistance, and advocacy at a systemic level, for more enlightened policies, respect of rights, or improved services. Three broad categories of self-help groups include those that are organized around a particular problem, such as bereavement or substance dependence, and focus on mutual support for individual recovery; those that are made up of ex-patients or survivors and provide mutual support but also emphasize systems issues and advocacy; and a third type of group that focuses on a particular disease or disorder, sponsoring research, education, and mutual support for people who have the disorder, with less emphasis on public policy or advocacy. Some groups bridge different sets of goals. All these groups were in some sense developed as viable alternatives to a mental health system that did not adequately address people's needs, or to fill in gaps in the system. A major reason for the formation of any such group is to provide members with peer support and to draw strength from numbers and the sense of a shared experience (Furlong-Norman, 1988).

The essential characteristics of self-help groups have been articulated both in the mental health self-help movement and in the general self-help arena. They include the self-definition of needs, equal power of members, mutual respect, a focus on shared experience, members' willingness to use their own experience as a basis for helping others, resources that are controlled by group members who plan and carry out programs, voluntary participation by members, autonomy, and responsivity to other special populations. Other benefits of self-help are important also: They offer tangible results to their participants, provide valuable forums for sharing information, and can provide participants with improved coping strategies. In this way, participants can act as role models for each other. Self-help groups are non-hierarchical and are generally informally operated, unlike more traditionally based services which tend to be bureaucratic and breed impersonal interactions (Gartner and Riessman, 1984; Silverman, 1980; White and Madera, 1992; Zinman et al., 1987).

Mutual help groups in general emphasize their independence from professional clinical services. There is no professional hierarchy, no bureaucratic policies or procedures to be observed, and the members of the group have full control over its activities. The only experts are the members, and their expertise derives from their own experience. The techniques of the groups rely strongly on role-modeling, mutual support, and shared problem-solving.

The first major development in self-help was Alcoholics Anonymous (AA), begun in 1935 by "Bill W." His work, along with the efforts of other pioneers of AA, was the cornerstone in developing the philosophy that people's reliance on professionals for treating major disorders was not sufficient, or even not needed (Bufe, 1991). Over time, millions of individuals have participated in AA, and many have found it to be highly successful in supporting and helping them as they recover from their addictions, although some people object to their philosophy or style of participation. The "twelve-step" model of AA has also been adopted by other organizations of people with habit disorders, to good effect.

Other mutual-help groups have been formed to enable individuals who have confronted specific life problems or crises to support each other. They include groups for those who have been bereaved, groups for women who have been victims of abuse, groups for single parents, and groups for people who have recently been divorced. Such groups, which are based on crisis theory and research on bereavement, focus on helping members cope with transitions (Silverman, 1966).

Consumers as Advocates and Service Providers

Two trends in the 1970s and 1980s prompted a change in attitude and policies towards consumer involvement: the emergence of self-help groups and larger consumer umbrella organizations, and an emphasis on consumer involvement incorporated into policy at the state and federal levels. Consumers have become vocal agents of change and active participants in the mental health system (Chamberlin et al., 1989; Chamberlin, 1990), have become involved in the planning, delivery, and evaluation of services throughout the country (Specht, 1988), and are viewed as an essential element in meeting the needs of persons with psychiatric disabilities. Consumer involvement rests on the principles of empowerment and the right to self-determination, and is upheld by the finding in a number of surveys that patients and their care providers often have very different priorities (e.g., Mitchell et al., 1983; Lynch and Kruzich, 1986). This movement has been reinforced by the rise of consumerism as a cultural phenomenon in recent years (Kopolow, 1979).

Consumers are involved in the mental health service system in two principal ways: through participation in self-help groups for mutual support and advocacy and as service providers, either independently or in collaboration with professionals.

Consumer Self-Help Organizations

In the 1970s a number of groups developed among former state hospital patients. These groups were initially small in size, their members united by their indignation over treatment received in the mental health system, and they generally took a militant stance against psychiatry. Some, such as the Network Against Psychiatric Assault (Hirsch et al., 1974) and Project Release, created the first opportunities for individuals to gather by themselves to provide each other with support and discuss issues such as civil commitment, involuntary administration of medications, and the right to treatment of persons confined in mental hospitals. These groups played a major role in helping consumer/survivors to organize for changes in an often oppressive system. Over time, with changes in federal law and the recognition of certain national trends, members began to work more collaboratively with the system, creating alternatives and establishing their own programs and initiatives (Furlong-Norman, 1988).

The National Mental Health Consumers' Association was formed in 1985. The difficulty of agreeing on the best approaches to advocacy in this highly charged arena was illustrated by the early breakaway of a group that became the National Alliance of Mental Patients, later renamed the National Alliance of Psychiatric Survivors. These two organizations shared many of the same objectives, but the Alliance of Psychiatric Survivors, as its name reflects, took a stronger position in opposition to all forms of involuntary treatment. Each of these organizations, however, served as an umbrella and support organization for the hundreds of consumer organizations that existed across the country. Today, both of these national organizations have ceased operations. The consumer movement does not have a single institutional voice, but is carried forward by a multitude of small groups across the country.

Nonetheless, certain consumer organizations have continued to be active in public advocacy. Their many activities include testifying before congressional committees on mental health issues, providing leadership in patients' rights issues before federal courts, providing technical assistance to protection and advocacy systems, and publishing newsletters and public education about mental illness and patients' rights through the media (Chamberlin et al., 1989).

Some examples of organizations formed to bring together people concerned about specific disorders include The National Depressive and Manic Depressive Association, formed in 1978, and the Depressive and Related Affective Disorders Association (DRADA), formed in 1986. Other examples are the Alzheimers Association, the Huntington's Disease Society of America, and the Anxiety Disorders Association. These groups spearhead efforts to increase understanding of and effective treatment for affective disorders through research, to destigmatize depression through public education, and to provide support to sufferers and their families.

Consumers as Service Providers

Judi Chamberlin's *On Our Own* (1978) was a catalyst for a major innovation which found expression in mental health service systems across the United States—the creation of consumer-operated programs and services. In the 1980s, the Community Support Program of the National Institute of Mental Health (NIMH), now of the Center for Mental Health Services (CMHS), increasingly acknowledged the growing and necessary involvement of consumers in the planning, delivery, and evaluation of programs and services. At the same time, mental health administrators and program managers became increasingly aware of the effectiveness of consumers working in the mental health field, partly because of the special qualities inherent in this unique pool of workers (Van Tosh, 1993). People with personal experience of mental illness have gradually become recognized as valuable contributors to the mental health system's workforce (Stroul, 1986; Specht, 1988; Furlong-Norman, 1988; Interagency Council on the Homeless, 1992; Nikkel et al., 1992; NASMHPD, 1989, 1993).

Van Tosh (1993) has articulated a number of ways in which consumers are specially equipped to provide mental health services. They are intimately familiar with many aspects of quality of care, the range of agencies, service models, housing opportunities, and other information. They are less likely to demand "compliance" with any or all services as a prerequisite for receiving other services, and often demonstrate great flexibility and patience in dealing with mentally disabled people. Consumers stress creativity in developing solutions based on the expressed preferences and identified needs of their clients, are less constrained by professional traditions, and are more amenable to alternative service approaches. They are able to tolerate unusual behaviors and do not feel compelled to maintain a professional distance (Besio and Mahler, 1993). Consumer workers are often willing to do more than what is routinely expected and to be flexible in the assignment of hours and tasks. Many possess the ability to identify effective practical interventions based on their own experiences. For example, consumer workers have acquired special knowledge about how to obtain resources. They are usually familiar with self-help groups, free health clinics, housing opportunities, and other services, having used them themselves. Because of their peer status, they are better able than professionals to establish rapport, act as role models for others, and raise their level of optimism towards recovery (Warner and Polak, 1993). Consumer workers are a major force in the elimination of stigma and discrimination, and they can assist in the development of greater sensitivity and skills among other workers (Besio and Mahler, 1993).

A variety of consumer-operated programs and services has been developed, staffed, and evaluated (Furlong-Norman, 1988; Barry, 1991). These services include drop-in centers, outreach programs for persons who are homeless and mentally disabled, peer companion programs, counseling and support services for patients being discharged from hospitals, businesses, housing programs, and many others (Mowbray and Tan, 1993; Shelton and Rissmeyer, 1989).

Primary consumers are becoming better organized year by year. Federally funded technical assistance centers such as the National Mental Health Consumers' Self-Help Clearinghouse and the National Empowerment Center use every means possible to disseminate information and promote communication and mutual support between and for consumers. They distribute newsletters and other information by mail, fax, or e-mail, organize conferences and teleconferences, and sponsor electronic bulletin boards. In addition, states have supported the creation of offices of consumer affairs within departments of mental health. Increasingly, they contribute forcefully and constructively to the mental health service enterprise.

Consumer Involvement in Research and Policy Development

More recently, consumer involvement has been extended to research and policy development, particularly in the area of mental health services. Former or current users of services have begun to participate in the development of research protocols to study innovative programs. Two major research centers have been federally funded to study self-help in mental health in addition to the two technical assistance centers operated by and for consumer/survivors to access information (Furlong-Norman, 1988).

The Family-Consumer Movement

Until relatively recently, families of psychiatric patients, devastated by the dreadful impact of misunderstood and maligned disorders, hardly dared speak up about their relatives, since they, themselves, were often thought to have brought on their relatives' conditions. When a few did speak up about lack of appropriate care and treatment at state or private facilities, such families were identified as troublemakers, uncooperative, lacking in insight, or pathologically dysfunctional. Others were afraid to speak out for fear their complaints might further jeopardize what comfort and access to treatment their ill relatives had. They quickly learned that complaining to officials about shoddy care-giving often brought retaliation against the ill relative.

With deinstitutionalization, the burden of daily care for severely disabled individuals has largely fallen on individual families (Hatfield, 1989; Cook et al., 1994). As many as two-thirds of patients released from inpatient care return to live with their families, who in many instances are expected to replace within their own homes, using personal resources, all of the things formerly provided in an integrated institutional care setting. Parents are the primary care-givers in over 60 percent of cases; most are women aged 65 years and older. Nearly one in three does not have another adult in the household able or available to assist in providing support, and 25 percent report that no other relative lives within an hour's drive.

The demands made on care-givers are great, as are their needs for support and assistance. In a recent survey, 60 percent indicated need for assistance in illness management, 70 percent indicated need for crises management assistance, 75 percent needed help with daily living skills, 65 percent indicated their relative required assistance in creating and maintaining social relationships, and 70 percent reported needing help in finding productive activities during the day (Steinwachs et al., 1992).

Families have organized for mutual support and advocacy. The major organization in the United States for families of mentally ill people is the National Alliance for the Mentally Ill (NAMI). More recently, The Federation of Families for Children's Mental Health has formed as an umbrella organization for many groups across the country that support families with mentally ill children.

NAMI was founded in 1979, in Madison, Wisconsin, with a declared mission for "the eradication of mental illness and improving the quality of life of those who suffer from these diseases." NAMI's policy agenda focuses on severe, persistent, disabling disorders, and the needs for systems of care for patients and support for care-givers. The national organization has been most effective in its ability to mobilize campaigns, such as the fight to preserve the NIMH Community Support Program when it was threatened with extinction by the Reagan Administration, and efforts to increase federal appropriations for research on severe disorders and to integrate NIMH within the National Institutes of Health. Their focus on remedying unmet needs is reflected in a variety of other advocacy initiatives, including federal legislation (P.L. 96–272) requiring states to develop comprehensive state plans for services for individuals with serious mental illnesses, and to require family and consumer participation on state advisory councils. NAMI also energetically campaigned alongside other advocacy groups to bring people with psychiatric disabilities under the protection of the 1990 Americans with Disabilities Act (ADA), which aims to ensure that people with mental illnesses are included in employment opportunity.

At the local level, AMIs have formed across the country, providing an ongoing focus on advocacy and education, fostering public support for increased mental health allocations and the transfer of funds from institutional to community care settings. Local alliances have developed a variety of support groups. Through a growing family of special interest networks they can link individuals with mental illnesses to their Consumer Council, sisters and brothers to their Sibling and Adult Children Network, families concerned about a child with a mental disorder to a Children and Adolescent Network, individuals of ethnic or minority heritage to a Multicultural Concerns Network, and so on. NAMI has 14 special networks of this sort.

Through collaborative efforts with psychiatrists in events such as Mental Illness Awareness Week, NAMI works to educate communities around the country. In order to provide advocates across the country with a useful aid to measure and evaluate services for their ill relatives, NAMI has published a biannual report, *Care of the Seriously Mentally Ill: A Rating of State Programs* (Torrey et al., 1990). These publications rank the states in terms of how well basic medical and social supports are provided to persons with severe mental illness. Another report, *Criminalizing the Seriously Mentally Ill: The Abuse of Jails as Mental Hospitals,* grew out of the finding that 40 percent of families surveyed reported that their ill relative had been arrested, in most cases for misdemeanors (Torrey et al., 1992).

In 1987, NAMI took the lead in founding the National Alliance for Research on Schizophrenia and Depression (NARSAD), an organization dedicated to raising private funds for research on serious psychiatric illness. Many eminent scientists support this effort, which annually funds a series of important research projects. In 1990, NAMI began administration of the Stanley Foundation Research Awards, which provide substantial grants for biomedical research both in the United States and abroad.

Forming Coalitions

Groups that advocate on behalf of psychiatric patients and psychiatric services have on occasions been frustrated to see their efforts fail because of a perception, or an allegation, that the various advocacy organizations, including professional organizations, failed to speak with a common voice, that sometimes their advocacy was directed in opposite directions, and that their cause was weakened by this disunity. Responses to these accusations have appeared in many arenas in the formation of coalitions to tackle specific issues (Ross, 1980). For example, a coalition was formed in Maryland to tackle the issue of discrimination in insurance coverage. The coalition included a variety of consumer groups and professional organizations that together brought this issue before the state legislature and succeeded in having passed a Mental Health Insurance Parity Bill, which requires that psychiatric services be paid for by insurers in essentially the same way that other medical services are paid for. The Maryland AMI could not have achieved this outcome alone. Nor could the local psychiatric association, or any one group. Together they were able to have legislation passed which set a new standard of fairness in health insurance.

This example serves to underline the interdependence of the mentally ill and those who provide services for them, and the need for close collaboration to achieve common goals. It serves also to emphasize that the days when patients were passive recipients of services are gone. The task of the community psychiatrist is to work collaboratively with the various groups of people in the community who have a major interest in the enterprise of mental health service provision, to see that resources are made available for the task and to ensure that services are provided in the best possible way.

References

Anthony, W.A., Cohen, M.R. and Farkas, M. (1990) *Psychiatric Rehabilitation.* Boston: Boston University Center for Psychiatric Rehabilitation.

Barry, D. (ed.) (1991) *Insites: The Robert Wood Johnson Foundation Program on Chronic Mental Illness.* 4(2):1–12.

Beers, C.W. (1907, 1981) *A Mind That Found Itself.* Pittsburgh: University of Pittsburgh Press.

Besio, S., and Mahler, J. (1993) Benefits and challenges of using consumer staff in supported housing services. *Hospital and Community Psychiatry,* 44:490–491.

Bufe, C. (1991) *Alcoholics Anonymous.* San Francisco, CA: Seeshop Press.

Chamberlin, J. (1990) The ex-patients' movement: Where we've been and were we're going. *The Journal of Mind and Behavior,* 11:323–336.

Chamberlin, J. (1978) *On Our Own.* New York: McGraw-Hill.

Chamberlin, J., Rogers, J., and Sneed, C. (1989) Consumers, families and community support systems. *Psycho-Social Rehabilitation Journal,* 12:93–106.

Cook, J.A., Lefley, H.P., Pickett, S.A., and Cohler, B.J. (1994) Age and family burden among parents of offspring with severe mental illness. *American Journal of Orthopsychiatry,* 66:435–447.

Fink, P.J., and Tasman, A. (eds.) (1992) *Stigma and Mental Illness.* Washington, D.C.: American Psychiatric Press.

Furlong-Norman, K. (ed.) (1988) *Community Support Network News.* 5(2):1–16.

Gartner, A., and Riessman, F. (1984) *The Self-Help Revolution.* New York: Human Services Press.

Hatfield, A.B. (1989) Serving the unserved in community rehabilitation programs. *Psychosocial Rehabilitation Journal,* 13(2):71–82.

Hirsch, S., Adams, J.K., Frank, L.R., Hudson, W., Keene, R., Krawitz-Keene, G., Richman, D., and Roth, R. (1974) *Madness Network News Reader.* San Francisco, CA: Glide Publications.

Interagency Council on the Homeless (1992) *Outcasts on Main Street: Report of the Federal Task Force on Homelessness and Severe Mental Illness.* Rockville, MD: National Institute of Mental Health.

Killilea, M. (1976) Mutual help organizations: interpretations in the literature. In Caplan, G., Killilea, M. (eds.), *Support Systems and Mutual Help: Multidisciplinary Explorations.* New York: Grune and Stratton.

Kopolow, L.E. (1979) Consumer demands in mental health care. *International Journal of Law and Psychiatry,* 2:263–270.

Lynch, M.M., and Kruzich, J.M. (1986) Needs assessment of the chronically mentally ill: practitioner and client perspectives. *Administration in Mental Health,* 4:237–248.

McHugh, P.R. (1992) Psychiatric Misadventures. *American Scholar,* 61:497–510.

Mitchell, J.E., Pyle, R.L., and Hatsukami, D. (1983) A comparative analysis of psychiatric problems listed by patients and physicians. *Hospital and Community Psychiatry,* 34: 848–849.

Mowbray, C.T., and Tan, C. (1993) Consumer operated drop-in centers: evaluation of operations and impact. *The Journal of Mental Health Administration,* 20:8–19.

NASMHPD (National Association of State Mental Health Program Directors) (1989) *Position Paper on Consumer Contributions to Mental Health Service Delivery Systems.* Alexandria, Virginia: NASMHPD.

NASMHPD (National Association of State Mental Health Program Directors) (1993) *Putting their money where their mouths are: SMHA support of consumer and family run programs.* Study #92-720. Alexandria, Virginia: NASMHPD.

Nikkel, R.E., Smith, G., and Edwards, D. (1992) A consumer-operated case management project. *Hospital and Community Psychiatry,* 43:577–579.

Parrish, J. (1989) The long journey home: accomplishing the mission of the community support movement. *Psychosocial Rehabilitation Journal,* 12:107–124.

Ross, C. (1980) Development of constituencies and their organizations: public policy formulation at the national level. In *Changing Public Policies of the Mentally Disabled.* Proceedings of the First Annual Fogarty Memorial Conference. Newport, Rhode Island: Ballinger Publishing Co.

Shelton, R., and Rissmeyer, D. (1989) Involving consumers in the discharge process. *Psychosocial Rehabilitation Journal,* 12:19–28.

Silverman, P.R. (1966) Services for the widowed during the period of bereavement. In *Social Work Practice.* New York: Columbia University Press.

Silverman, P.R. (1980) *Mutual Help Groups: Organization and Development.* Beverly Hills, CA: Sage.

Specht, D. (1988) *Highlights of the Findings of a National Survey on State Support of Consumer/Ex-patient Activities.* Holyoke, MA: Human Resource Association of the Northeast.

Steinwachs, D.M., Kasper, J.D., and Skinner, E.A. (1992) Patterns of use and costs among severely mentally ill people. *Health Affairs,* 11(3):178–185.

Stroul, B. (1986) *Models of Community Support Services: Approaches to Helping Persons with Long Term Mental Illness.* Rockville, MD: National Institute of Mental Health Community Support Program.

Torrey, E.F., Flynn, L., and Wolfe, S. (1990) *Care of the Seriously Mentally Ill.* Washington, D.C.: NAMI/The Public Health Research Group.

Torrey, E.F., Flynn, L. and Wolfe, S. (1992) *Criminalizing the Seriously Mentally Ill.* Washington, D.C.: NAMI/The Public Health Research Group.

Utah Alliance for the Mentally Ill (1989) Unpublished report of Mental Illness Awareness Week survey.

Van Tosh, L. (1993) *Working for a Change: Employment of Consumers/Survivors in the Design and Provision of Services for Persons Who Are Homeless and Mentally Disabled.* Rockville, Maryland: Center for Mental Health Services.

Warner, R., and Polak, P. (1993) *An Economic Development Approach to the Mentally Ill in the Community.* Rockville, MD: National Institute of Mental Health.

White, B.J., and Madera, E.J. (1992) *The Self-Help Sourcebook: Finding and Forming Mutual and Self-Help Groups.* New Jersey: St. Clares-Riverside Medical Center.

Zinman, S., Harp, H., and Budd, S. (1987) *Reaching Across.* Sacramento, CA: California Network of Mental Health Clients.

13

The Mental Health System and the Law

JEFFREY S. JANOFSKY

Perhaps more than any other field within psychiatry, community psychiatry relates closely to the law and the courts in a number of ways. Public programs receive their mandate from legislated governmental policies, which are in turn strongly influenced by the actions of the courts. The care of psychiatric patients has traditionally been accepted as a public responsibility. Public laws are invoked to provide for psychiatric care, to regulate the manner in which it is provided, and to protect the interests and rights of those who receive care. The disturbed behavior of psychiatric patients may cause them to commit antisocial or criminal acts. Every modern country addresses these issues within its system of laws. This chapter deals with United States law in relation to the mentally ill, but it will be found that, while details may vary, at least within the English-speaking nations the underlying principles are similar everywhere.

The Role of the Legislatures and Courts in Deinstitutionalization

Before 1946 the responsibility for treatment of the mentally ill resided with the states, and most patients with chronic mental disorders were treated at large state hospitals (Grob, 1991). The passage of the National Mental Health Act[1] in that year ended this federal inactivity. The Act, among other provisions, made grants to states to assist the establishment of treatment and evaluation centers dealing with the diagnosis, treatment, and prevention of psychiatric disorders. Funding for inpatient institutional care and treatment was specifically excluded. The modern community psychiatry movement was thus legislatively born. In 1954 the momentum for legislative action switched back to the states when New York passed the Community Mental Health Services Act. The state would reimburse localities for the provision of, among others, outpatient psychiatric clinics. Other states soon followed, and by 1967, 27 states had passed community mental health legislation (Blain, 1975). In 1956, for the first time in the twentieth century, public mental hospital populations began to shrink rather than grow. That same year, Title V of the Health Amendments Act of 1956 allocated seed money for pilot projects to improve outpatient mental health care.[2] With the passage of Title II of the Community Mental Health Centers Act in 1963, the federal government for the first time provided funds both for capital costs and for direct funding of outpatient mental health services.[3]

With the passage of these federal and state laws it was expected that the Community Mental Health Centers would facilitate discharge from state hospitals and reintegrate chronically institutionalized psychiatric patients into the community. Unfortunately, as one critic pointed out, by 1975 "only 10 percent of all patients seen at Community Mental Health Centers were diagnosed as schizophrenic" (Torrey, 1983). Schizophrenia was the leading chronic mental disorder on inpatient state psychiatric wards.

A series of court decisions contributed to correcting this imbalance, shifting the emphasis for public sector treatment of the seriously mentally ill to outpatient care, and indirectly increasing the percentage of patients with major mental illness treated in CMHCs. In *Lake v Cameron*[4] in the U.S. Court of Appeals for the District of Columbia, Judge Bazelon ruled that the state should "bear the burden of exploration of possible alternatives to commitment" as a requirement for a legally valid civil commitment statute. In 1974, this obligation was further amplified in *Lessard v Schmidt*[5] when Wisconsin's involuntary civil commitment statute was adjudicated unconstitutional, in part because it failed to "require those seeking commitment to consider less restrictive alternatives to commitment." These alternatives included "voluntary court-ordered outpatient treatment" among other treatments.

Another major milestone that affected community mental health treatment occurred in 1972 when for the first time a U.S. Federal court found a constitutional right to treatment for committed inpatients in state facilities. *Wyatt v Stickney*[6] originated as a class action suit on behalf of involuntarily committed patients at Bryce State Hospital in Tuscaloosa, Alabama. The Federal court found that Alabama's failure to provide minimal inpatient treatment was a violation of the Fourteenth Amendment to the United States Constitution. The Court appended a detailed appendix in its opinion enumerating "minimal Constitutional standards for adequate treatment of the mentally ill." The Alabama State Hospital system was eventually placed in receivership, and a Federal master was appointed to spend the money required for these minimal standards to be attained. One of these standards in *Wyatt* was the right of involuntarily committed patients to be placed in "the least restrictive condition necessary to achieve the purposes of commitment."

While the above referenced cases referred specifically to involuntarily committed inpatients, they are all vitally important to the CMHC movement. They established the legal basis for moving the focus of care whenever possible out of restrictive hospitals. Outpatient treatment in a CMHC has frequently been argued to be the least restrictive alternative for patients with chronic mental illness, and states thus came under increased pressure to provide this alternative.

Competency, Informed Consent, and Advance Directives

Competency

In community mental health settings with their high prevalence of very ill patients, a correspondingly high risk exists that patients' ability to make rational and reasoned decisions regarding their own health care will be impaired. Mere refusal of recommended treatment, however, does not make a patient incompetent. The Supreme Court in *Cruzan v Director, Missouri Department of Health* declared that the United States Constitution provides "that a competent person has a constitutionally protected liberty interest in refusing unwanted medical treatment. . . ."[7] All adult patients are presumed competent to make medical treatment decisions for themselves. In this respect, mentally ill persons are not different, in the eyes of the law. Particularly in the light of the assertive and intensive approaches increasingly employed in community mental health practice, psychiatrists must be aware of the complex issues involved.

While technically *competency* is a legal term, and only a judge can declare a patient legally incompetent, physicians frequently assess patients' capacity to make informed decisions about their health care. This capacity is often termed *clinical competency* or *medical capacity*. In the present discussion, the terms *competence* and *competency* are used to refer to such clinical capacity as assessed by physicians, rather than to a legal status pronounced by a judge. Questions about a patient's competence usually arise in the clinical setting when the patient, health care provider, and family cannot agree on the best course of action. In this situation, the health care provider's first responsibility is to clarify the nature of the problem, for it may not be one of competency at all. In the process of clarification, the health care provider should think clinically before thinking legally. Thinking clinically often reveals that what appears to be a problem in competency is actually a problem in communication (e.g., the patient or family does not understand the patient's fears) or a problem in relationships (e.g., the health care provider has slighted the patient, whose response is to frustrate the health care provider's efforts; a disagreement between the patient and family has more to do with preexisting quarrels than with the patient's current medical situation). In most cases, members of the treatment team are able to recognize and address such issues; if resolution of the problem proves difficult, consultation with a forensic psychiatrist may be useful.

Even when it is clear that the patient's competence to make medical decisions is impaired, health care providers should still first think clinically. This is important because the first question to be answered in the assessment of competence is: "Competent to do what?" While there are many types of competency defined by law including competency to be executed, the community mental health care provider will usually be asked to assess a patient's capacity to give consent to medical treatment.

Informed Consent

Since the early twentieth century American physicians have had to ask their adult patient's permission before proceeding with a medical or surgical procedure. In 1914, Judge Cardoza wrote in *Schloendorff*, "every human being of adult years and sound mind has a right to determine what shall be done with his own body, and a surgeon who performs an operation without his patient's consent . . . is liable in damages."[8] Under *Schloendorff*, however, physicians merely needed to ask their patient's permission to proceed, and had no duty to explain the procedure in detail. It was not until the end of World War II and the Nazi doctors' war crime trials that the doctrine of *informed* consent began to evolve, first in human subjects research and then in clinical care. The Nuremberg Military Tribunal held that:

> The voluntary consent of the human subject is absolutely essential. This means that the person involved should have the legal capacity to give consent; should be so situated as to be able to exercise free power of choice without the intrusion of any element of force, fraud, deceit, duress, over-reaching or other coercion; and should have sufficient knowledge and comprehension of the elements of the subject matter involved as to enable him to make an understanding and enlightened decision.[9]

The modern doctrine of informed consent has come to mean that a patient's consent to a medical procedure must be knowing, competent, and voluntary. The patient must be presented with and understand what the physician intends to do, and what are the risks, benefits, and alternatives. At first physicians were obligated to communicate as much data about the proposed treatment as was the normal standard of professional practice among other physicians.[10] Since 1972, in some jurisdictions, physicians have been obligated to disclose what a hypothetical, reasonable patient would find necessary to make an adequate informed decision.[11] A patient may well have the capacity to understand and decide about a straightforward, safe, minor treatment, but not a complex, risky, major one. Judgments about competence are therefore made in a context that includes not only the patient's mental state, but also the nature of the decision to be made.

Whenever the assessment of incompetence is undertaken, a thorough history is required, as is examination of the patient's mental state. The goal here is to document phenomena (e.g., coma, delusions, hallucinations, dementia) that might affect the patient's capacity to make the decision in question. A quantitative test of cognitive functioning, such as the Mini-Mental State Exam (Folstein et al., 1975) should be part of this evaluation. Several commentators have suggested that the clinical evaluation of competency to give informed consent should also include an assessment of whether the patient:

1. actually evidences a choice;
2. evidences a choice with a reasonable outcome;
3. has a factual understanding of the proposed treatment, including its benefits, risks, and alternatives;

4. applies rational reasoning; and
5. appreciates the consequences of the decision.

(Roth et al., 1977; Appelbaum and Roth, 1982). On the basis of these data, the psychiatrist makes a judgment as to the person's competence to make the specific decision regarding psychiatric treatment.

In the CMHC setting serious illness may frequently interfere with patients' ability to make rational and reasoned decisions regarding their own health care. Such patients may be truly clinically incompetent. In the absence of evidence of dangerousness, which would permit use of involuntary treatment procedures, mental health care providers have five choices:

1. Take no action until the patient returns to competency. Such a course is most useful when the patient is suffering from a disorder that waxes and wanes, like bipolar disorder, and the patient is not a danger to himself or others.
2. Physically force the patient to take the treatment without consent. This course is only legally and ethically permissible when an acute emergency exists. It is seldom applicable in the outpatient setting and generally requires that a patient be transported to an emergency facility.
3. Petition the court to appoint a guardian to make treatment decisions for an incompetent patient. The appointment of a guardian is both time-consuming and expensive, but assures that an incompetent patient's rights are protected. At a guardianship hearing mental health workers may be asked to give their opinion regarding the patient's diagnosis and ability to make rational decisions regarding treatment, and about the risks, benefits, and alternatives of the treatment being proposed.
4. Some jurisdictions may allow health care providers to use less formal means by allowing a substituted decision maker to act on behalf of patients who are clinically assessed as unable to make informed health care decisions. The applicability of such substituted decisions statutes varies widely from jurisdiction to jurisdiction, and appropriate legal advice should be obtained before attempting their use.
5. If the patient has a previously appointed guardian of the person or a previously appointed health care agent under an advance directive, the health care provider should read the guardianship or advance directive document to see if it allows the guardian or health care agent to consent in place of the incompetent patient. Consultation with an attorney may be useful when the document is ambiguous.

The *Cruzan* decision also makes it clear that different states may set different standards as to how a substituted decision maker should exercise medical decision-making for an incompetent patient. Some states have chosen a "subjective standard" where the substitute decision maker reflects what the incompetent patient would have done under the same situation had he or she been competent. Other states use an objective "best interest" standard allowing the substitute decision maker to make decisions about treatment based on what most people would decide in a similar situation. Still other states use a combination of both standards.

Advance Directives

Advance directives, also called durable powers of attorney for health care, are legally binding documents that allow competent patients to document which medical procedures they would want to have done should they become incompetent in the future. Two general types of advance directives exist: instruction directives and proxy directives. Instruction directives allow competent patients to tell their doctors, and the world in general, what their health care choices are, should they not be able to make those choices clear in the future. Proxy directives designate a third party to make treatment decisions on a patient's behalf should the patient become incompetent at some point in the future. Proxy directives can be very general, giving the third party total discretion, or, when combined with an instruction directive, limited by the caveats in the instruction directive.

Given the Supreme Court's *Cruzan* decision, it is imperative that patients make advance directives regarding future medical treatment before they become unable to make such decisions for themselves. This is particularly true in the community mental health setting where patients may either have waxing and waning illnesses, like bipolar disorder, or chronically progressive illnesses, like dementia. Thomas Szasz, an "anti-psychiatrist" and an opponent of involuntary treatment, proposed that advance directives be used by currently competent psychiatric patients to resist involuntary treatment (Szasz, 1982). Other commentators have noted that advance directives could be used by a currently competent patient to request psychiatric treatment that the patient might refuse if symptomatic (Appelbaum, 1991). While no state has specifically legislated a psychiatric advance directive for these purposes, at least two states, New York[12] and Maryland,[13] have passed authorizing statutes for medical advance directives that are written broadly enough to include psychiatric advance directives.

Discussion with a patient about advance directive options gives the mental health care provider further opportunity to clarify aspects of treatment and to maximize the patient's autonomy. Even if the patient chooses not to write an advance directive, the discussion itself may aid the treatment alliance.

Voluntary Hospitalization and Treatment

For the past 30 years, psychiatrists have attempted to maximize voluntary admissions to psychiatric hospitals and minimize involuntary admissions. They have done this by attempting to persuade patients who initially refused psychiatric hospitalization to come into the hospital voluntarily. They have also maximized voluntary admission by allowing patients who may not have been fully capable of making an informed decision about admission to sign in voluntarily if that patient gave no indication of being unwilling to be a patient in the hospital. That is, psychiatrists have allowed patients to *assent* to be voluntary patients when they may not have been competent to give *fully informed consent* to hospitalization as voluntary patients.

The 1990 Supreme Court case *Zinermon v Burch*[14] calls this practice into question. David Burch, later diagnosed as suffering from paranoid schizophrenia, was found wandering along a Florida highway, bruised, bloody, and disoriented. He was taken to a mental health center, where he was found to be hallucinated and confused. He thought he was in heaven. Florida law requires that a voluntary patient must make application by "express and informed consent." Burch signed in voluntarily to the center and then 3 days later signed in voluntarily to a state hospital. There was no inquiry as to his competence made at either facility. Burch remained hospitalized for 5 months without a review of his voluntary status. He later sued, claiming that he was not competent to sign in voluntarily to the hospital. His suit was dismissed at the trial court level. Burch appealed and his case was subsequently heard by the U.S. Supreme Court. The Supreme Court decided the case on a technical legal issue unrelated to the issue of voluntary psychiatric hospitalization. However, the court commented that by not formally assessing Burch's competency to be admitted voluntarily to a psychiatric hospital, the state deprived Burch of a substantial liberty interest.

The decision in *Zinermon* means that, at least in states whose voluntary admission statutes require an assessment of competency, patients must be assessed for their capacity to understand the voluntary admission process before being admitted voluntarily. If the patient lacks the capacity to make an informed decision about voluntary hospitalization and meets the legal criteria for involuntary hospitalization, then the patient should be admitted involuntarily. It is unclear, however, how nondangerous patients who assent but lack the capacity to give informed consent to voluntary admission should be handled. A state's guardianship or substituted consent procedure could be used, but some states specifically exclude psychiatric admission from guardianship or substituted consent statutes. An attorney familiar with local mental health care law should be consulted.

The Right to Refuse Anti-Psychotic Medications

The doctrine of informed consent has governed the parameters of the physician-patient relationship when a physician suggests that a patient begin a new treatment. Voluntary psychiatric inpatients and outpatients have always had the same rights, at least in theory (Appelbaum, 1988). Prior to the 1970s, however, involuntary psychiatric inpatients were thought to have no right to refuse anti-psychotic medications or other treatments, and their competency to refuse based on informed consent criteria was not even assessed. This made logical sense at a time when involuntary commitment laws were based solely on the presence of a mental disorder and a need for treatment. It would have been illogical for patients to be able to refuse the very treatments that could help them improve and be discharged from hospital. When involuntary civil commitment statutes began to be rewritten in the 1970s to require a showing of dangerousness rather than a need for treatment, however, it could logically be argued that states had to show some additional reason why the patient should be forced to take medication.

In 1975 Massachusetts, under the *Rogers* decision, became the first state to prohibit forced anti-psychotic treatment of involuntarily committed patients, except in emergencies, without specific procedural safeguards.[15,16] *Rogers* held that refusal can only be overridden at a procedurally rigorous judicial hearing where a patient's clinical competency is determined. If the patient is found incompetent, the judge decides whether, if competent, the patient would have accepted the treatment. If the patient is found competent, or if the judge decides an incompetent patient would, if competent, have refused the treatment anyway, the patient is allowed to continue to refuse medication.

Hoge and colleagues prospectively studied a large sample of psychiatric patients in Massachusetts who had refused anti-psychotic medication (Hoge et al., 1990). Medication-refusing patients were found to be significantly more psychiatrically ill than non-refusing control patients, and to not have had a corresponding anti-Parkinsonian drug prescribed (presumably resulting in uncomfortable extrapyramidal side effects). Patients who refused had almost a doubling of hospital length of stay and were significantly more likely to be secluded, to require restraint, or to engage in more assaultive and threatening behavior than non-refusing patients. Most patients who initially refused anti-psychotic medication finally agreed to accept medications voluntarily, and 23 percent of patients who refused had medications discontinued by their doctors. Only 18 percent of patients eventually reached a final judicial review, and *all* patients who did were ordered by the judge to take medication.

Since the *Rogers* decision in Massachusetts, different states have adopted widely varying methods to address procedurally how involuntarily committed patients should be allowed to refuse psychiatric treatment. Some states have chosen to follow the *Rogers* rights-driven model, while other states have adopted a more treatment-driven clinical review panel model in which an independent clinical panel addresses the appropriateness of the prescribed medication without addressing competency at all (Appelbaum, 1988).

Confidentiality and the Duty to Warn

General Principles

Psychiatric patients have traditionally assumed that whatever they told a mental health care provider in therapy would be kept confidential. Jerome S. Beigler, M.D., the then Chair of The American Psychiatric Association's Committee on Confidentiality, observed, "As asepsis is to surgery, so is confidentiality to psychiatry."[17] Over the years, however, the position of absolute confidentiality in psychotherapy has eroded because of the underlying tension between a patient's right to confidentiality and the state's need to protect the general community welfare.

To fully understand this area, one must first understand the difference between *confidentiality* and *privileged communications.* Confidentiality is most generally de-fined as the right of an individual to have communications that are imparted in con-fidence, not to be revealed to a third party. It is derived from the underlying ethical code of medicine and the more recently defined constitutional right to privacy. The concept of privileged communications is a narrow offshoot of the right to confiden-tiality. Privileged communication applies *only* in judicial settings, such as courtrooms, and the extent of privilege is limited by law. An individual (patient) has a testimonial privilege when he has the right to bar another person (mental health professional) from testifying in court based on information that person has gained from contact with him. Different jurisdictions have different laws regarding whose communications are privileged. In some jurisdictions, for example, communications with physicians in general are privileged. In other jurisdictions communications with psychiatrists and other mental health professionals are privileged, but not communications with other physicians and health professionals. Some jurisdictions have no health care provider privilege statute at all. Finally, there are many exceptions to privilege statutes, and the trial judge is the final arbiter of whether privilege applies in a partic-ular case.

A mental health professional's first indication that a third party wants the patient's record may be when the mental health professional is served with a subpoena re-questing the patient's records or even requesting the therapist's presence in court. Even if the therapist feels the patient's treatment may be privileged, the subpoena should *not* be ignored. Contact the patient to see if the patient is represented by his own attorney. If so contact the patient's attorney and discuss the matter. The attorney may decide it is in the patient's best *legal* interest for the patient to waive testimonial privilege and for the therapist to testify on the patient's behalf (remember the testi-monial privilege is the patient's, and the patient may choose to waive the privilege when it is in his own best interest). Before agreeing to do so, the therapist should decide whether it is in the patient's best *clinical* interest to provide such testimony. If the patient's clinical and legal interests diverge, then the therapist should meet with the patient and his attorney to discuss the risk and benefits of the therapist's providing testimony. If the patient does not have an attorney, then the CMHC attorney should be contacted to help the patient assert testimonial privilege.

While the above analysis applies to facts that the patient tells a therapist in treat-ment and to clinical diagnostic and treatment opinions, it does not force the therapist to perform evaluative services or answer legal questions that are not a part of ongoing treatment. For example, a therapist may be asked or even ordered by the court or an administrative agency to answer a question regarding a patient's ability to act as a parent (in a custody matter) or a patient's criminal responsibility at the time of a prior crime. If such issues are not related to the patient's current treatment, the therapist has every right not to perform such evaluative services and should never do so if such an evaluation would interfere with ongoing treatment. The correct response would be to inform the court that the therapist does not have an opinion on the matter in question "to a reasonable degree of medical certainty [probability]."

Specific Exceptions

While, in general, mental health professionals have a duty to keep what their patients tell them confidential and to use that information only in the best interests of the patient, in most jurisdictions mental health professionals now have an affirmative duty to *breach* confidentiality in two specific situations: (1) when there is suspected child abuse, and (2) when the patient threatens to harm another person.

All states now require mental health professionals, when acting in a professional capacity, to report patients to a designated state agency if they believe that patient is physically or sexually abusing a child (Malia, 1990). This trend in the law does protect children, but creates major problems for the treatment of patients with the diagnosis of pedophilia. Self-referrals to one clinic that treated paraphilia dropped to zero after a mandatory reporting law was passed in Maryland (Berlin et al., 1991). Mental health workers in community psychiatry should be sensitive to this issue. It is important to inform patients as soon as the issue of possible child abuse comes up in treatment that the therapist has an affirmative duty to breach confidentiality should the patient admit to harming a child. This is especially important as most patients expect absolute confidentiality in the mental health setting and may not be aware of the provider's duty to breach confidentiality under certain circumstances.

Mental health professionals have always had a duty to take action to prevent their patients from harming themselves or others. Traditionally, if mental health care providers failed in this duty, the mental health care provider could be sued for malpractice by the patient. Prior to the 1970s, however, mental health care providers owed no duty to third-party victims injured by their outpatients. This changed in 1974 after the case of *Tarasoff v Regents of University of California*[18] was decided. After several appeals, the *Tarasoff* case established that physicians and psychologists in California owed a duty to protect potential victims injured by their patients, and that physicians or psychologists who failed in this duty could be sued by the victim. The court in *Tarasoff* ruled that ''the public policy favoring protection of the confidential character of patient-psychotherapist communications must yield to the extent to which disclosure is essential to avert danger to others. The protective privilege ends where the public peril begins.''[19] This radical change in liability for physicians and psychologists caused tremors throughout the health care community. While originally only applicable to California physicians and psychologists, the *Tarasoff* doctrine of duty to third parties has been accepted by many other jurisdictions in the United States in various forms either through judge-made law or through specific statute. It has been specifically extended to psychotherapists in general in at least one jurisdiction.[20] Some states have limited mental health care providers' duty to specific, foreseeable, or identifiable victims.[21] Other jurisdictions have vastly broadened the duty to include either a psychiatric patient's unintentional harm done to another[22] or to the public in general when a therapist knew or should have known of a patient's dangerous propensities.[23] At least one other state, Ohio, imposes no *Tarasoff* duty at all.[24] It is vital that community mental health workers be aware of their legal duty to their patients' potential victims in the jurisdiction where they work.

Again, community mental health workers should think clinically before thinking legally. Good clinical practice—including a thorough clinical assessment of the patient, obtaining consultation when necessary, and selecting, implementing, and documenting a clinical course of action—will solve most *Tarasoff* problems without resorting to legal consultation. Appropriate clinical assessment includes taking a thorough history and mental status examination, assessing the reasons for the patient's violent thoughts or behavior and what specific victim or victims the patient threatens to harm, and collecting data from as many outside informants as possible. Clinical interventions may include changing the patient's medications, changing the type of therapy by involving the family members or possibly the intended victim in the treatment, hospitalizing the patient, or notifying the intended victim and/or the police of the patient's threats. Most important, the mental health care provider should clearly document this assessment and intervention process and the specific reasoning that supports that clinical decision.

Based on population data alone, the best predictor of general future violent behavior in both mentally ill and non–mentally ill populations is a past history of violent behavior. Attempts to link the presence of mental disorders in general, or specific mental disorders such as schizophrenia, with increased risk of violent behavior in populations are inconclusive (Monahan and Steadman, 1983; Cirincione et al., 1992). Recent preliminary epidemiological work, however, has demonstrated a positive relationship between the presence of "thought/control-override symptoms" (thought insertion, paranoid, and thought transference delusions) and assaultive behavior toward others (Link and Stueve, 1994). Thought/control-override delusions were felt to be better predictors of violence than other psychotic symptoms alone.

The clinician, however, is not attempting to predict the population risk of violent behavior in general, but rather whether a specific patient will or will not commit a future violent act. Jurisdictions with *Tarasoff* duties that limit clinicians' duty to predict their patients' future violent behavior to situations where the patient threatens a specific or reasonably foreseeable victim acknowledge the difficulty mental health professionals have in accurately predicting their patients' future violent acts. Jurisdictions that would impose a higher legal duty for physicians to protect the world in general from their patients' future violent actions ask the clinician to perform what may be an impossible task.

Negligence and Community Practice

Criminal law asks to what extent, if any, has the defendant injured society and what sentence, if any, is necessary to *punish* the defendant. In contrast civil law asks to what extent, if any, has the defendant injured the plaintiff and what remedies, if any, are appropriate to *compensate* the plaintiff for his loss. Negligence, a specific type of civil law action, occurs when a person unintentionally causes harm to another when certain specific conditions are met. A person is guilty of committing a negligent act when that person *d*eviates from a *d*uty which *d*irectly causes *d*amages (the four *d*'s of negligence). Malpractice is an example of a specific type of negligence where a health care provider, who owes a duty of good care to a patient, breaches that duty, causing the patient harm. To prove malpractice the patient must show that the patient entered treatment with the health care provider, therefore establishing a duty of care. The patient must then prove the provider deviated from that duty by showing that the provider did not follow the established standard of care. The patient must then prove that this deviation directly caused the patient's damages and then must quantify those damages, which can include physical or psychological injury, lost wages, lost property, or pain and suffering.

There is little hard reliable data regarding types of malpractice actions against psychiatrists. In community settings, providers who treat many patients on antipsychotic medications are perhaps more vulnerable than other psychiatrists to claims of malpractice alleging failure to give adequate informed consent for neuroleptic medication resulting in tardive dyskinesia. The doctrine of informed consent has already been generally explained. Claims of negligent failure to obtain informed consent for neuroleptic use begin by alleging that the physician failed to inform the patient adequately of the risks, benefits, and alternatives of neuroleptic therapy. The patient may allege that although the information was given, the patient was not capable of understanding it. Finally, the patient might contend that the consent obtained was not voluntary.

To inform the patient fully, the physician must be aware of the latest data available regarding the association between tardive dyskinesia and neuroleptic use. The American Psychiatric Association's 1992 Task Force Report on tardive dyskinesia thoroughly reviews these issues and makes the following recommendations:

1. Review indications for neuroleptic drugs and consider alternative treatments when available.
2. Educate the patient and his or her family regarding benefits and risks. Obtain informed consent for long-term treatment, and document it in the medical record.
3. Establish objective evidence of the benefit from neuroleptics, and review it periodically (at least every 3–6 months) to determine ongoing need and benefit.
4. Utilize the minimum effective dosage for chronic treatment.
5. Exercise particular caution with children, the elderly, and patients with affective disorders.
6. Examine the patient regularly for early signs of dyskinesia, and note them in the medical record.
7. If dyskinesia does occur, consider an alternative neurologic diagnosis.
8. If presumptive tardive dyskinesia is present, reevaluate the indications for

continued neuroleptic treatment and obtain informed consent from the patient regarding continuing or discontinuing neuroleptic treatment.

9. If a neuroleptic is continued, attempt to lower the dosage.

10. If dyskinesia worsens, consider discontinuing the neuroleptic or switching to a new neuroleptic. At present, clozapine may hold some promise in this regard, but it is important to stay alert to new research findings.

11. Many cases of dyskinesia will improve and even remit with neuroleptic discontinuation or dosage reduction. If treatment for tardive dyskinesia is indicated, utilize more benign agents first (e.g., benzodiazepines and tocopherol), but keep abreast of new treatment developments.

12. If movement disorder is severe or disabling, consider obtaining a second opinion.

Community Psychiatry and the Criminal Justice System

Deinstitutionalization and the changes in civil commitment standards that have made it more difficult to involuntarily hospitalize patients have sometimes resulted in a revolving door between community services, inpatient psychiatric units, and jails. Civil commitment laws based on the police powers theory, which requires a patient be dangerous to self or others before involuntary hospitalization can be initiated, have virtually usurped the prior civil commitment standard based solely on a patient's "need for treatment" as defined by a mental health professional. Thus, chronically mentally ill patients may become noncompliant with outpatient treatments and medication, leading to relapse. At that point they may not be dangerous to themselves or others and thus not meet modern civil commitment criteria. In some cases, when the patient's symptoms manifest themselves in antisocial behavior, the patient may be incarcerated for petty crimes. Formerly many of these patients might have been hospitalized rather than incarcerated. Thus, community psychiatry interacts more frequently than ever before with the criminal justice system.

Patients who are arrested may avail themselves of the insanity plea or other defenses based on lack of mental capacity. A psychiatrist may be asked to provide records or even to testify at the hearing where criminal responsibility will be determined. Patients who are adjudicated insane or not criminally responsible may be released, after a period of hospitalization, to the community. Many such patients will be conditionally released with stipulations that they maintain psychiatric treatment, refrain from using alcohol or illicit drugs, and take prescribed medications (Bloom et al., 1991). Alternatively, patients who are arrested may plead guilty and receive "psychiatric probation." In this alternative patients charged, usually with minor crimes, either plead or are found guilty and are given probation while serving minimal or no jail time, with the special condition that the patient must accept psychiatric treatment and recommended medications.

Treating insanity acquitees on conditional release or patients on "psychiatric probation" places mental health workers in the unfamiliar position of acting as both an agent for the patient and an agent for the state. It is vital for every professional worker in this situation to explore such agency issues with their patients. If a patient has previously been found to be not guilty by reason of insanity, and has now been released for outpatient treatment, or alternatively if a patient has been referred for "psychiatric probation," the mental health worker should explore the limits of confidentiality with the patient before collecting data or beginning treatment. The patient who has been referred by the courts must understand that anything mentioned in treatment might be revealed to a third party. At the same time, the mental health professional should make it equally clear that an attempt will be made to maintain confidentiality in the therapeutic relationship as much as possible, and that confidentiality will only be breached when required by the court conditions mandating treatment. For example, a mental health professional might be mandated under a probation or conditional release agreement to report whether a patient is coming to treatment, taking prescribed medications, or using illicit drugs or alcohol, but not mandated to reveal other aspects of treatment to any third party.

Psychiatric Impairment and Disability

Mental health care providers are frequently asked by various state and federal agencies to provide assessments of their patient's mental disorder and ability to work. These assessments are required before patients may receive funding through state and federal entitlement programs.

To be effective in assisting their patients in this area, mental health care providers must understand the language used in these settings. *Impairment* is defined as an alteration of an individual's health status that is assessed by medical means. *Disability* is defined as an alteration of an individual's capacity to meet personal, occupational, or social demands or to meet statutory or regulatory requirements. Disability is assessed by non-medical means. The evaluation of impairment for all medical specialties has been formalized in the *Guides for the Evaluation of Permanent Impairment, 4th edition* (American Medical Association, 1993). Impairment in a functional area does not necessarily amount to a disability, however. For example, consider two patients, each with a 100 percent impairment of the little finger of the left hand. If one patient is a laborer, his level of disability, that is, his inability to carry out his job with his impairment, will be zero. However, if the other patient is a concert pianist, that same impairment will cause total disability.

Unfortunately, the correlation between impairment and disability for psychiatric conditions is usually less clear. Medically determinable impairments in thinking, affect, intelligence, perception, judgment, and behavior can be assessed by direct observation, a formal mental status examination, and psychological testing. However, current research in psychiatry finds little relationship between psychiatric signs and symptoms and subsequent disability. Hence, for psychiatry, there is no direct link between impairment and disability. To bridge this gap, the Social Security Administration, which is responsible for management of federal entitlement programs in the

United States, has identified four areas of functional limitations that must be taken into consideration to assess the severity of psychiatric impairment (Social Security Administration, 1994). These four areas are (1) assessment of activities of daily living; (2) social functioning; (3) concentration, persistence, and pace; and (4) decompensation in work or work-like settings (failure of adaptation to stress).

To assess activities of daily living, the mental health care provider needs to assess the patient's ability in self-care and hygiene, communication, ambulation, travel, sexual function, and sleep, and to judge the quality of these activities by their independence, appropriateness, and effectiveness. To assess social functioning, the patient's capacity to interact appropriately and communicate effectively with others should be assessed. Impairment in this area is manifested by altercations, evictions, job firings, and social isolation. When a health care provider assesses a patient's concentration, persistence, and pace, the health care provider needs to note the patient's abilities to sustain focused attention long enough to permit a timely completion of tasks. It is important to point out that a patient who appears to concentrate adequately on a mental status examination or in a psychological test situation may not do so in a real-life work situation. Finally, a patient's ability to adapt to stress needs to be assessed. The patient's inability to adapt to stress is manifested by exacerbation of signs and symptoms with accompanying difficulty in maintaining activities of daily living and social functioning, or maintaining concentration, persistence, and pace in the setting of increased stress. Common stressors on the job include decision-making, attendance, scheduling, completion of tasks, and interaction with peers and others.

The mental health care provider needs to take these impairments into consideration and rate the patient's impairments on a scale ranging from nonexistent to severe. Once the mental health care provider completes the impairment rating, the evaluating agency will apply such data to that agency's definition of disability. To be disabled under Social Security criteria, for example, requires that the patient have the "inability to do any substantial activity by reason of any medically determinable physical or mental impairment which can be expected to result in death or which has lasted or can be expected to last for a continuous period of not less than twelve months."

To complete an adequate psychiatric impairment assessment, mental health care providers should take the patient's usual psychiatric history and mental status examination, emphasizing data that elucidates the four impairment points noted above. A formulation should link the patient's subjective historical statements with objective mental status exam findings. Finally, those objective findings need to be related to the impairment categories noted above.

References

American Medical Association (1993) *Guides for the Evaluation of Permanent Impairment, 4th edition.* Chicago: American Medical Association.

American Psychiatric Association: (1992) *Tardive dyskinesia: A task force report of the American Psychiatric Association.* Washington, D.C.: APA Press.

Appelbaum, P.S., and Roth, L.H. (1982) Competency to consent to research: A psychiatric overview. *Archives of General Psychiatry,* 39:951–958.

Appelbaum, P.S. (1988) The right to refuse treatment with antipsychotic medications: Retrospect and prospect. *American Journal of Psychiatry,* 145:413–419.

Appelbaum, P.S. (1991) Advance directives for psychiatric treatment. *Hospital and Community Psychiatry,* 42:983–984.

Berlin, F.S., Malin, H.M., and Dean, S. (1991) Effects of statutes requiring psychiatrists to report suspected sexual abuse of children. *American Journal of Psychiatry,* 148:449–453.

Blain, D. (1975) Twenty-five years of hospital and community psychiatry: 1945–1970. *Hospital and Community Psychiatry,* 26:605–609.

Bloom, J.D., Williams, M.H., and Bigelow, D.A. (1991) Monitored conditional release of persons found not guilty by reason of insanity. *American Journal of Psychiatry,* 148:444–448.

Cirincione, C., Steadman, H.J., Robbins, P.C., and Monahan, J. (1992) Schizophrenia as a contingent risk factor for criminal violence. *International Journal of Law and Psychiatry,* 15:347–358.

Folstein, M.F., Folstein, S.E., and McHugh, P.R. (1975) Mini-mental state: A practical method of grading the cognitive state of patients for the clinician. *Journal of Psychiatric Research,* 12:189–198.

Grob, G.N. (1991) From hospital to community: Mental health policy in modern America. *Psychiatric Quarterly,* 62:187–212.

Hoge, S.K., Appelbaum, P.S., Lawlor, T., *et al.* (1990) A prospective, multicenter study of patients' refusal of antipsychotic medication. *Archives of General Psychiatry,* 47:949–956.

Link, B.L., and Stueve, A. (1994) Psychotic symptoms and the violent/illegal behavior of mental patients compared to community controls. In Monahan, J., Steadman, H.J. (eds.), *Violence and Mental Disorder: Developments in Risk Assessment.* Chicago: University of Chicago Press.

Malia, T.R. (1990) Validity, construction, and application of statutes limiting physician-patient privilege in judicial proceedings relating to child abuse or neglect. *American Law Reports,* 44:649–667.

Monahan, J., and Steadman, H.J. (1983) Crime and mental disorder: An epidemiological approach. In Tonry, M., Morris, N. (eds.), *Crime and Justice: An annual review of research,* 4:145–189.

Roth, L.H., Meisel, A., and Lidz, C.W. (1977) Tests of competency to consent to treatment. *American Journal of Psychiatry,* 134:279–284.

Social Security Administration (1994) *Disability Evaluation Under Social Security.* SSA Publication No. 64-039.

Szasz, T.S. (1982) The psychiatric will: a new mechanism for protecting persons against "psychosis" and psychiatry. *American Psychologist,* 37:762–770.

Torrey, E.F. (1983) *Surviving Schizophrenia.* Philadelphia: Harper and Row.

Legal References

1. P.L. 79-487.
2. P.L. 84-911.
3. P.L. 88-164.

4. *Lake v Cameron*, 364 F.2d 657 (D.C. Cir. 1966).

5. *Lessard v Schmidt*, 349 F.Supp 1078 (E.D. Wis. 1972), *vacated and remanded*, 414 U.S. 473 (1974), *on remand*, 379 F.Supp. 1376 (E.D. Wis. 1974, *vacated and remanded on appeal*, 421 U.S. 957 (1975).

6. *Wyatt v Stickney*, 325 F.Supp. 781 (M.D. Ala. 1971), 344 F.Supp, 373 (M.D. Ala. 1972), *aff'd sub nom, Wyatt v Aderholt*, 503 F.2d 1305 (5th Cir, 1974).

7. *Cruzan v Director, Missouri Department of Health*, 497 U.S., 110 S. Ct. 2841, 111 L Ed 2d 224 (1990).

8. *Schloendorff v Society of New York Hospital*, 211 N.Y. 125 (1914).

9. *Trials of War Criminals Before the Nuremberg Military Tribunal*, 2:181–182, 1947.

10. *Nantanson v Kline*, 186 Kan. 393, 350 P2d 1093 (1960).

11. *Canterbury v Spence*, 150 U.S. App. D.C. 263, 464 F2d 772 (1972).

12. N.Y. Pub Health Law, Art 29-C (1991).

13. Health-General Article 5-601 to 5-618, Maryland Annotated Code.

14. *Zinermon v Burch*, 110 S.Ct. 975 (1990).

15. *Rogers v Okin*, 478 F.Supp 1342 (D. Mass., 1979).

16. *Rogers v Commissioner*, 390 Mass. 489, 458 N.E.2d 308 (1983).

17. *Citizens Privacy Protection Act: Hearings Before the Subcommittee on the Constitution of the [Senate] Committee on the Judiciary*, 95th Cong., 2d Sess. 223, 255 (1978).

18. *Tarasoff v Regents of University of California*, 13 Cal.3d 177, 118 Cal.Rptr. 129, 529 P.2d 553 (1974), reheard *en banc* 17 Cal.3d 425, 131 Cal.Rptr. 14, 551 P.2d 334 (1976).

19. *Tarasoff v Regents of University of California*, 17 Cal.3d 425 at 442, 131 Cal.Rptr. 14, 551 P.2d 334 (1976).

20. *Peck v The Counseling Service of Addison County, Inc.,* 146 Vt. 61.499 A2d 435 (1985).

21. Courts and Judicial Proceedings 5-316, Maryland Annotated Code.

22. *Peterson v State*, 100 Wash. 2d 421, 671 P2d 230 (1983) (*en banc*).

23. *Lipari v Sears*, 497 F.Supp 185 (1980).

24. Ohio Rev. Code Ann. 5122.34 (Supp 1990).

III

Methods

14

The Outpatient Clinic

GEETHA JAYARAM

This chapter describes the structure, functions, and scope of an outpatient clinic within a psychiatric service system. Over three decades the outpatient clinic has evolved from being a free-standing clinical unit to being a hub in the network of services that comprises a comprehensive psychiatric service system. Since the inception of the federal community mental health centers in the 1960s, outpatient clinics and the community mental health movement as a whole have had to adapt to changes in legislation, politics, evolving financing mechanisms and humanitarian efforts (Hadley and Culhane, 1993). They have also had to contend with major expansion of programs and staffing, and with evolving concepts in treatment of the mentally ill. In treating chronic mental illnesses, the emphasis has shifted from inpatient to outpatient settings, and cost containment has become a major objective (Greene and De La Cruz, 1981; Gallant, 1983). Rapid treatment and curtailed lengths of inpatient stay, with greater fiscal incentives to shift care and cost to the outpatient sector as rapidly as possible, is the trend everywhere, so that hospitalization is recommended only as a last resort. Community mental health centers have responded to this challenge by offering comprehensive and continuous care through an array of ambulatory services (Lewis et al., 1989).

The Clinic within a System of Care

Within the network, referrals to the outpatient clinic are received from inpatient units, emergency services, private practitioners, social service or law enforcement agencies—or individuals may be self-referred or brought by family members, friends, or neighbors. In turn, the clinic interacts with other components of the service network, such as psychosocial rehabilitation programs, vocational programs, housing committees, and home-based care providers. Together these components devise a coordinated plan of treatment and rehabilitation which is individualized for each patient and which organizes and directs care. The plan is examined and updated periodically to evaluate progress; it serves to anchor treatment and to provide a synopsis of the patient's treatment profile.

The outpatient clinic has thus developed into a treatment-provision and coordination center for most patients within the service system, and it is greatly improved in its ability to structure and manage psychopharmacological treatments, liaison activities, linkages with inpatient units, and case-management and treatment approaches that address the needs of individuals with varying degrees of disability. In addition to the universal professional goals of providing services of the highest quality, a system-oriented outpatient treatment program has additional priorities arising from its mission, embodied in the concepts of accessibility and continuity of care (Bennett and Freeman, 1991).

Accessibility

Accessibility may be considered in geographic, cultural, and financial terms. Barriers to geographic accessibility include not only distance, which is a particular problem in rural areas, but also lack of transportation. Siting an outpatient center should take into consideration the difficulties that patients will experience in traveling to their visits. Not only the existence of public transportation is important, but the frequency of services can have an impact on utilization (Breakey and Kaminsky, 1982). Cultural accessibility becomes a relevant issue when providing for services to minority groups (Adibempe, 1994) if the clinic is located in a neighborhood where they feel ill at ease. Recruiting bilingual therapists for the clinic staff improves responsiveness to the population served. Financial accessibility is a consideration in fee-for-service systems, where individuals may not have insurance to pay for treatment, or may not have cash for a co-payment, where that is required. For that reason, community programs where fees are required, but which have a mandate to serve their catchment area population, must provide some type of sliding scale of fees so that inability to pay does not present a barrier to access.

Continuity of Care

Continuity of care is generally accepted as highly important in the longitudinal treatment of a person with a chronic illness (Bachrach, 1981). Continuity of care can imply continuity of provider of care or continuity of treatment planning (Bey et al., 1972). In many cases an outpatient treatment provider has a better longitudinal perspective on the patient and the illness than anyone else who may come in contact with that person as he or she moves through the system. A case manager, likewise, maintains close contact with a client over time, but is unlikely to be as familiar with the details of the patient's medical and psychiatric history. It is important, therefore, that an outpatient clinic have mechanisms in place to ensure that when a patient enters or leaves the program there is opportunity for exchange of information with other treatment providers, assuming the patient gives consent. When a patient in the outpatient clinic is temporarily being treated elsewhere, such as in an emergency service, a crisis program, or an inpatient unit, the outpatient therapist keeps closely in touch with the treating team, providing information and insights that will assist the team and maximize continuity (Rubin, 1978).

Service Delivery

Services provided in a public sector outpatient clinic give priority to treatment and management of severely mentally ill patients whose illnesses require long-term care (Kantor et al., 1978; Sheldon, 1964) but also address the needs of community residents requiring short-term treatment for a variety of disorders. Catchment area populations differ in ethnic and socioeconomic characteristics. Treatment, however, is similar in concept, the focus being on reduction of symptoms, preventing relapses, maximizing functional capacities, and decreasing number of hospitalizations (Turner and Wan, 1993). When a chronically mentally ill patient drops out of treatment, it is the responsibility of the therapist to ensure all efforts at outreach have been made to reengage the patient in treatment, or to transfer the care to an outreach program (Lurigio and Lewis, 1989).

Intake

The process of intake is crucial to ensure smooth entry for the individual into treatment and to utilize manpower most efficiently. The intake worker in most cases provides the first interface between the clinic and the prospective patient. He or she thus has an extremely important public relations role, encouraging people to take advantage of available services, diffusing stigma, and facilitating access. The intake worker's responsibility is not only to screen all calls for service, but to prioritize care to those who need it most urgently. Thus individuals who are judged to be dangerous to themselves or others, or who require detoxification, are referred to an emergency service or admitted for inpatient treatment without delay. When outpatient treatment is most appropriate, the intake worker directs patients to the most appropriate caregiver, either another agency or an individual therapist within the clinic. The handling of intake with empathy, skill, and sensitivity requires an experienced staff member who is committed to the goals of the center, without conflicting interests.

Developing the most appropriate treatment strategies for patients depends on intake policies and protocols that streamline service delivery. Certain prospective patients may have priority, such as those about to be discharged from inpatient treatment, or homeless individuals. Other cases require special procedures. For instance, in dealing with patients referred from the criminal justice system, part of the intake procedure will be proper documentation, contact with parole or probation officers, and evaluating legal charges as they relate to illness.

The intake process balances maintaining a waiting list of patients seeking treatment with directing acutely ill patients to emergency care or for crisis outreach. Patients residing within the catchment area have priority. From time to time, the intake worker and clinic director may have to assess the pulse of the community and its changing needs: for example, whether the number of homeless patients referred is on the increase, whether emergency services for clinic patients are appropriately utilized or abused, or whether large numbers of patients are inappropriately referred to the clinic who may be better served elsewhere.

Unfortunately, according priority to the care of seriously ill populations at times deprives less ill patients of much-needed attention for disorders related to marital, occupational, family, or relational problems, or personality disorders, causing delays or diversion of such patients to other providers of treatment. Inability to afford private care may forestall their treatment elsewhere also. Non-medical clinic therapists are skilled in treating such patients and enjoy a diversity in case-mix which is important for staff retention. The clinic director must therefore assist the intake worker to regulate patient flow into the clinic to preserve balance. For in-depth reading on structuring services in a community clinic, the reader is directed to other sources (Hershorn, 1993; Rossman et al., 1979; Ruiz and Tourlentes, 1983; Tollington, 1969).

Networking and Liaison

Active liaison is essential to provide comprehensive, continuous treatment, to facilitate transfer of patients between agencies within the service system, and to coordinate changing levels of need. Specific staff members within the clinic serve as liaisons with other service components, such as inpatient units, psychosocial programs, substance abuse programs, emergency departments, and primary care physicians in the community. The clinician in charge of liaison needs to play an active role in linking the treatment organizations and should not merely pass information back and forth. An active liaison role includes continuous reassessment of system needs, troubleshooting, setting specific targets, and anticipating obstacles to integration of services. The liaison person focuses primarily on system issues, to ensure smooth collaboration, in contrast to case managers, who focus on the needs of individuals, ensuring that the system functions effectively for a specific person. Liaison efforts take place at the individual therapist's level also, in relation to treatment of his or her own patients.

Liaison between service components is particularly important in dealing with issues of co-morbidity. For example, in addressing the needs of dually diagnosed individuals with mental illness and substance dependence, cross-training of clinicians is necessary for staff members who are trained in either type of service provision but not in the other (Chapter 27). Close integration between service systems is also vital in providing general health care for psychiatric patients (Barnes et al., 1994; Chapter 20).

The Psychiatrist in the Multidisciplinary Team

The psychiatrist's role as a leader in community mental health administration has diminished. The central role of the psychiatrist as clinical leader is generally accepted, however, although boundaries between disciplines and hierarchies are less clear than formerly.

The introduction of psychotropic medications as one of the greatest advances in modern psychiatry enabled the shifting of care for schizophrenic and bipolar patients to community-based settings and ambulatory programs. Over the last two decades, as community outpatient programs have focused more specifically on the needs of more severely ill patients, the need for expertise in the treatment of major mental illnesses has been more widely appreciated and psychiatrists more actively involved (Torrey, 1986).

A primary task for the field continues to be that of defining a clear role for psychiatrists, avoiding role diffusion, establishing responsibilities for community psychiatrists that utilize all aspects of their training, underscoring the medical contributions of the discipline, and promoting team approaches with other disciplines (Ribner, 1980; Knesper, 1981). Medical hierarchies are less powerful in community mental health centers than in hospitals; the psychiatrist is indispensible and brings special skills to the team, but is a peer with members of other disciplines. He or she must therefore be flexible and bring an attitude of mutual respect, a willingness to learn from others, and an attitude of cooperation and mutual support—attributes that are assets in the private sector as much as in the public sector. Psychiatrists assume an active teaching role in disseminating medical information to their colleagues in an appropriate and acceptable manner that promotes team work. The goals are to enhance the knowledge and expertise of non-medical therapists in the clinic, promote a greater understanding of medical and psychiatric concepts and methods, increase the team's skill levels in a variety of areas, and enable them to be effective physician extenders. Clinic therapists, who may come from professional backgrounds in psychology, social work, counseling, or nursing, are primarily responsible for implementing treatment plans. Their cooperation with other staff members, willingness to be educated, and genuine interest in their patients are essential to their effective functioning. Poor team work always impacts negatively on treatment outcome.

As a leader of the clinical team, a psychiatrist must be expert in the maintenance of seriously ill patients in an ambulatory setting, sophisticated in pharmacological treatments, and creative in strategizing care to prevent relapses and rehospitalizations. The psychiatrist is often called on to educate patients about medication side-effects and to converse with family members or caretakers, who provide essential information on prodromal symptoms, responses to medications, and compliance with medication regimens. Psychiatrists must acquaint themselves with low-dose and maintenance strategies for psychotropic medications. Many outpatient clinics are expert in the management of clinic sub-populations. Psychiatrists may therefore be required to play a role in managing lithium clinics, geriatric clinics, clinics for the treatment of long-term schizophrenia, or clinics for HIV-related disorders. A physician in this setting must thus have a broad range of skills in treating several categories of patients. Both parallel models, in which psychiatrists and therapists carry individual and at times overlapping caseloads, as well as collaborative models of teamed visits, exist in clinics.

There are potential problems in collaboration among disciplines. Non-medical therapists may view their task as exclusively the provision of psychotherapy, avoiding a broader understanding of the impact of medications and medical problems in the treatment of psychiatric illness and on the process of psychotherapy also. Short-sighted psychiatrists may go along with this perception, thinking that this will protect their unique role as the medical expert. Ultimately the psychiatrist's effectiveness is enhanced, however, and his or her sphere of influence increased, by fostering the development of expert teams that can treat large numbers of patients effectively and efficiently.

Non-Medical Psychiatric Therapists

Although their specific roles may vary from clinic to clinic, good therapists in community mental health clinics bring a variety of skills to the task. They carry sizable caseloads, which nowadays consist largely of seriously mentally ill patients. Therapists are the primary clinicians for their patients and provide many services, ranging from the practice of individual psychotherapy, group therapy, substance abuse counseling, family therapy, and a variety of case management functions, to medication management under the supervision of a psychiatrist.

Managing a therapist's caseload requires balancing numbers of intakes and discharges, and skillful appointment scheduling. Besides continually evaluating need for continuity of care and frequency of visits for each patient, every therapist balances time constraints against acuity of patient needs. The more successful a therapist is in retaining chronically ill patients in treatment, the more rapidly his or her caseload becomes full. On the other hand, clinics with a service responsibility to a specific population are obligated to accept new individuals for treatment. Caseloads therefore tend to expand beyond the capacity of the therapist to provide optimal care. Supervision by the clinic's medical director is crucial and necessary to ensure that clinicians maintain a proper balance in their caseloads.

Discharge decisions are made jointly by the therapist and treating physician and require careful consideration. In situations where a patient has unilaterally ceased coming to the clinic, the therapist should offer outreach by letter or in person prior to discharge, or use a crisis outreach worker to ascertain that the patient is not ill and in need of acute intervention.

Population Focus

It is essential that the staff of a community outpatient clinic should be aware of patients' cultural identities and of their cultural reference groups. It is a generally accepted rule that the staff of the clinic should include a mix of therapists and physicians in terms of both ethnicity and sex, thereby enhancing patient comfort as well as affording better communication and greater sensitivity to the patients' personal concerns. Bilingual therapists enhance the process of treatment of language minorities, promoting access to and retention in therapy (Gaw, 1993; Chapter 11).

Quality Assurance

Certain concepts from business and industry have been brought into health care. Of these, the one that has greatest impact on cinical practice is quality assurance. The basic concept is that of self-examination for improvement of performance, but it has lent itself to some gimicry, with a proliferation of variants, such as "Quality Improvement" or "Continuous Performance Improvement" (Horn and Hopkins, 1994). Quality assurance activities are required by third-party regulatory bodies such as the state mental health administration or the Joint Commission for Accreditation of Health Care Organizations (Ruiz and Tourlentes, 1983). The American Psychiatric Association guidelines for practice in community mental health centers and the Manual of Psychiatric Quality Assurance issued by the American Psychiatric Association Committee on Quality Assurance in 1992 are available for guidance (Mattson, 1992).

The Joint Commission on Accreditation of Health Care Organizations now requires a 10-step model to be in place in outpatient programs. Their standards require that there is a clear hierarchy of responsibility and reporting. Assignment of quality assurance tasks must be ongoing. A key activity in any quality assurance program is the medical records review or audit, in which records are examined for clinical pertinence and quality, completeness, and timeliness. When accomplished at least quarterly, this procedure greatly increases awareness and quality of documentation. Audits may be performed by a committee of peers, or in rotation by all members of a center's staff. Audits should be performed using a standardized form, with appropriate feedback and a requirement for correction of deficiencies. The latter part of the audit process tends to be the weakest link in the chain, but is the most useful in accomplishing change and must not be overlooked.

Credentialing and privileging is another aspect of quality assurance, similarly performed by a committee of senior staff with the center director. The credentialing process employs standard procedures for assessing credentials and assigning privileges to perform specific procedures. Specific skills to be assessed might include group therapy, family therapy, or substance abuse treatment. The committee reviews the clinician's training and supervision records, licensing, and certification and takes into consideration continuing education requirements. Credentials need not be updated more frequently than annually.

Another aspect of quality assurance is the systematic review of incidents or clinical misadventures that occur in the clinic, for the purpose of improving methods and avoiding similar incidents. A committee of the clinical directors of the clinic, all of those involved in the clinical incident, and, if possible, an outside expert, convene to review the events, the responses of staff, and the outcome. A report is prepared, sharing any new insights or recommendations with the clinic staff.

Risk Management

Risk management involves the training of staff in avoiding those situations which might place patients at risk or which may place the clinician or the clinic itself at risk of legal liability. Staff must be informed about medico-legal matters such as the laws of confidentiality, duty to warn, issues of informed consent, the rights of patients, and involuntary committment laws. They should be skilled in dealing with threatening or violent behavior. All clinicians must be fully aware of the importance of good recordkeeping. A systematic program of education in these areas should be provided.

Program Evaluation

Program evaluation within an outpatient clinic is focused on review of organizational structure and function in order to efficiently and effectively deliver service with minimal disruption (Hargreaves and Attkisson, 1978; Schulberg, 1981). Systematic data collection is a basic first step and is generally required by regulation. Management information systems or clinical information systems are easily implemented, although ensuring that data are accurately and systematically entered is more difficult. Busy clinicians are often, for good reason, committed more to direct patient care than to "paperwork," whether it be medical records or management data. Incentives or strict supervision may help to ensure that data are submitted promptly and accurately. Computer terminals for each therapist may simplify the process and expedite data entry.

Program evaluation is not only concerned with productivity, but also with processes and outcomes of care. The evaluator must have an ability to fully appreciate clinicians' needs and should not be directly involved in patient care in order to objectively effect necessary changes through the director of the clinic. It is possible through continuous evaluation to identify limitations in service delivery, gaps in the care of specific populations, or underutilized services (Williams and Williams, 1986; Donlon and Rada, 1976).

The Limitations of Outpatient Treatment

Increasingly complex cases are being successfully managed in ambulatory settings. Nevertheless, outpatient clinics have their limitations, and in certain circumstances more intensive, supportive, or controlled approaches are needed. This situation arises (1) when outpatient medication management fails because of poor response, poor compliance, or untoward or toxic reactions; (2) when a crisis occurs in the patient's life that causes a relapse of psychotic symptoms despite energetic treatment; or (3) when a patient is dangerous or threatening to self or others.

In some cases where a person is experiencing a major relapse of an illness, inpatient treatment is the only option. The current inpatient treatment philosophy is to admit patients for brief periods of time to resolve crises only, after which patients are rapidly returned to the community support system. In some cases, additional resources can be mobilized to assist the patient and the support system to cope with the crisis without admitting the patient to hospital. Alternative approaches to dealing with crises include referral to an emergency service or a mobile crisis team and case management approaches. In the longer term, if a person is not being successfully treated in the outpatient clinic, mobile treatment services may be indicated.

Lessons for the Private Sector

Many similarities exist between privately and publicly funded clinics. With rapid changes in a competitive marketplace, and with corporatization of health care, skills necessary to manage a public sector outpatient clinic are easily transferrable to the private sector (Drucker, 1990). Both aim for cost-effective management, and increasingly both are turning to capitation funding. On one hand, financial control may be more easily maintained in a private clinic, with integrated management, fewer contentions about authority, and less disparity between clinical and administrative hierarchies. On the other hand, community mental health centers have always operated under budgetary restrictions and have consciously promoted efficiency in treatment. Today, both use the team approach to maximize efficiency. Although fewer or no demands exist in a private clinic to provide reports to public authorities, the increasing presence of managed care is acutely felt by private practitioners to have the same qualities as a burdensome bureaucracy. Accountability to the individual patient is emphasized more in a private setting; accountability to a community is at the center of public programs. Comprehensive, integrated systems of care are not yet widespread in private insurance or care management systems but are certainly possible. With profit as a primary objective for private organizations, it is doubtful whether too many will be eager to duplicate services available at community mental health centers until the proper incentives are put in place. As the private-public distinction blurs, however, private sector organizations will increasingly turn to the experience of the public sector gained from several decades of thought, experience, teamwork, and research.

Conclusion

This chapter describes current concepts in the design, function, and mission of an outpatient community mental health clinic. In the future, the corporatization of health care in the United States and the inevitable emergence of capitated systems will have significant influence on community-based care. For an outpatient clinic to survive in a fully competitive, vertically integrated system of care, it will have to have several distinguishing attributes: skilled, efficient staff; low cost, maximum coverage; and the ability to operate within fixed prospective payments as fee-for-service models disappear.

References

Adibempe, V.R. (1994) Race, racism, and epidemiological surveys. *Hospital and Community Psychiatry,* 45:27–31.

Bachrach, L. (1981) Continuity of care for chronic mental patients: a conceptual analysis. *American Journal of Psychiatry,* 138:1449–1456.

Barnes, H.N., O'Neill, S.F., Aronson, M.D., and Delbanco, T.L. (1994) Early detection and outpatient management of alcoholism: A curriculum for medical residents. *Journal of Medical Education,* 59:904–906.

Bennett, D.H., and Freeman, H.L. (1991) *Community Psychiatry.* London: Churchill Livingstone.

Bey, D.R., Chapman, R.E., and Tornquist, K.L. (1972) A lithium clinic. *American Journal of Psychiatry,* 129:468–470.

Breakey, W.R., and Kaminsky, M.J. (1982) An assessment of Jarvis' Law in an urban catchment area. *Hospital and Community Psychiatry,* 33:661–663.

Donlon, P., and Rada, R.T. (1976) Issues in developing quality aftercare clinics for the chronic mentally ill. *Community Mental Health Center Journal,* 12:29–36.

Drucker, P.L.D. (1990) *Managing the Non-Profit Organization: Principles and Practices.* New York: Harper Collins.

Gallant, D.M. (1983) Outpatient treatment: community and private practice support systems, *Journal of Clinical Psychiatry,* 44(6):15–22.

Gaw, A.C. (1993) *Culture, Ethnicity and Mental Illness.* Washington, D.C.: American Psychiatric Press.

Greene, L.R., and De La Cruz, A. (1981) Alternative to and transition from full-time hospitalization. *Community Mental Health Center Journal,* 17:191–202.

Hadley, T.R., and Culhane, D.P. (1993) The status of community mental health centers for ten years into block grant financing. *Community Mental Health Journal,* 29:95–102.

Hargreaves, W.A., and Attkisson, C.C. (1978) *Evaluation of Human Service Programs,* p. 305.

Hershorn, M. (1993) The elusive population: characteristics of attenders versus non-attenders for community mental health center intakes. *Community Mental Health Journal,* 29(1): 49–57.

Horn, A.D., and Hopkins, D.S.P. (1994) *Clinical Practice Improvement: A New Technology for Developing Cost-Effective Quality Health Care.* New York: Faulkner and Gray.

Kantor, L.E., Kaursch, D.F., and Smith, L. L. (1978) Development of an aftercare program in a non-metropolitan area. *Community Mental Health Journal,* 14:46–53.

Knesper, D.J. (1981) How psychiatrists allocate their professional time: implications for educational and manpower planning. *Hospital and Community Psychiatry,* 32:620–624.

Lewis, D.A., Shadis, W.R. Jr., and Lurigio, A.J. (1989) Policies of inclusion and the mentally ill: long-term care in a new environment. *Journal of Social Issues,* 45(3):173–186.

Lurigio, A.J., and Lewis, D.A. (1989) Worlds that fail: a longitudinal study of urban mental patients. *Journal of Social Issues,* 45(3):79–90.

Mattson, M.R. (1992) *Manual of Psychiatric Quality Assurance.* Washington, D.C.: American Psychiatric Association.

Ribner, D.S. (1980) Psychiatrists and community mental health: current issues and trends. *Hospital and Community Psychiatry,* 31:338–341.

Rossman, B.B., Hober, D.I., and Ciarlo, J.A. (1979) Awareness, use, and consequences of evaluation data in a community mental health center. *Community Mental Health Center Journal,* 15:7–16.

Rubin, A. (1978) Commitment to community mental health aftercare services: staffing and structural implications. *Community Mental Health Center Journal,* 14:199–208.

Ruiz, P., and Tourlentes, T.T. (1983) Community Mental Health Centers. In Talbott, J.A.,

Kaplan, S.R. (eds.), *Psychiatric Administration: A Comprehensive Text for the Clinician-Executive,* p. 103.

Sheldon, A. (1964) An evaluation of psychiatric after-care. *British Journal of Psychiatry,* 110: 662–667.

Schulberg, H.C. (1981) Outcome evaluations in the mental health field. *Community Mental Health Center Journal,* 17(2):132–142.

Tollinton, H.J. (1969) The organization of a psychotherapeutic community. *British Journal of Medical Psychology,* 42:271–275.

Torrey E.F. (1986) Management of chronic schizophrenic outpatients. *Psychiatric Clinics of North America,* 9(1):143–151.

Turner, J.T., and Wan, T.T.H. (1993) Recidivism and mental illness: the role of communities. *Community Mental Health Journal,* 29(1):3–14.

Williams, M.E., and Williams, T.F. (1986) Evaluation of older persons in the ambulatory setting. *Journal of the American Geriatric Society,* 34(1):37–43.

15

The Psychotherapy of Schizophrenia

MARY C. EATON

The powerful impact of psychoactive drug therapy on the course of schizophrenia has mitigated the devastation of the disease, but has often resulted in inattention to patients' psychotherapeutic needs. People with schizophrenia represent a major portion of patients treated in community mental health clinics and their illnesses are usually lifelong. Because of the severity of the illness, and the fact that combining pharmacologic with psychotherapeutic interventions produces the best outcome, the role of psychotherapy in the treatment of schizophrenia deserves attention.

Within psychiatry there has been a historical rift between medical and psychological treatment approaches. Early in the century, in the absence of other effective measures, psychotherapy was enlisted to treat a putative psychologic cause of schizophrenia. The introduction of psychotropic medications in the 1950s showed dramatic efficacy in reducing symptoms of a condition that was being increasingly appreciated as biological in origin. Psychologically oriented—especially psychoanalytically oriented—therapists, concerned not to suppress meaningful psychic material, rejected medical treatment and continued on their psychological course, while others, persuaded by psychopharmacology, embraced what was characterized as a "medical" model. Experience, however, proved what is now generally accepted, that interweaving pharmacological treatment with skilled supportive psychotherapy, provided by the psychiatrist or, more often, the non-physician therapist, best supports the patient's course.

This chapter addresses the experience of the person with schizophrenia in the era of biologic treatment and considers the place and conduct of psychotherapy in contributing to improved treatment outcome. First, however, because older psychological theories of schizophrenia have historical importance and continue to influence thinking among professionals and lay people alike, the history of treatment is briefly reviewed.

Historical Setting: Psychological Perspectives

In the late nineteenth and early twentieth centuries, Sigmund Freud's theories about the psychosexual bases of psychoses and neuroses set the stage for a psychological approach to mental disturbance. Great interest was engendered in psychological treatment with a hope that the many forms of emotional and mental suffering could be treated by psychoanalysis. In the case of schizophrenia, however, Freud considered the psychosis to be underlain by a narcissism so severe as to be untreatable by analysis. The schizophrenic individual was thought to have withdrawn libidinal attachment from the outside world, directing it inward, so that he was theoretically insufficiently connected to things or people outside himself to profit from psychological treatment (Freud, 1914). By the 1940s, the work of Heinz Hartmann (1939), Frieda Fromm-Reichmann (1948), and others expanded on Freud's original theories. Severe psychiatric disturbance continued to be conceived as deriving from profound injury to the infant's early attachments (Bowlby, 1953; Sullivan, 1953). However, several theoretical developments influenced thinking about therapy. Human development was increasingly viewed as continuing beyond the critical first 6 years. Relationships in addition to the early parental ones were appreciated as influencing personality structure and psychic conflict (Sullivan, 1953).

Adolf Meyer, whose orientation was more neurobiological and humanistic than theoretical, encouraged treating the patient with schizophrenia in as normal a fashion as possible. Outpatient, community-based care was preferred to the then-standard long-term inpatient stays. Patients lived at home or elsewhere in the community, while visiting their doctors at the community hospital. Physicians were trained to know and understand their patients, not only in terms of symptoms, but as people with whom they would be working over many years. In addition to the psychiatrist, a social worker was an essential part of Meyer's model. The social worker visited patients and their families in their homes to better understand day-to-day needs and provide support, in coordination with the psychiatrist's care of the patient (Meyer, 1950).

Another psychological perspective attracted attention in following decades, that of communication theorists, who, intrigued with what they considered to be distorted symbolic processes in families of schizophrenics, developed several notions about causation. The predominance of arbitrariness and inconsistency over reason and reality in dyadic and family relationships was thought to result in schizophrenia in a family member (Bateson et al., 1956; Lidz et al., 1957; Lidz et al., 1958; Laing and Esterson, 1971).

One consequence of these psychological theories was to pathologize and blame the family. If an offspring developed schizophrenia it was an indictment of the family, a prejudice that followed in large part from professionals' assumptions, in the absence of a disease perspective, that all psychopathology was psychologically caused. As a consequence, the family was denied help and information in understanding their relative's condition and excluded from the treatment process. Thus schizophrenia was not only devastating in its own right, but was frequently associated with guilt, shame, and alienation.

The rapid action and relative efficacy of the neuroleptics introduced in the 1950s quickly made medication the preferred treatment in the state hospitals and practices of general psychiatry. In the dominant psychoanalytic practices, however, drugs were viewed as anathema to "real treatment" since analytic therapy sought to understand the psychological meanings of symptoms, not to suppress them with medications. Two camps developed: the biological and the psychodynamic.

The Role of Psychotherapy in a Biologic Era

In time a more balanced view has emerged of schizophrenia as a biological illness with a strong genetic component to its etiology, often with far-reaching effects on the individual's capacities. While medications are an essential feature of treatment, there is a better appreciation of the importance of supportive psychological treatments and practical interventions in addition to medication therapy in reducing relapse (Hogarty et al., 1974; Vaughn and Leff, 1976; Falloon et al., 1982; Hogarty et al., 1986). The most knowledgeable authorities on treatment efficacy, the patients themselves, attest to the importance of the therapeutic relationship in helping them to live with an unpredictable and deeply disruptive illness (May, 1968; Ruocchio, 1989).

For many patients, schizophrenia is either turbulent or boring. While acute episodes often raise the greatest attention, the quiet struggle with negative symptoms, medication side effects, and residual positive symptoms is what, to a large extent, characterizes "normal life" for the patient. Schizophrenia and its treatment attack motivation, interest, and often the capacity to think and feel deeply, leaving in their wake apathy and mental inactivity. A sophisticated, flexible psychotherapy responsive to the multifaceted nature of the illness, together with an appreciation of the person affected, is needed to support an optimum course for the patient.

The Psychiatrist and the Non-Physician Therapist

The roles of therapist and psychiatrist may be embodied in the same person. However, in community psychiatry the psychiatrist and non-physician therapist often work side by side as colleagues. The psychiatrist is the expert in psychopharmacology and medical care, and experienced in the practice of psychiatry. The non-physician therapist is on the front line with the patient. In addition to having skills and experience in psychotherapy, the therapist needs to be proficient in the diagnosis and signs of mental illness, psychopharmacology, and the assessment of side effects. The psychiatrist and therapist have unique as well as overlapping expertise. Bringing their knowledge and observations to bear in a genuine collaboration can improve the accuracy of diagnostic and treatment decisions, enrich the understanding of the patient and the therapy, and provide a high standard of patient care.

Collaboration with the Multidisciplinary Team

Often the support patients need exceeds what can be provided in the clinic. Case managers, psychosocial rehabilitation counselors, board-and-care providers, and housing counselors are among those who may be providing essential supports to the patient. Other important sources of care are inpatient services, and emergency room and crisis bed staffs. The therapist's relationship with other providers of care should be positive and collaborative, with the aim of sharing relevant information for ongoing diagnostic purposes, practical problem-solving, and treatment planning.

As community psychiatry seeks to respond to the multiple needs of patients, there is a tradeoff of benefits between patient confidentiality and information sharing. Certainly privacy has more meaning to some patients than others, and some situations demand more information sharing than others. In giving or receiving patient information, consent is required and patients should be included or informed as much as possible about the purpose of the communication and what is being communicated.

General Considerations in Treating Schizophrenia

Schizophrenia varies in its manifestations, and similarly, the experience of the illness varies with the person who has it. In addition to the familiar syndrome that defines it—hallucinations, delusions, thought disorder, and the like—there are other aspects of the illness that have important implications for treatment.

Vulnerability to Stress

''Stress'' deserves clarification. It is not an event in itself, but the outcome of an event or circumstance impinging on the individual. Hence the result depends on the severity of the stressor, its meaning to the person affected, and such qualities as the impressionability, coping mechanisms, resilience, and support in the individual affected.

Relapse or setbacks in a schizophrenic illness are frequently associated with stress (Zubin and Spring, 1977; Falloon et al., 1982; Weinberger, 1987; Malla et al., 1990). Sources of stress commonly include riding a bus, being in a crowd, dealing with strangers, or handling disagreements; also, major life events such as a marriage, a new job, or loss of a family member can be quite stressful. An event that might simply annoy or excite someone who is not ill can affect a person with schizophrenia severely.

For example, a difficult boss or cliquish co-workers can trigger paranoid responses. Negative or neutral interactions on the job may precipitate uneasiness in the affected person, quickly leading to hallucinations of personal, derogatory comments interspersed in others' conversation. Laughter, the way a chair is positioned or papers stacked, an irritable co-worker, can elaborate the paranoid perceptions. The accumulation of such experiences may result in inappropriately expressed anger and job loss.

When a patient's symptoms increase, it is important to consider the context in which this has happened. Sometimes understanding the context of the stress, as well as planning how to contain, reduce, or circumvent the stressful event, can provide sufficient therapeutic benefit to ride out the exacerbation. At other times, a temporary medication increase is advisable, depending on the seriousness of symptoms and the patient's coping abilities. Anticipating potentially stressful circumstances can guide prophylactic measures such as not reducing an asymptomatic patient's medication when he or she is about to return to work.

Emotional Flattening

Some people with schizophrenia may seem to care little about the things or people around them. One reason that emotional flattening occurs may be that a florid episode is so devastating to one's sense of self and of what was known and trusted, that the result is a certain self-protectiveness and disengagement from the rest of the world. Emotional flattening or incongruity may also be traced to disorganized thinking, biologically induced changes in the experience of feelings and ideas, negative symptoms, or persistent paranoia (Andreasen, 1994).

Depression and Suicide

A number of people with schizophrenia manage to be ill and proceed in recovery, including periodic relapses, with striking indifference to what has befallen them. However, depression and demoralization are not uncommon and are usually implicated in suicides when they occur. Patients can develop despair as a reaction to a first episode, to relapse, or to persistent symptoms. Depressed mood or ideas, agitation, irritability, and/or vegetative changes may also indicate the coexistence of an affective illness.

Epidemiological studies show that patients with schizophrenia are at two to three times greater risk for suicide than the general population (Tabbane et al., 1993; Shuwall and Siris, 1994). The most vulnerable period is in the first two years following initial hospitalization (Sorenson and Knight, 1986), and suicide completers tend to be better educated, with higher pre-morbid achievement, and higher awareness of their psychopathology (Drake et al., 1986; Westmeyer et al., 1991). Additional risk factors include abrupt worsening of mental status, especially command auditory hallucinations to kill oneself (Yasuda, 1992); social isolation coupled with changed mental status and suicidality; and a history of previous suicide attempts (Drake et al., 1986). Hopelessness may be the ultimate cutting edge of a decision for suicide and should be assessed judiciously (Drake et al., 1986).

The patient's signs and complaints of depression must be heeded so that appropriate interventions may be employed, including supportive therapy, antidepressant medication, increase in neuroleptic dose and/or therapeutic placement (full or partial hospitalization, referral to a crisis bed, or staying with a supportive friend or relative). On the other hand, many a veteran of clinical practice has encountered a patient's calculated suicidal threat aimed at bringing about hospitalization to escape a legal or social obligation, or simply to relieve discomfort. Appreciation of the patient's endowments, personality, circumstances, psychotic symptomatology, mood state, and outlook will contribute to accuracy of disposition.

Impaired Integrative Capacity

In schizophrenia, not only is there loss of what was accustomed, but also the tools used to encode, decipher, and organize information are impaired. Throughout treatment the effect of thought disorder, paranoia, loosened associations, and altered meaning of symbols on the individual's capacity to integrate information of even the simplest kind needs to be appreciated.

An example of impaired integration is afforded by a severely ill patient who could not bring together customary cues and associations to solve the seemingly simple problem of catching the bus home. As he came to one of the streets along the way, the one-way street sign was pointed in the direction opposite his destination. Perplexed, he stood for a long while looking at the one-way sign, then looking at the street. Finally he found a solution by facing in the direction of the sign while walking backwards for the four blocks it took to get to his stop. The experience was so fraught with ideas of reference and foreboding that he did not leave the house again for two weeks.

Because of the impaired integrative capacity, a great deal of time in therapy is given to issues of daily life, reality-testing, and problem-solving. Demands on the patient—such as waking up in the morning, getting the children off to school, keeping appointments, listening to voices, remembering to take medicine—may hang in disarray in the patient's mind, badly impeding purposeful, organized behavior. In therapy, the patient and the therapist repeatedly spend time articulating the disarray, structuring it, and increasing the patient's organization and mastery.

Personality

While personality may suffer extensively in schizophrenia, it is rarely if ever totally masked. Often traits of personality have an important effect on the individual's adjustment to his illness and progress in treatment. Recognizing and working with individual personality strengths and vulnerabilities is an integral part of the treatment. Personality affects the way symptoms are reported, the way medicines are taken, the nature of the patient's relationships, the utilization of psychotherapy and rehabilitation services, daily adjustment, and life achievements.

Like knowledge of symptoms, appreciation of personality dimensions contributes to accuracy in assessment and intervention. An obsessional patient's anxiety over loss of control can be overwhelming and may be defended against by denial. However, supporting his tendency to intellectualize by helping him describe and order his experience, helping him identify problems of logic in psychotic thinking, and introducing scientific concepts of the origin of the disorder can provide a means for him to recover some control, and enough insight to cooperate in treatment. Another person who is less analytical or distressed by the meaning of changed experience to his sense of self derives greatest benefit from a direct, simple explanation of his illness, what medicine to take, what side effects to anticipate, and when his next appointment will be. A histrionic, self-dramatizing patient, directed by emotional responses, requires a combination of compassion and definition, understanding and firmness. Where the schizoid patient is best approached with simplicity, mildness, and reserve, an angry, suspicious patient with a background of abuse may require firm demonstration that he is taken seriously and that his therapist will see to his care with authority.

In addition, understanding personality as it interfaces with illness is often invaluable in making judgment calls over such matters as hospitalization, assessment of disability, or response to threatening behavior. For example, the evaluation of disability or need for hospitalization in an antisocial individual presenting with complaints of hallucinations and paranoia is best made with a careful assessment of motive. The dangerousness of an immature individual given to tantrums and bombastic threats when unstable may be assessed with less alarm than that of another symptomatic individual whose menacing behavior is associated with a past history of violence.

Comorbidity: Alcohol and Other Substance Abuse

''Dual diagnosis'' of substance use and mental illness presents major challenges to community psychiatry. A conservative estimate of lifetime prevalence of alcohol and/ or drug abuse among people with schizophrenia is 47 percent (Ziedonis and Fisher, 1994). Comorbidity of substance abuse and illness is associated with treatment noncompliance, increased frequency of relapse and hospitalization, and greater utilization of health and social services (Wolpe et al., 1993; Ziedonis and Fisher, 1994). Patients with substance abuse and dependence, past or present, are more likely to commit suicide or be involved in homicidal or violent behavior than non-users (Hendin, 1986).

Even though some patients recognize personal costs of their substance abuse— such as depression, paranoia, legal problems, and losing possessions or self-regard— denial at one level or another is a prominent obstacle to treatment. Patients often deny or minimize their substance use for reasons ranging from sociopathy to shame. In the initial evaluation and subsequently, it is important to learn about patients' past and present substance use for the same reasons that it is important to inquire about health history, current physical conditions, and medications. Motivation for substance use such as self-medicating or social acceptance, frequency of use, cost, and how the patient pays for his habit should be investigated. Toxicology screens should be considered for use at evaluation along with baseline blood work, as well as when patients are unstable, and randomly for known abusers. The results and purpose of screens, such as understanding contributions to mental status changes and making appropriate treatment decisions, should be shared with the patient.

Drug and alcohol treatment programs in the United States are in many cases separate from mental health programs and are frequently hesitant or unequipped to serve people with comorbid psychiatric illnesses. As funding for treatment programs is curtailed, options are further restricted. Increasingly, community psychiatry programs recognize the need to offer drug and alcohol treatment services for dually diagnosed individuals within their own purview (Ziedonis and Fisher, 1994; Chapter 25).

Mental Retardation and Schizophrenia

Persons with significantly limited intellectual capacity may have more difficulty than others in responding adaptively to their illness and treatment. Even without illness, people with global intellectual deficits are at a disadvantage in handling the complexities of modern life. Individual adjustments may be made in such forms as stubbornness or deceitfulness, but while understandable, the adaptive efficacy of these strategies is limited. The presence of an illness that distorts perception and impairs thinking further limits understanding and adaptation. Not surprisingly, it has been argued that cognitive impairment may be a significant contributor to disability among patients with schizophrenia (Schretlen et al., 1994).

The intellectually limited or retarded patient must be listened to with as much or more care than any other patient, so that both his symptoms and what is important to him are understood. The therapist will be most helpful by using simple sentences, avoiding complex ideas, providing repetition, and showing interest in the patient. Patients in even the moderate range of mental retardation can be reliably diagnosed with standard tools (Meadows et al., 1991), and pharmacologic treatment is the same as for any other patient. Dependency is usually greater among the retarded patients so that the therapist may need to have more frequent contacts with family or surrogate for illness management and support. Day programs and sheltered employment designed for people with intellectual disability can be excellent resources for patients and their families.

Course of Illness and Rate of Improvement

It is essential for both the therapist and the patient to remember that recovery often takes a long time. Getting over the acute phase may be accomplished in a few weeks or months, but getting "back on one's feet" may take years. Along the way there will be plateaux of no change, and setbacks or relapses, and these should be put in perspective as they occur. Patients and their families should be helped with a realistic time perspective and should understand that convalescence is a necessary part of the recovery process. This is not to suggest that patients should be protected from activity or responsibility, only that the rate of improvement may be slow. For example, in the area of work, recovery may start with a few basic household tasks. In time the patient may be ready to add outpatient occupational therapy, a rehabilitation or educational program, or to engage more in the community with the help of a case manager. Some patients enroll in job training programs while others seek work directly. Without an appreciation of the long time needed for progress, patients and their families may become discouraged and settle for an outcome that falls well short of what is possible. The therapist's quiet and enduring optimism about the patient and his or her progress and achievements are key to successful therapy and good outcome.

The Therapeutic Relationship

The relationship between patient and therapist is often one of the few constants in the patient's life. It is this relationship that endures over the years, helping the patient to live with and adapt to the vicissitudes of chronic illness. In the absence of a cure for schizophrenia, and with imperfect treatments to control it, it is often the therapeutic relationship that keeps the patient connected to treatment, and that adds humanity to a life overshadowed by a dehumanizing illness.

Effective clinicians vary in their personal styles, formulations, and treatment decisions. Regardless of these differences, treating the patient with regard and dignity is essential to developing a productive working relationship. The therapeutic relationship is of utmost importance for enabling the patient to bring his strengths to bear on his life and illness, to accept help in analyzing his difficulties and to make decisions, report symptoms, and cooperate more fully in treatment. With a relationship of trust, a poorly compliant patient may consent to accept intramuscular neuroleptic injections or a demoralized patient may find hope; a delusional patient may agree to a medication change despite his paranoia, or may surrender a weapon because he now feels safe. In addition, a good working relationship can be an invaluable support to family members or surrogates who find they are no longer alone in coping with the effects of their relative's illness and have someone to call in times of need.

With few exceptions, psychosis is isolating. The patient is estranged from customary meaning and experience and from other people who understandably shrink from his peculiar, often disturbing behavior. While he may be absorbed in his psychosis—angry, fascinated, frightened, or elated—he is also quite alone with it. Empathy is a powerful tool in penetrating the patient's isolation, making a connection, and eliciting illness phenomena. Empathy should not be confused with overidentification or effusive support. Empathy calls on intellectual and intuitive capacities, as well as a knowledge of disease process in order to approximate the cognitive and emotional experience of the patient. From a position of empathy, the clinician can maintain an informed and sensitive correspondence between the patient's raw experience and diagnostic and treatment considerations.

The utility of empathy can be seen in working with very ill patients, where empathic consonance with the patient's state can allow the therapist to meet the patient on his own ground. Empathy lends receptivity to the therapist's listening, which in turn enables relevant responses to the patient. As the patient sees that he is heard, he will begin to speak more openly. Likewise, in even the most thought-disordered patient, some thread of meaning is usually detectable with unhurried listening and occasional elucidating reflections of the patient's productions. Such connection is usually met with enthusiasm in the patient who is accustomed to people walking away from his babble, and the patient may himself be relieved at a more lucid expression of his own thoughts.

Finally, in addition to serving diagnostic and treatment decisions, empathic listening can make a connection between the therapist and the patient which is humanizing in the face of an often dehumanizing illness, can counteract shame, and may serve to increase the patient's investment in getting better.

Practical Issues of Therapy

The following suggestions are based on assumptions that psychotherapy is a long-term undertaking and that one of its functions is to promote the patient's functioning and sense of himself as a reasonably confident, competent individual.

Getting to Know the Patient

Careful history-taking enables the therapist to learn about the patient's life in detail. Usually the patient appreciates the therapist's rigor in inquiring about his personal and family background. With the patient's permission, interviewing a family member provides important additional information (see below).

Following the history-gathering, the therapist moves into less formal conversation, ranging in topics from symptomatology to how the patient spent the day yesterday. By listening for and inquiring about details of the patient's life, the therapist communicates a sense of interest in the patient, which in turn helps the patient to feel more interesting himself. Over time, the therapist comes to know likes and dislikes and details of the patient's daily life, relationships, and personal expectations. In helping to promote conversation, the therapist may also contribute his own experience, in a manner aimed at enhancing the patient's interest but not burdening him with personal information. In this process of "getting to know the patient," the patient in turn can identify with his therapist, providing important ballast and expanded sense of self.

The Family

Patients do not live in vacuums, and in general the family should be invited to a session near the beginning of treatment. "Family" may be a close relative, a friend, or a board and care provider. Before talking to family members, the therapist obtains the patient's permission, which is usually granted when the purpose is explained. The patient should understand that a family meeting is a way of helping the therapist get to know the patient better, and that this is a general, not a personal, discussion. Family members can give additional background information, including family history of illness and premorbid adjustment, and can describe their perception of how things have been going along at home. Consent is required, and the patient should choose whether he wants to be part of the session or have the family seen separately.

The goal in meeting the family, in addition to gathering information, is to establish a friendly acquaintance, educate the family about illness and treatment, and demonstrate accessibility should the family need to contact the therapist. On occasion, a family wants no involvement. More often, though, the family may suffer considerable emotional strain arising out of their relative's illness and may carry misinformation. Among other things, they may feel angry, guilty, stigmatized, helpless, or confused. Illness education—what schizophrenia is, how it is treated, how it may affect their relative's functioning now and later on, and what the therapist and others involved in care are prepared to do—can be immensely supportive to the family as well as helping the family support their relative's treatment and adjustment. Repeated meetings may be elected to review progress at home and solve problems of daily life. Psychoeducation and problem-solving family treatment models combined with standard neuroleptic medication have demonstrated significantly reduced relapse rates as compared to non-family treated patients (Falloon and Pederson, 1985; Hogarty, et al., 1986).

Establishing a Proper Distance

Many schizophrenic patients have difficulty in dealing with close relationships. Whether this is a primary psychological feature of schizophrenia or a function of impaired integrative capacity, or of paranoia, it is essential for the practitioner to be mindful of the patient's need for boundaries.

While a friendly position is desirable in the therapist, and while sharing over impersonal matters such as hobbies can be quite valuable in building a relationship, the therapist is responsible for neither neglecting nor smothering the patient. A calm, friendly attitude, which is at the same time professional, is reassuring to the patient. An excess of spontaneity, self-revelation, time, or personal investment can result in empathic failure. Sensitivity to the somewhat fragile issue of closeness can produce a robust, non-burdening relationship that enhances the patient's sense of self and self-esteem.

Understanding without Collusion

Demonstrating understanding of and interest in the patient's psychotic experience is important not only in ensuring that the patient knows he is taken seriously, but also in developing a conversation that may reveal additional material, such as a full-blown delusion. Discussion of delusions or hallucinations with acutely ill patients may lead to the problem of demonstrating understanding on the one hand, without seeming to collude with the patient over his symptoms on the other. While this is sometimes a delicate task, the solution lies in validating what is real to the patient, that is, his *experience* of his symptoms, while not endorsing the symptoms as real themselves. The therapist and patient can agree on the patient's experience although their interpretations of the experience can differ.

When to introduce the concept of illness as an alternative explanation for the patient's experience is a matter of judgment. Some patients are sufficiently ambivalent about their delusions that early on the therapist can ally himself with the questioning side and can introduce some reality-testing for the patient's consideration. Some patients are perplexed and overwhelmed and are relieved by an illness explanation in the first interview. Still others are severely anxious and wary, requiring more time to form a relationship before entertaining alternative ways of interpreting phenomena. For virtually all patients, a full acceptance of the idea of illness takes time and work, and their ambivalence about the veracity of experience may persist well after a degree of insight has been developed.

Length of Sessions

The optimal time and frequency of visits is a function of the patient's tolerance for therapy and what is needed to get the job done (symptom management, solving daily life problems, dealing with depression or ennui, characterological issues, etc.). A half hour every week, every other week, or less frequently, is often satisfactory, while some patients will use an hour a week. The frequency and length of visits commonly changes over time, but should be based on several considerations: the acuity or quiescence of the illness, the severity of environmental stressors, the patient's level of distress and desire for therapeutic contact, the stage of treatment, and the therapist's and patient's consensus on what is useful.

Silences

Lengthy silences should be avoided. They threaten patient boundaries and the organization of the patient's thinking, as well as potentiate paranoia. Pauses are acceptable, but the therapist must be able to ensure safety by talking easily with the patient over neutral as well as emotive material.

Simple Achievements

Patients drift off or get distressed when the therapist talks too much or speaks in complex sentences or makes the visits too long. Ideas should be presented in small, manageable packages because the illness frequently challenges attention and the ability to integrate new information. The patient's ability to experience a good conversation is an accomplishment in itself and enhances self-esteem. If a problem is solved or an issue is addressed, so much the better. Gains are made in small steps.

Compliance

Compliance with medication is an issue for psychotherapy because it is so much a product of the patient's attitudes toward the illness, the desire for control over personal destiny, and the therapeutic relationship. While medication compliance is essential to improving the course of illness, consistent, accurate medication use is often not easy to achieve even in cooperative patients. In a study of 20 schizophrenic outpatients on once-a-day dosing, most patients (80 percent) made errors in their pill-taking 40 to 80 percent of the time (Kapur et al., 1991). Compliance is affected by comorbid drug addiction (Wolpe et al., 1993), problems of communication, patient satisfaction with care-givers, inclusion in treatment decisions, and knowledge of the purposes of medications prescribed (Lee et al., 1992; Imanaka et al., 1993; Morris and Schulz, 1993; Mayer and Soyka, 1992), all of which may be understood in terms of the patient's need for autonomy, choice, and trust. Taking medication frequently has symbolic meaning: "I am sick, I will always have an illness." Not taking medicine, conversely, can convey the sense: "I am well." Consistent, accurate pill-taking can be difficult to achieve when patients suffer from disorganized thinking and behavior, when they or someone close to them thinks they should not be taking medicine, when they have been well for a period of time and assume they no longer need medicine, or when they are acutely ill and develop paranoid ideas about the pills they take.

Being on the front line, therapists also need to be alert to side effects which the patient may not be able to pinpoint but which could result in noncompliance, and to bring these to the psychiatrist's attention for evaluation. The therapist's ability to recognize side effects and to report them to the psychiatrist can lead to improved medication management, resulting in the patient's increased comfort, improved functioning, and greater compliance with the treatment plan.

Humor

For patients, being able to experience humor and engage with another in a humorous exchange is of inestimable value. Particularly when it is the patient's humor which guides the exchange, humor turns the present from drab to interesting, engenders a sense of liveliness, and helps the patient to recover a sense of self. Schizophrenia, once treated, is not in the majority of cases an enlivening experience, whereas humor is, and in turn serves self-esteem.

Dependency

Whether explicit or implicit, the patient's dependency on the therapist is a matter of fact. Some patients will be distressed by this, others will exploit it. Given the character, the chronicity, and the irregular course of the illness, it is right, not wrong, for the patient to depend on others. The patient quite properly depends on the therapist to listen, help solve problems, and provide reason, support, and authority. In times of psychiatric instability and high stress, the need to depend on the therapist may be great, while at other times, the need is small. As in many relationships, the principle guiding a healthy balance between dependency and independence is for the therapist to provide support and intervention where needed, but to refrain from doing for the patient what he can do for himself. Dependency is a fluid, changing aspect of the therapeutic relationship best managed with periodic reflection on the contributions of the patient, the illness, the social environment, and the patient-therapist relationship.

Conclusion

As schizophrenia has come to be appreciated as an illness affecting the brain, the role of psychotherapy has shifted from attempting to unravel a presumptive psychological cause to supporting the person in his treatment and adaptation. Because schizophrenia attacks virtually every aspect of thinking, feeling, and functioning, and because it is a lifelong condition, resort to a purely biological approach is rarely sufficient to support optimal course or individual integrity. The time will likely come when enough is understood about pathology, mechanism, and treatment that schizophrenia will take its place alongside such historical blights as smallpox and polio. Until that time, however, an intelligent, informed, supportive psychotherapy combined with skillful use of biologic interventions appear to provide the most effective and humane treatment of a truly challenging disease.

References

Andreasen, N. (ed.) (1994) *Schizophrenia: From Mind to Molecule.* Washington, D.C.: American Psychiatric Press.

Bateson, G., Jackson, D., Haley, J., and Weakland, J. (1956) Toward a theory of schizophrenia. *Behavioral Science,* 1:251–264.

Bowlby, J. (1953) Some pathological processes set in train by early mother-child separation. *Journal of Mental Science,* 99:265–272.

Drake, R.E., Gates, C., and Cotton, P.G. (1986) Suicide among schizophrenics: A comparison of attempters and completed suicides. *British Journal of Psychiatry,* 149:784–787.

Falloon, I.R.H., Boyd, J., McGill, C., Williamson, M., Razani, J., Moss, H., and Gilderman, A. (1982). Family management in the prevention of exacerbations of schizophrenia: A controlled study. *New England Journal of Medicine.* 306:1437–1440.

Falloon, I., and Pederson, J. (1985) Family management in the prevention of morbidity of schizophrenia: the adjustment of the family unit. *British Journal of Psychiatry,* 147: 156–163.

Freud, S. (1914) On narcissism: An introduction. In *Standard Edition. Vol. 14* (ed. and trans. Strachey, J., 1957), pp. 67–102. London: The Hogarth Press.

Fromm-Reichmann, F. (1948) Notes on the development of treatment of schizophrenics by psychoanalytic therapy. *Psychiatry,* 11:263–273.

Hartmann, H. (1939; trans. 1958) *Ego Psychology and the Problem of Adaptation.* New York: International Universities Press.

Hendin, H. (1986) Suicide: A review of new directions in research. *Hospital and Community Psychiatry,* 37:148–154.

Hogarty, G.E., Anderson, C.M., Reiss, D.J., Kornblath, S.J., Greenwald, D.R., Javna, C.D., Madonia, M.J., et al. (1986) Family psychoeducation, social skills training, and maintenance chemotherapy in the aftercare treatment of schizophrenia: 1. One-year effects on a controlled study on relapse and expressed emotion. *Archives of General Psychiatry,* 43:633–642.

Hogarty, G.E., Goldberg, S.C., Schooler, N.R., Ulrich, R.F., et al. (1974) Drug and sociotherapy in the aftercare of schizophrenic patients: 1. Two-year relapse rates. *Archives of General Psychiatry,* 31:603–618.

Imanaka, Y., Araki, S., and Nobutomo, K. (1993) Effects of patient health beliefs and satisfaction on compliance with medication regimens in ambulatory care at general hospitals. *Nippon Eiseigaku Zasshi [Japanese Journal of Hygiene],* 48:601–611.

Kapur, S., Ganguli, R., Ulrich, R., and Raghu, U. (1991) Use of riboflavin as a marker of medication compliance in chronic schizophrenics. *Schizophrenia Research,* 6:49–53.

Laing, R.D., and Esterson, A. (1971) *Sanity, Madness, and the Families of Schizophrenics* (2nd ed.). New York: Basic Books.

Lee, S., Wing, Y.K., and Wong, K.C. (1992) Knowledge and compliance towards lithium therapy among Chinese psychiatric patients in Hong Kong. *Australian and New Zealand Journal of Psychiatry,* 26:444–449.

Lidz, T., Cornelison, A., Fleck, S., et al. (1957) The intrafamilial environment of schizophrenic patients. II. Marital schism and marital skew. *American Journal of Psychiatry,* 114:241–248.

Lidz, T., Cornelison, A., Terry, D., et al. (1958) Intrafamilial environment of the schizophrenic patient: VI. The transmission of irrationality. *Archives of Neurological Psychiatry,* 70:305–316.

Malla, A.K., Cortese L., Shaw, T.S., and Ginsberg, B. (1990) Life events and relapse in schizophrenia. A one year prospective study. *Social Psychiatry and Psychiatric Epidemiology,* 25:221–224.

May, P.R.A. (1968) *Treatment of Schizophrenia.* New York: Science House.

Mayer, C., and Soyka, M. (1992) Compliance in schizophrenic patients with neuroleptics—an overview. *Fortschritte der Neurologie-Psychiatrie,* 60:217–222.

Meadows, G., Turner, T., Campbell, L. Lewis, S.W., Reveley, M.A., and Murray, R.M. (1991) Assessing schizophrenia in adults with mental retardation. *British Journal of Psychiatry,* 158:103–105.

Meyer, Adolph. (1950) *Collected Papers of Adolph Meyer. Vol. IV.* Baltimore: Johns Hopkins University Press.

Morris, L.S., and Schulz, R.M. (1993) Medication compliance: The patient's perspective. *Clinical Therapeutics,* 15:593–606.

Ruocchio, P.J. (1989). How psychotherapy can help the schizophrenic patient. [Patient essay.] *Hospital and Community Psychiatry,* 40:188–190.

Schretlen, D., Jayaram, G., Gallucci, G., Bobholz, J.H., and Eaton, W. (1994) Screening for cognitive impairment in an urban community mental health clinic. In revision, The Johns Hopkins University.

Shuwall, M., and Siris, S.G. (1994) Suicidal ideation and postpsychotic depression. *Comprehensive Psychiatry,* 35:132–134.

Sorenson, S.B., and Knight, K. (1986) Suicide in schizophrenia [letter]. *Journal of Clinical Psychiatry,* 47:570–571.

Sullivan, H.S. (1953) *The Interpersonal Theory of Psychiatry.* New York: W.W. Norton.

Tabbane, K., Joober, R., Spadone, C., Poirier, M.F., and Olie, J.P. (1993) Mortality and cause of death in schizophrenia. Review of the literature. *Encephale,* 19:23–28.

Vaughn, C.E., and Leff, J.P. (1976) The influence of family and social factors on the course of psychiatric illness: a comparison of schizophrenic and depressed neurotic patients. *British Journal of Psychiatry,* 129:125–137.

Weinberger, D. (1987) Implications of normal brain development for the pathogenesis of schizophrenia. *Archives of General Psychiatry,* 44:660–669.

Westermeyer, J.F., Harrow, M., and Marengo, J.T. (1991) Risk for suicide in schizophrenia and other psychotic and nonpsychotic disorders. *Journal of Nervous and Mental Disorders,* 179:259–266.

Wolpe, R.R., Gorton, G., Serota, R., and Sanford, B. (1993) Predicting compliance of dual diagnosis inpatients with aftercare treatment. *Hospital and Community Psychiatry,* 44: 45–49.

Yasuda, M. (1992) A clinical study of suicidal behavior in schizophrenic patients. *Seishin Schinkeigaku Zasshi [Japanese Psychiatry and Neurology],* 94:135–170.

Ziedonis, D.M., and Fisher, W. (1994) Assessment and treatment of comorbid substance abuse in individuals with schizophrenia. *Psychiatric Annals,* 24:477–483.

Zubin, J., and Spring, B. (1977) Vulnerability—a new view of schizophrenia. *Journal of Abnormal Psychology,* 86:103–126.

16

Assertive Community Treatment

ANNELLE B. PRIMM

Since the 1960s numerous psychiatric outreach and home care programs have been developed. Of these the Training in Community Living model, developed in Madison, Wisconsin (Stein and Test, 1980, 1985), has become the most highly recognized and frequently imitated model.

Mobile treatment, assertive community treatment, and *continuous care teams* are synonymous, referring to a type of care and treatment provided to the severely and persistently mentally ill that incorporates mobility, assertiveness, and continuity. *Assertive outreach* and *assertive (or intensive) case management* employ similar methods and have similar goals, but assertive community treatment differs in that psychiatrists' services are a built-in feature of the model and do not have to be brokered from other sources. In this chapter, the terms *Assertive Community Treatment* (ACT), *Training in Community Living* (TCL), *Mobile Treatment,* and *Program for Assertive Community Treatment* (PACT) will be used interchangeably to describe the model of care that incorporates outreach and care in the patient's own environment, with case management functions provided by teams in which the inclusion of a psychiatrist is a key feature.

ACT responds to three mental health service priorities: maintaining patients in the least restrictive environment; preventing the revolving door syndrome of preventable rehospitalization; and providing continuity of care. The creation of mobile treatment as a concept stems from the recognition that patients with severe and persistent mental illness are at high risk for relapse and are often unable to benefit from treatment services that are passive, static, and disjointed. Mobile treatment teams provide ongoing, community-based intensive care and outreach to severely mentally ill patients in their homes and in any other community environment as needed. Care is provided by a team of clinicians, including psychiatrists, who take ongoing responsibility for assertively addressing a variety of patient needs. Such needs extend from psychiatric care to medical care, entitlements, food, shelter, clothing, recreation, and rehabilitation.

As integral members of the mobile treatment team, psychiatrists visit patients in the home and at various locations in the community. Without the active involvement of a psychiatrist, patients who refuse to visit an outpatient mental health center are at risk of not receiving necessary psychiatric treatment with proper continuity of care (Reding et al., 1994). Thus, the presence of a psychiatrist on the team is a practical feature that facilitates treatment and continuity.

A considerable literature has developed in the area of home-based outreach services in general (Braun et al., 1981; Davis et al., 1972; Fenton et al., 1979; Friedman et al., 1960; Langsley and Kaplan, 1968; Pasamanick et al., 1967; Witheridge et al., 1982) and Assertive Community Treatment specifically (Bond et al., 1988; Hoult et al., 1983; Jerrell and Hu, 1989; Marks et al., 1988; Primm and Houck, 1990). Mobile treatment programs have been evaluated in randomized controlled trials and found to be effective along a number of dimensions, including reduced hospitalization, improved symptomatology, increased compliance, and enhanced quality of life (Hoult and Reynolds, 1984; Muijen et al., 1992; Stein and Test, 1980; Burns and Santos, 1995).

The model has been adapted to many different geographical locations in urban, suburban, and rural environments. Adaptations to densely populated, urban catchment areas—like the COSTAR program (Community Support, Treatment and Rehabilitation) in East Baltimore, The Thresholds Bridge program in Chicago, and programs in London and Sydney, New South Wales—face the challenge of addressing the problems of the severely mentally ill in an environment of economic deprivation and related social disorganization. The unemployment, poverty, crime, and substandard housing associated with urban areas all create extra hurdles for the severely mentally ill and their helpers. Assertive community treatment teams practicing in these areas must be that much more adept at finding scarce resources and being tenacious advocates for their patients.

The fewer the systems boundaries, and the more integrated within a comprehensive service network, the easier it is for an ACT team to maintain patients in treatment. The services that facilitate ongoing care include psychiatric and residential rehabilitation programs, adult psychiatric outpatient clinics, day hospitals and inpatient programs, occupational therapy, 24-hour psychiatric emergency services, and medical services. The availability of such resources extends the capacity to provide comprehensive care to the patients. In addition, service network components have become important sources of patient referral to outreach programs. As state hospitals downsize, mobile treatment services become a ready source of intensive outpatient care for deinstitutionalized patients.

Implementation

The following constitute the important elements of mobile treatment practice that give the model utility and potency in meeting the varied needs of the seriously mentally ill.

Flexibility

A key benefit of the mobile treatment model is that patient characteristics and need dictate the type and degree of service provided, and thus services are tailored to the patient in an individualized fashion. The mobile treatment team can formulate and carry out the treatment plan to meet an array of patient needs in a way not possible in conventional settings. For example, visit frequency, duration, or intensity may be adjusted according to patient stability or need for crisis prevention or intervention. The type of services and number of services applied may also be varied to meet patient need, including mental status examinations, medication checks, supportive or insight-oriented psychotherapy, couples or family therapy, and group psychotherapy.

Home Visiting and Community Outreach

The capacity to be flexible regardless of patient location is another asset of assertive community treatment. Such flexibility is not easily accomplished in more traditional outpatient treatment settings where clinicians must adhere to rigid schedules and are expected to stay within the four walls of an office setting. Mobile treatment patient visits occur in the office, in the home, in institutions, in fast food restaurants, or even on the street. Any location in the community serves as a potential locus for patient assessment and treatment. The capacity to do outreach in any environment increases the likelihood that the patient will remain in treatment.

Home visiting affords the care provider an inside view of the patient's micro-environment. Treatment plans can be specifically tailored to the needs of the patient. Treatment can be more effective when a provider can see firsthand how a home situation affects clinical state.

Mobility

In instances where public transport cannot be used, automobiles and vans for transporting larger groups of patients are indispensable. Staff should maintain up-to-date driver's licenses and may choose to do home visiting in their own cars; however, any transporting of patients must be done in a program-procured and insured vehicle. Although most patients will need transportation and accompaniment to appointments and other business, patients are encouraged to be independently mobile by walking when appropriate or by using public transportation once they are motivated to learn how to do so. For those patients unable or unwilling to be independently mobile, it is the responsibility of the team to transport the patient to the program office setting to conduct necessary business there.

Twenty-Four-Hour Availability

The needs of the chronically mentally ill do not conform to the hours of the typical business day and thus dictate that 24-hour services be established. Crises that could potentially lead to rehospitalization have a chance of resolution with round-the-clock response capacity. Some mobile treatment programs provide 24-hour availability of face-to-face contact. For those programs that provide on-site services 8:30 A.M. through 5 P.M., weekdays only, patients and families access staff by telephone at night and on weekends via a pager system. For emergencies, psychiatrists are available by beeper 24 hours a day with emergency services providing backup for crises that cannot be handled by telephone.

Mobile treatment team members spend time during the day with patients anticipating crises and implementing crisis prevention strategies. Focusing on prevention of crises lowers the likelihood that a crisis will occur unexpectedly overnight and on weekends and holidays. Access to communication with providers on a 24-hour basis is particularly reassuring to patients and significant others who know support is available regardless of the day or time at which the need for assistance arises.

Small Caseloads

In the TCL model, clinicians perform therapist and case manager roles simultaneously, carrying ideal caseloads of 10 patients. Limited caseload size permits clinician flexibility in a way not possible in traditional clinics where caseloads average between 50 and 100. In the mobile treatment setting, clinicians can see patients for extended periods if necessary and provide the kind of attention needed to teach daily living skills. Clinicians are also able to reprioritize agendas and address patient needs on demand if patients visit unexpectedly or are in crisis.

Due to fiscal constraints and other pressures over time, caseloads per clinician in the original PACT program expanded to an average of 18 patients (Thompson et al., 1990). Programs providing similar services are at risk for the same consequence. Fiscal limitations on additional staff hiring has dictated that there be increased clinician caseloads and/or considerable patient turnover in order to make room for other patients in need of mobile treatment services.

Continuity of Care

Bacharach (1981) describes continuity of care as ''a process involving the orderly, uninterrupted movement of patients among the diverse elements of the service delivery system.'' ACT teams commit themselves to follow patients on an ongoing basis regardless of the time of day, location, or clinical state of the patient. The team takes primary responsibility for patient care and makes a concerted effort to follow the patient regardless of the circumstances, an additional important element in continuity (Torrey, 1986).

Even when a patient is hospitalized, mobile treatment clinicians visit the patient and consult with the inpatient treatment team. Continuity of care is maintained through the regular presence of the clinician on the inpatient unit. In some programs, clinicians and psychiatrists take on a secondary role regarding patient care on the inpatient unit. The inpatient treatment team has direct control of hospital length of stay, placing the mobile team at a relative disadvantage in terms of maximizing the efficiency of the hospitalization. However, the input of clinicians is valued and provides important patient care information to the inpatient unit, thereby indirectly minimizing length of stay. The use of readmission and discharge diaries were found to be helpful in managing lengths of stay of patients in Britain (Marks et al., 1994).

In contrast, some assertive community treatment teams have sole responsibility for inpatient care when the patient is hospitalized, thus providing a seamless clinical service (Fenton et al., 1979; Hoult et al., 1983; Muijen et al., 1992). In outreach programs such as the Daily Living Programme in London, patient care was the primary responsibility of the outreach team even when the patient was hospitalized (Muijen et al., 1992).

As demonstrated in the evaluation of TCL programs, outcomes of reduced hospitalization and improved social and vocational functioning in experimental groups endure as long as the patient continues to receive mobile treatment (Stein and Test, 1980; Hoult et al., 1983). Once the experimental treatment is withdrawn, patients revert to old patterns of recidivism and functional marginality. Based on these findings, COSTAR, in Baltimore, initially practiced with the understanding that once patients were identified as meeting criteria for mobile treatment services they would always be eligible for them in some form, even if at lower frequency or intensity as they stabilized over time (Primm and Houck, 1990). However, such a practice is unlikely to continue in an environment of restricted fiscal resources and increasing demands for mobile treatment patient slots.

Patient satisfaction with mobile treatment (Olfson, 1990) and resistance to the prospect of transitioning to mainstream services may warrant continuation of mobile treatment services even in the face of considerable improvement and attainment of treatment plan goals. During their tenure in mobile treatment, many patients have experienced greater stability and sense of well-being than they have had in their lifetimes, although this has not been a universal finding (Olfson, 1990). Patients are understandably reluctant to sacrifice their achievements in exchange for becoming a mobile treatment graduate while risking the loss of stability and comfort in treatment. Some programs, including The Bridge and COSTAR, have attempted to transfer patients from the mobile treatment model to a traditional outpatient clinic. Even when patients were selected on the basis of willingness to receive services in a different treatment setting and achievement of short- and long-term treatment goals including treatment compliance, appointment-keeping, and independence in basic living skills, success in returning to less intensive treatment models was not universal. After experiencing initial periods of tenure and stability in conventional treatment, some began to attend erratically and relapse. Hospitalization and re-enrollment in mobile treatment followed, confirming the need for a policy of ongoing, long-term involvement with the mobile treatment program (Dincin et al., 1993).

Brief Outreach

Within a mental health service network, certain patients need a safety net as they make the transition from assertive community treatment to traditional outpatient care.

Also, patients in outpatient or day hospital programs who may be at risk of dropping out of treatment, but who do not need long-term mobile services, may similarly benefit from a brief period of extra support and assistance. This type of safety net or extra support can be provided by a *brief outreach team* that provides temporary help with restoring and maintaining treatment plans, compliance with medications, appointment keeping, escorting, and other forms of practical help when a patient is unable or unwilling to come on their own for clinic or day hospital services. Thus, contact with the referring clinician can be reestablished and a crisis averted without resorting to hospitalizing the patient or placing him or her in the long-term care of the mobile treatment service.

Another use of brief outreach is the identification of those patients who will need longer term mobile treatment. For instance, persons who continue to need outreach services beyond a limited service period may be referred to long-term mobile treatment.

Multidisciplinary Teams

The team approach in mobile treatment brings many advantages. It affords the patient a treatment plan that represents the integration of different perspectives in team treatment planning meetings. The greater the spread of disciplines represented, the potentially richer and better informed is the treatment plan. At COSTAR, the professionals represented on the team include psychiatrists, nurses, social workers, rehabilitation specialists, and psychologists. The team approach allows all staff to become familiar with patients' personal assets, resources, and problems, facilitating interchangeability of staff in the event of clinician absence and turnover. The familiarity of patients with clinicians other than their own primary clinician eases anxiety and allows treatment to proceed in an uninterrupted fashion when the primary therapist is not available (Primm and Houck, 1990).

Regardless of discipline, mobile treatment clinicians should be prepared to perform a basic set of functions. Witheridge (1989) has outlined a broad job description for assertive community treatment workers that includes a set of eleven functions and expectations: (1) identifying members of the target population; (2) engaging new participants; (3) conducting assessments and planning interventions; (4) assuming ultimate professional responsibility; (5) home visiting; (6) attending to the concrete details of everyday life; (7) providing assistance and training in the patient's own environment; (8) arranging for medical services; (9) providing interagency resource brokering and advocacy; (10) facilitating necessary readmissions and working with inpatient staff; and (11) working in partnership with families.

Certain personal characteristics and attitudes that exemplify a successful mobile treatment clinician are traits that are inherent to the individual and cannot easily be taught (Witheridge, 1989). Staff often select themselves; however, great care should be taken to expose potential mobile treatment clinicians to the full scope and various roles and expectations of the job. It is helpful to have prospective staff share a day with the mobile treatment team before committing themselves to employment. Team member selection must take into consideration maturity, energy, enthusiasm, experience with the severely mentally ill, and comfort with confronting the hardship of others.

At COSTAR, during early morning team meetings the agenda of the day is mapped out and patient needs and crises are anticipated. In addition, there is a weekly round during which all patients are discussed at greater length. The round is organized to monitor certain critical indicators including at-risk status for incarceration, psychiatric and medical hospitalization, and homelessness. The team tracks these categories as a group on a weekly basis, documenting the strategies that will be carried out to prevent the occurrence of institutionalization or homelessness. Over time, clinicians become adept at predicting the at-risk state of individual patients by the reemergence of certain signs, symptoms, or behaviors. As a result, the team can adjust its treatment plan to prevent an unwanted outcome in a quicker, more focused manner.

The Daily Living Programme (Marks et al., 1994) and COSTAR have relied heavily on psychiatric nurses who at any given time constitute at least half of the clinical staff. Nurses, often pairing with clinicians in other disciplines, manage medications and therapeutic monitoring, administer injections, and assist in the recognition and treatment of acute and chronic medical conditions, particularly hypertension and diabetes mellitus (Primm and Houck, 1990). Their knowledge of health promotion information has benefited patients in areas such as nutrition, safe sexual practice, and prenatal care. A social work presence brings valuable input regarding social systems, benefits, entitlements, and development of resource bases, both intra- and extra-institutional. Social workers share knowledge with all staff so that non–social work staff become savvy about these issues. Along with psychologists, social workers have also promoted extensive utilization of individual, group, couples, and family therapy, adding a socialization and relationship-building dimension to patient offerings.

In contrast to other assertive community treatment programs, COSTAR has chosen not to employ paraprofessionals as clinicians. Although paraprofessionals have been known to be helpful in obtaining resources for patients and performing basic functions such as providing transportation and teaching basic living skills, they are not usually able to provide quality clinical observation without having had professional training and experience. A professional clinician can conduct case management activities while assessing mental status or performing supportive psychotherapy. The performance of dual roles by professionals is a better use of resources. As a result, COSTAR personnel costs are higher, but this is an expenditure with high return on the investment.

On the other hand, paraprofessionals may have greater appeal to patients because they are able to create a more peer-like relationship with less social distance. Such relationships may help to generate more patient cooperation and active participation in treatment. Dixon and colleagues describe the use of consumers as team members in their work with Assertive Community Treatment Team for the severely mentally ill homeless in Baltimore (Dixon et al., 1994). Consumer advocates serve in supportive and advocacy roles for patients in a flexible manner. Although there are numerous questions and boundary issues surrounding their involvement in a multidisciplinary treatment team, they bring an important perspective. Consumer advocates provide insight and knowledge regarding the survival skills needed by a mentally ill person who is homeless. They also teach others how to utilize the mental health system and other public resources.

Establishing a family-like environment in a mobile treatment office can disarm some of the most reluctant patients so that they may engage mobile treatment services with enthusiasm and even visit the office on a regular basis. Clerical staff help to create a comfortable, user-friendly atmosphere. Clerical staff, serving as receptionists and registrars, should be hired based on their experience working with the severely mentally ill and/or their possession of excellent communication and interpersonal skills. In addition to handling paper work and providing telephone reception, clerical staff can help maintain a warm milieu by the way they greet and interact with patients both in person and over the phone. Clerical staff are often able to provide perspectives on patient behavior based on patient trust and comfort with them. At times, clerical staff are privy to information that patients do not share with their therapists. As a result, the team can solicit the input of clerical staff at appropriate times. Clerical staff are truly seen as adjunct team members.

It is important to organize opportunities for continuing education for the team on topics such as psychiatric treatment, psychopharmacology, mobile treatment techniques, and specialized services for patients with problems that are difficult to treat, such as those with dual diagnoses. The intimate nature of assertive community treatment work dictates that staff have an opportunity to discuss the full range of social and community psychiatry topics and related issues such as stigma, race, class, and culture in the context of community mental health service provision.

The Role of Psychiatrists

Mobile treatment multidisciplinary teams are generally led by psychiatrists who carry a number of roles and responsibilities (Olfson, 1990). Establishing the direction of mobile treatment services, leading the decision-making process regarding programmatic issues, and providing administrative supervision are key functions. Clinical supervision of team members through team conferences and individual meetings provides opportunities to teach the basics of providing mobile treatment to the severely mentally ill. Maintaining ethical standards in treatment and understanding legal issues related to patient care represent another dimension of the psychiatrist's role.

Clinically, psychiatrists must be prepared to perform evaluations readily in any setting as necessary: in a car, in the home, in a restaurant, wherever the patient can be engaged. The psychiatrist, like all team members, must be ultimately flexible and ready to reprioritize when a rare opportunity arises to see a patient who has been difficult to find. Psychiatrists are also needed to communicate with other physicians involved in patient care. This is crucial when confronting medical problems where mutual awareness of treatment plans, laboratory studies, diagnoses, and prognoses is key.

The psychiatrist leads the team making final decisions while maintaining an open-minded approach to incorporating the ideas of others into the treatment plan. The psychiatrist must also recognize and respect the autonomy of staff. Team members have to act independently particularly in crisis situations, conferring with other staff and soliciting supervision at a later time. However, more seasoned clinicians require less supervision.

Mobile treatment interventions are more likely to succeed when team members know the psychiatrist has listened and considered their point of view. A dogmatic, dictatorial approach from the psychiatrist is counterproductive. The staff act as the eyes and ears of the psychiatrist. The psychiatrist must learn to trust the judgement of clinicians regarding individual patients when appropriate as the psychiatrist cannot expect to have intimate knowledge of every detail of each patient. The psychiatrist, therefore, relies heavily on the clinician for information and ongoing assessment as well as the clinician's ability to discern which problems or side effects need the psychiatrist's attention. Encouragement of treatment planning creativity and innovation in team members benefits the program, the staff, and the patients.

Psychiatrists who practice mobile treatment have a role to play in training psychiatric residents in this type of care-giving. Exposure to home-visiting provides residents with a realistic view of how their patients live and how environment influences mental status (Reding et al., 1994). With supervision, residents can overcome the fears of performing mobile outreach, appreciate the value of a home visit in uncovering otherwise unavailable information, and learn to tailor patient interventions to patient needs.

Case Management

Inherent in the mobile treatment provider role is the provision of case management services including assessment, linking, monitoring, relationship formation, support, outreach, referral, crisis intervention, medication monitoring, brokering, coordination, planning, and advocacy. These functions constitute an amalgam of the clinical and brokering models of case management (Bachrach, 1989). Case management also implies that providers assist patients in developing basic living skills. The use of acronyms can be helpful in providing a standard format for conceptualizing patient needs and organizing the documentation of patient contacts and interventions. The acronym SHARES is used by COSTAR clinicians to remember Symptoms, Housing, Activities of daily living, Recreation, Employment, and Significant others. (Primm and Houck, 1990). Programs may adopt their own mnemonic to address the full range of tasks performed by the mobile treatment team.

Under the *symptom* category, clinicians assess psychiatric and physical status, package and/or administer medications to facilitate patient compliance, and assist patients in obtaining medical care and maintaining care of physical problems. Assisting

patients with medical care is particularly important since the majority of the chronically mentally ill are known to have high rates of chronic medical illness and to neglect
physical upkeep and medical follow-up (Roca et al., 1987). Accompanying patients
on medical visits, providing important historical information to medical personnel,
and assisting patients with carrying out medical treatment plans can potentially lead
to reduced morbidity and mortality among this medically vulnerable group.

In addressing *housing* concerns, patients are assisted in locating and maintaining
safe housing. The severely and persistently mentally ill are at high risk for becoming
homeless. COSTAR provides 24-hour telephone access to patients, families, and land-
lords in order to assist with problem solving and avert crises and hospitalization. In
addition, assistance is provided with developing skills of *activities of daily living* in
areas including, but not limited to upkeep of personal hygiene and grooming, housekeeping, menu planning, shopping, laundering, parenting, budgeting, and money management.

Recreation activities constitute an important part of quality of life. Social gath-
erings are convened, and several groups meet weekly to provide a recreation function
or socialization opportunity. The encouragement of social reintegration plays an important role in maintenance of stability in severely and chronically mentally ill patients.

Employment encompasses a range of activities including outpatient occupational
therapy, prevocational programs, psychosocial rehabilitation, and competitive or volunteer employment. Patients should be encouraged to involve themselves in some
form of structured, productive activity commensurate with their level of functioning
and degree of motivation.

Within the category of *significant others,* support, psychoeducation, and counseling for family and other persons close to the patient are a necessity. A patient cannot
be insulated from the problems facing those persons living in the same home environment; thus, such problems have a direct impact on patient care. It is, therefore,
important that the team assist significant others with problem solving and find ways
of sharing the burden of involvement with a severely mentally ill person. Families
find it comforting that mobile treatment programs provide quick response to crises
through 24-hour telephone availability.

Assertiveness

Severely mentally ill patients, by virtue of the symptoms of their illness, are at times
unwilling to accept psychiatric treatment in any form, or are unable to come forward
for care independently. Thus, the ability to perform assertive outreach is an integral
part of mobile treatment. Care providers do not passively wait for patients to appear
for treatment or to request services. Rather, patient needs are anticipated and acted
upon without patient initiation. Inherent in assertiveness is mobility, the ability to go
out by car or van to see the patient in any location. When patients initially refuse
clinical services through home visiting and outreach, assertive strategies can be em-

ployed. The patient can be wooed with whatever resources or services he or she values. In the early phases of contact, obtaining benefits, upgrading housing, or procuring food may have greater value to the patient than actual treatment. Persistence is important, particularly when patients initially reject the mobile treatment provider. It is important to keep coming back to try to penetrate patient resistance. Patients do, of course, have the ultimate right to refuse treatment.

In some programs, all patients must assent to mobile treatment, particularly when the state does not have an outpatient commitment statute allowing forced outpatient care. In some states outpatient commitment laws permit forced treatment in the community, and mobile treatment is necessary to carry it out. In states without involuntary outpatient treatment, mobile treatment teams must use persuasion and assertiveness to pursue a trusting alliance with patients quickly in order to engage them in treatment as soon as possible. If patients refuse all contact and resources after several attempts, providers retreat and wait to be recontacted in the future, sometimes with the knowledge that the patient is seriously ill but not dangerous to a point where involuntary admission would be justified.

Safety

When teams work in urban catchment areas plagued with poverty and crime, managers and staff must be concerned about safety. Home visiting is potentially dangerous, but risk can be minimized by taking appropriate precautions. Effective safety measures include dressing inconspicuously, removing medical attire such as white coats, avoiding attention-getting jewelry, carrying essentials such as medication paraphernalia in small pouches, conducting most home visits during morning hours, and telephoning in advance so that patients, families, and neighbors are alert to the arrival of home visitors. Staff are vigilant about being aware of any suspicious-looking activity and avoid areas that appear unsafe. Home visiting in pairs on the first home visit and subsequent visits brings added security when the safety of an area is in question.

When patients are discovered to be hostile or threatening at the time of a home visit, clinicians should not try to establish control in the situation or restrain a patient. Instead, safe practice dictates that staff leave the premises as soon as possible. In some cases, it may be necessary to call police to initiate civil commitment procedures so that the patient may be safely evaluated at the nearest emergency room. Abiding by these basic rules, a mobile treatment provider can avoid preventable incidents.

Outcomes

Findings in the majority of controlled evaluations of mobile treatment programs applied to a broad spectrum of severely mentally ill patients reveal favorable results in a number of domains (Burns and Santos, 1995). It is not clear which specific features are responsible for these outcomes, but the amalgam of the elements of assertive community treatment forms a product that has been shown to generally increase longevity of community tenure and improve clinical, social, and rehabilitative status. A delineation of experimentally demonstrated gains follows by category.

Hospitalization

A common yet problematic index of outcome in evaluations of mobile treatment programs is psychiatric hospitalization. Its common forms of measure are number of hospitalizations, duration or length of stay, and number of bed days.

The main randomized investigations of TCL programs are those in Sydney, Australia, Wisconsin, and London. In these studies, patients eligible for hospital admission were randomly assigned to either an experimental group that received mobile treatment or a control group that received hospitalization followed by standard outpatient treatment. The study subjects were continued on this regime for periods of between one and two years.

The evaluation of the Wisconsin TCL program was the first to demonstrate that the experimental group experienced significantly fewer psychiatric hospital bed days than controls (Stein and Test, 1980). The Australian TCL program achieved results indicating reductions in both number and duration of hospital stays (Hoult and Reynolds, 1984). A combination of favorable outcomes regarding hospitalization was shown in the evaluation of The Daily Living Programme in London. Lengths of stay were shorter and bed days were fewer with no real difference noted in overall number of hospitalizations between the experimental and control groups (Marks et al., 1994).

All related gains in community tenure in the experimental group were lost after discontinuation of the TCL programs in all three sites, resulting in increased rates of hospitalization, number of bed days, and lengths of stay. Such degeneration illustrates that if such gains are to be sustained, assertive community treatment must be maintained.

Family Burden

Caring for a severely mentally ill person has often been seen as a burden on the family. Patients enrolled in assertive community treatment programs who experience increased community tenure potentially pose a greater disruption to their families. Reduction of family burden has often been seen as a potential favorable outcome of mobile treatment through the psychoeducation and support provided to families and significant others. Family burden scales have been developed to measure the amount of burden imposed on families of patients enrolled in community care services (Grad and Sainsbury, 1968; Pai and Kapur, 1982).

The Wisconsin and Sydney TCL programs do not indicate an actual reduction in the impact on the family of the severely mentally ill enrolled in mobile treatment programs; however, no increase in family burden over conventional office-based care was demonstrated (Reynolds and Hoult, 1984; Test and Stein, 1980). If relative satisfaction can be construed as an index of family burden, it may be meaningful that the significant others of the Daily Living Programme enrollees indicated a significantly greater degree of satisfaction than the relatives of controls (Marks et al., 1994).

Psychiatric Symptom Level

Comparison of the Wisconsin experimental and control groups regarding their performance on various clinical rating scales reveals overall greater symptom improvement in the experimental group (Stein and Test, 1980). Subjects of the Daily Living Programme showed slight improvements in psychiatric symptoms 20 months postbaseline (Marks et al., 1994), and the Australian research documented less symptomatology among subjects in the TCL group (Reynolds and Hoult, 1984).

Social Adjustment

Analysis of data from Wisconsin and Australia confirms that patients enrolled in assertive community treatment programs have enhanced levels of social functioning (Hoult et al., 1983; Marks et al., 1994; Stein and Test, 1980). An evaluation of the social behavior and quality of social networks of COSTAR patients revealed that longer periods of COSTAR contact were associated with less social behavior problems and greater quantity and quality of social networks (Thornicroft and Breakey, 1991).

Patient Satisfaction

Patients of TCL programs in Australia, London, and Wisconsin were significantly more satisfied with their care than patients in conventional care (Hoult et al., 1983; Marks et al., 1994; Stein and Test, 1980). Stein and Test's work showed that on subjective measures of quality of life, members of the experimental group experienced a greater sense of overall well-being than did controls (Stein and Test, 1980).

Functional and Occupational Status

The Wisconsin group found that patients receiving assertive community treatment were unemployed for shorter periods and earned more through competitive employment than did controls (Stein and Test, 1980). Occupational measures were not obtained for the Daily Living Programme. Results from Australia revealed no difference in employment among recipients of community care compared with controls; however, global functioning did show greater improvement (Hoult et al., 1983).

Cost

The initial evaluation of the Wisconsin TCL program found that when financial and social costs were assessed, mobile treatment was no more costly than conventional treatment (Weisbrod et al., 1980). In their economic analysis of the Daily Living

Program in London, Knapp and colleagues (1994) found that the mobile program was significantly less costly than standard hospital and outpatient treatment. The principal savings accrued from the marked reduction in inpatient utilization that is possible with ACT, and more than compensated for the additional cost of the intensive staffing of the program itself. Knapp and his colleagues noted that there was no evidence of additional costs to other agencies, which might have compensated for the health service cost reduction.

Conclusion

Assertive community treatment is a brand of outreach aimed at the severely and persistently mentally ill that carries persuasive experimental evidence of improvement of overall clinical and social outcome. It accomplishes these improvements and maximizes community tenure through the deployment of a treatment team that provides long-term, assertive, round-the-clock, mobile, flexible psychiatric treatment and case management services. The psychiatrist presence on the treatment team guarantees that case management and treatment services remain cohesive and coordinated.

References

Bacharach, L.L. (1981) Continuity of care for chronic mental patients: a conceptual analysis. *American Journal of Psychiatry,* 138:1449–1456.

Bacharach, L.L. (1989) Case management: toward a shared definition. *Hospital and Community Psychiatry,* 40:883–884.

Bond, G.R., Miller, L.D., Krumweid, R.D., and Ward, R.S. (1988) Assertive case management in three CMHCs: a controlled study. *Hospital and Community Psychiatry,* 39:411–418.

Braun, P., Kochansky, G., Shapiro, R., Greenberg, S., Gudeman, J.E., and Shore, M.F. (1981) Overview: deinstitutionalization of psychiatric patients, a critical review of outcome studies. *American Journal of Psychiatry,* 136:736–749.

Burns, B.J. and Santos, A.B. (1995) Assertive community treatment: An update of randomized trials. *Psychiatric Services,* 46:669–675.

Davis, A.E., Dinitz, S., and Pasamanick, B. (1972) The prevention of hospitalization in schizophrenia: five years after an experimental program. *American Journal of Psychiatry,* 42: 375–388.

Dincin, J., Wasmer, D., Witheridge, T.F., Sobeck, L., Cook, J., and Razzano, L. (1993) Impact of assertive community treatment on the use of state hospital inpatient bed-days. *Hospital and Community Psychiatry,* 44:833–838.

Dixon, L., Krauss, N., and Lehman, A. (1994) Consumers as service providers: the promise and the challenge. *Community Mental Health Journal,* 30:615–625.

Fenton, F.R., Tessier, L., and Streuning, E.L. (1979) A comparative trial of home and hospital psychiatric care. One year follow-up. *Archives of General Psychiatry,* 36:1073–1079.

Friedman, T., Rolfe, P., and Perry, S. (1960) Home treatment of psychiatric patients. *American Journal of Psychiatry,* 135:592–593.

Grad, J., and Sainsbury, P. (1968) The effects that patients have on their families in a community-care and a control psychiatric service: A two-year follow-up. *British Journal of Psychiatry,* 114:265–278.

Hoult, J., and Reynolds, I. (1984) Schizophrenia: a comparative trial of community-oriented and hospital-oriented psychiatric care. *Acta Psychiatrica Scandinavia,* 69:359–372.

Hoult, J., Reynolds, I., Charbonneau-Powis, M., Weekes, P., and Briggs, J. (1983) Psychiatric versus community treatment: the results of a randomized trial. *Australian and New Zealand Journal of Psychiatry,* 17:160–167.

Jerrell, J.M., and Hu, T.W. (1989) Cost-effectiveness of intensive clinical and case management compared with an existing system of care. *Inquiry,* 26:224–234.

Knapp, M., Beecham, J., Kostogeorgopolou, V., Hallam, A., Fenyo, A., Marks, I.M., Connolly, J., and Muijen, M. (1994) Service use and costs of home-based versus hospital based care for people with serious mental illness. *British Journal of Psychiatry,* 165:195–203.

Langsley, D.G., and Kaplan, D.M. (1968) *The Treatment of Families in Crisis.* New York: Grune and Stratton.

Marks, I., Connolly, J., Muijen, M., Audini, B., McNamee, G., and Lawrence, R.E. (1994) Home-based versus hospital care for people with serious mental illness. *British Journal of Psychiatry,* 165:179–194.

Marks, I., Connolly, J., and Muijen, M. (1988) The Maudsley Daily Living Programme: a controlled cost-effectiveness study of community-based versus standard in-patient care of serious mental illness. *Bulletin of the Royal College of Psychiatrists,* 12:22–24.

Muijen, M., Marks, I., Connolly, J., Audini, B., and McNamee, G. (1992) The Daily Living Programme preliminary comparison of community versus hospital-based treatment for the seriously mentally ill facing emergency admission. *British Journal of Psychiatry,* 160:379–384.

Olfson, M. (1990) Assertive community treatment: an evaluation of the experimental evidence. *Hospital and Community Psychiatry,* 41:635–641.

Pai, S., and Kapur, R.L. (1982) Impact of treatment intervention on the relationship between dimensions of clinical psychopathology, social dysfunction and burden on the family of psychiatric patients. *British Journal of Psychiatry,* 12:651–658.

Pasamanick, B., Scarpitti, F.R., and Dinitz, S. (1967) *Schizophrenics in the Community.* New York: Appleton-Century-Crofts.

Primm, A.B., and Houck, J. (1990) COSTAR: Flexibility in urban community mental health. In Cohen, N.L. (ed.), *Psychiatry Takes to the Streets,* pp. 107–120. New York: The Guilford Press.

Reding, K.M., Raphelson, M., and Montgomery, C.B. (1994) Home visits: psychiatrists' attitudes and practice patterns. *Community Mental Health Journal,* 30:285–296.

Reynolds, I., and Hoult, J.E. (1984) The relatives of the mentally ill: a comparative trial of community-oriented and hospital-oriented psychiatric care. *Journal of Nervous and Mental Disease,* 172:480–489.

Roca, R.P., Breakey, W.R., and Fischer, P.J. (1987) Medical care of chronic psychiatric outpatients. *Hospital and Community Psychiatry,* 38:741–745.

Stein, L.I., and Test, M.A. (1980) Alternative to mental hospital treatment. I. Conceptual model, treatment program and clinical evaluation. *Archives of General Psychiatry,* 37:392–397.

Stein, L.I., and Test, M.A. (1985) *The Training in Community Living Model: A Decade of Experience.* San Francisco: Jossey-Bass.

Test, M.A., and Stein, L.I. (1980) Alternative to mental hospital treatment, III. Social cost. *Archives of General Psychiatry,* 37:409–412.

Thompson, K.S., Griffith, E.E.H., and Leaf, P.J. (1990) A historical review of the Madison model of community care. *Hospital and Community Psychiatry,* 41:625–633.

Thornicroft, G., and Breakey, W.R. (1991) The COSTAR Programme: 1: improving social networks of the long-term mentally ill. *British Journal of Psychiatry*, 159:245–249.

Torrey, E.F. (1986) Continuous treatment teams in the care of the chronically mentally ill. *Hospital and Community Psychiatry*, 37:1243–1246.

Weisbrod, B.A., Test, M.A., and Stein, L.I. (1980) Alternative to mental hospital treatment. *Archives of General Psychiatry*, 37:400–405.

Witheridge, T.F. (1989) The assertive community treatment worker: an emerging role and its implications for professional training. *Hospital and Community Psychiatry*, 40:620–624.

Witheridge, T.F., Dincin, J., and Appleby, L. (1982) Working with the most frequent recidivists: A total team approach to assertive resource management. *Psychosocial Rehabilitation Journal*, 5:9–11.

17

Emergency Services in the Community Psychiatry Network

MARK N. MOLLENHAUER
MICHAEL J. KAMINSKY

The Federal Community Mental Health legislation of the 1960s and 1970s mandated a psychiatry emergency service (PES) as one of the five basic components of the Community Mental Health Center (P.L. 88–164, 1963; P.L. 94–63, 1975), recognizing that hospital emergency departments had not traditionally responded adequately to the emergency mental health needs of communities. Since that time, clinical practice and legislation have further shaped and refined the role of the PES in the community system. The emergency service plays several broad roles: It is a high-volume point of entry into the service system; it is a back-up for other services outside their normal working hours; and it advocates for patients and for the mental health system itself with somatic physicians and other service agencies. All these roles depend on an experienced and well-trained staff that can make accurate psychiatric diagnoses, can understand the whole patient in terms of the social context from which she or he springs, and can use the community service network to develop an effective treatment plan for the patient. The resources needed to meet these requirements are costly and are most efficiently focused at one site rather than being distributed and duplicated throughout the community, especially since the narrowing of the CMHC mission during the 1980s (Hillard, 1994). The PES is where resources such as psychiatric and medical expertise, properly trained security staff, seclusion rooms, and 24-hour staffing are based. With these resources, and a collaborative relationship with a general emergency medicine department, the PES is able to respond instantly to behavioral emergencies of any magnitude. For the responses to be effective in the long term, the PES must be aware of and connected to the rest of the community network and must also be familiar with the life of the community it serves: its culture, its structure, its needs, its resources, and its temperament (Huffine and Craig, 1974).

The PES is part of a complex and sometimes poorly integrated set of medical, social, and law-enforcement systems. Even when it is functioning at its best, certain difficulties are inherent. Breakdowns are liable to occur in service integration and coordination; some patients may misuse the system; and the PES may be unable to meet all the non-psychiatric needs of its patients or to work effectively with other treatment providers within the system.

Over the past few years, health care delivery and reimbursement have changed because of budget constraints and the implementation of managed care methods. These changes have affected the practice of emergency psychiatry, primarily by directing more patients to effective, innovative, and intense outpatient treatments, rather than to inpatient treatment settings (Lazarus, 1993a). Most recently, as the PES has become a fully realized component of the community network, it has spread outside the walls of the hospital, taking its services onto the streets in the form of mobile crisis services (Wellin et al., 1987).

The Need for Emergency Services

To understand the diverse aspects of the function of the PES, it is first necessary to understand why it exists, and whom it serves. Although a psychiatric emergency is ultimately defined by the patient and his community, it usually involves a dangerous or distressed patient manifesting a behavioral disturbance that cannot be or has not been dealt with in a less intensive setting, such as the clinic or the home. The PES manages patients with such behavioral emergencies and plans the treatment of these patients once the immediate crisis has passed.

Three distinct constituencies benefit from the PES: the community, the community health network, and the patient. The PES serves the community by treating people with changes in mental life who can be dangerous or disruptive to families, neighborhoods, or workplaces. It serves the community mental health network by treating patients who are unwilling to be treated or who are unmanageable in other settings. Also, patients may experience crisis at times when the community mental health network is otherwise unable to respond effectively or efficiently, so that the emergency service provides the only resource. The PES serves patients not only by relieving distress and suffering, but also by protecting them from themselves, since while they are mentally disturbed they may make decisions or take actions they will later regret.

The PES serves three groups of patients: people with severe mental illness, people with extreme personality vulnerabilities, and people with somatic illnesses who manifest psychiatric symptoms.

Severe Mental Illness

Patients with severe mental illnesses are seen in the emergency service when their symptoms become too distressing or too dangerous to themselves or others. In the midst of major mental illness, whether chronic or acute, they may not be able to make informed, appropriate decisions about major life matters, including their health care. Instead, their decisions may be based on colorations of mood, delusional belief systems, or input from hallucinations. Risk may arise from errors of omission, as in failing to look both ways before crossing the street or being unable to eat or bathe, or from errors of commission, as in assaulting family members or attempting suicide. People with chronic mental illness may make poor decisions even when they are not in the severest extremes of illness. For example, a person with schizophrenia may have poor judgment as a result of baseline thought disorder or disorganization.

Patients with severe mental illnesses may avoid other psychiatric treatment and end up in the PES for that reason, or they may be brought there because they cannot safely be managed elsewhere. They may divert themselves from the community network as a result of culture, prejudice, and life experience, or of illness itself. Some patients and their care-givers may come from a social context in which traditional medical treatment is eschewed or mistrusted, or may have had a bad experience in the system, or may doubt psychiatry's efficacy. Others may deny the reality of the illness, or believe that help is not possible. Thus people may avoid the psychiatric treatment network until a crisis or the severity of the illness drives them to the emergency department of the hospital, viewed by many people, particularly in disadvantaged urban populations, as a source of primary care and a problem solver for a variety of human service needs. The PES then, despite the efforts to direct patients to less intensive and less costly alternatives, often becomes the first point of contact for acutely ill psychiatric patients.

Emergency services in many jurisdictions are designated by law as as the appropriate agencies to take clinical control when patients with severe mental illness lose control of their own behavior. Under involuntary treatment statutes individuals with severe mental illness can be coercively brought into treatment when they behave dangerously—usually by the police, friends, or family. In this situation the PES is a universally available and easily accessible setting in which patients in any mental state and of any degree of dangerousness may be contained, managed, and treated (Gillig et al., 1990).

The unpredictable behavior and dangerous decisions that bring a patient into treatment continue to affect his care even when he is in the treatment setting. Violence may be directed toward health care workers just as much as anyone else. A delusional patient may feel threatened by all, and therefore may act against any. Similarly, a severely disturbed patient who was judged to be at risk of suicide at home or in the street, continues to be at risk of attempting suicide while sitting in a waiting room. A standard outpatient clinic often cannot provide the support and tight control needed in this situation, so that these patients are directed to the PES for their initial evaluation.

Personality Disorders

Some patients with personality disorders come to the PES as a result of poor coping skills, inability to evaluate options, exaggerated dependency needs, hopelessness, or despair. For example, a young person with dramatic and narcissistic traits might impulsively attempt suicide after a romantic disappointment, not pausing to think that he or she might die as a result, or that life is full of contingencies and options if he or she did not attempt self-harm. Patients such as these require support, remoralization, and crisis management. This can be done well in the intensive setting of a PES and may avert or shorten inpatient admission.

Some other patients with personality disorders who present to the PES may be pathologically extroverted: they are present-oriented to a degree that interferes with their functioning. They "live for the moment" and act on impulse. They do not tolerate frustration well and seek immediate gratification. Problems may arise for them in the PES because of conflicts of expectations: They may seek care in the PES with the goal of obtaining physical comfort through pharmacologic or other means, while their care providers have other goals related to health and quality of life. The clinicians seek not merely to ease the pain of the moment, but to provide assistance to the individual in developing his own coping strategies for future well-being. Present orientation in absence of planning leaves these patients impulsive and vulnerable to active self-harm or to harmful situations. This often includes the use of drugs and alcohol, which lead to both physical illnesses such as AIDS or hepatic cirrhosis, and to secondary mental illnesses, such as drug-induced mood disorders or psychotic syndromes.

Pathologically extroverted patients often demonstrate a series of paradoxes that complicate their care. They may feel disenfranchised while at the same time acting entitled or demanding. They may mistrust the health care system while at the same time demanding that the health care system take care of them. They may be unaware and be unwilling to be made aware of the consequences of their behaviors for themselves, for other individuals, and for society as a whole, yet this awareness may be the best thing for them. Impulsivity and low frustration tolerance, which lead to dissatisfaction with life and demoralization, may in some patients lead to abuse of mood-altering drugs, which can complicate the clinical picture by inducing drug-related depressive syndromes indistinguishable from idiopathic mood disorders. At other times, patients may merely claim symptoms of mood disorders to achieve their goals of comfort. Providers must start with the presumption that any threats of suicide are genuine, but keep in mind that threats may be manipulative, aimed at achieving only the goal of comfort. Distinguishing malingered from genuine mood disorders requires an extended and complete evaluation of the patient, including information gathered from outside sources.

Somatic Illnesses with Psychiatric Symptoms

A third major category of patients who present themselves to the PES are those with psychiatric symptoms resulting from somatic illness. Patients in this category can be initially directed to psychiatrists because their symptoms are not at first recognized to be those of a somatic disorder. A careful diagnostic evaluation by the emergency psychiatrist is needed to establish that there is an underlying physical illness, and to redirect the patient to the most appropriate medical treatment. Mistakes in triage may begin with the patient, for example, where someone beginning to become delirious from psychotropic medications assumes the medication is ineffective and begins to take larger doses, only to make the symptoms worse. In another case, a psychiatric patient may be aware that the symptoms are not typical of his or her psychiatric disorder, but the primary medical doctor or the emergency department physician may not heed this information or may ignore the possibility that a change in mental state is due to "medical" problems rather than to a primary psychiatric disorder.

Medical illnesses presenting with mental status changes such as delirium, confusion, or stupor, or occurring in a person with psychosis or severe personality disorder, may place the person at risk directly, because of metabolic or structural disturbance, or indirectly, because of the poor judgment and inattention that result. Thus, in caring for patients with mental status changes due to medical problems, the emergency team faces the same difficulties as in the care of the severely mentally ill. Often the emergency physician or primary medical doctors do not appreciate that a medical treatment plan that would be reasonable and appropriate for a patient with intact cognition will fail in one who is confused, deluded, or impulsive. Thus, though the care of these medically ill patients is not, strictly speaking, within the purview of psychiatry, advocacy for them must be. The PES clinician must be able to recognize when psychiatric symptoms reflect an underlying medical condition, argue persuasively for its treatment, and fight off efforts to construe the problems as primarily psychiatric. The source of the problems cannot be discerned, and the proper care cannot be determined, however, until a complete evaluation is done, including history, physical examination, appropriate laboratory tests, psychiatric history, and mental state examination.

Functions of the Emergency Service

Point of Entry

Patients with psychiatric needs arrive in an emergency facility for a variety of reasons. Whatever their original reason for presentation, when their psychiatric problems become apparent, they will be directed to the psychiatric service. The psychiatric team must assess the presenting problem, but must go beyond immediate treatment to take the long view of the person's needs, including the correct disposition within the mental health care system for a definitive response to the person's treatment. Some patients have little insight into their psychiatric treatment needs and would not otherwise seek out psychiatric treatment, were they not referred by the emergency medical staff (Ellison and Wharff, 1985; Craig et al., 1974.) In communities where there may be little access to primary care, including primary psychiatric care, people may not come into treatment until a crisis occurs for themselves, their families, or the community. The PES is often the component of the community network that is able to meet this need for immediate treatment by being prepared for the intensity of the crisis and can also establish a definitive ongoing treatment plan within the mental health system.

Even in the midst of crisis, there is variation in patients' insight and desire for treatment. At one end of the spectrum are those who want psychiatric help but know no other way to get it than to come to the general hospital emergency department. In the middle of the spectrum are people with psychiatric problems who may pass through a general emergency department for somatic complaints and are referred to a PES when their psychiatric symptoms or signs are discovered by emergency physicians. Finally at the opposite end of the spectrum are patients who are unaware of any disturbance or are unwilling to be treated. They may be brought in for evaluation by the police, by friends or by family.

Maximum Intensity Available at All Hours

The PES should be designed to deal with any intensity of behavioral disturbance at any hour of the day or night. This allows the rest of the community network to focus its energies on ongoing treatment provision, to adhere more closely to regular schedules of daily work, and not to have to allocate its resources to anticipating behavioral emergencies. Since the PES must sustain vigilant watchfulness at all hours and be prepared to deliver clinical care of any level of intensity at any hour, it can also stand in for other components of the community system during off-hours. To fulfill this system function, linkages with other system components are vitally important for information sharing. Case managers, therapists, and other care providers, who have expert longitudinal knowledge of their patients, should be accessible 24 hours a day to provide background information to the emergency team, and the emergency team must make use of this availability.

Advocacy

Dealing with the acute psychiatric manifestations of physical illness puts the PES in frequent contact with somatic physicians and the medical system as a whole, and therefore allows it to be an advocate for the patient and for the psychiatric system. Thus, it may be the PES that reminds somatic physicians that patients with histories of psychiatric illness may also have physical illnesses that must be treated, or that in spite of behavioral disturbances or disorganization of thinking, psychiatric patients deserve respect and adequate medical treatment. The PES may further remind the medical community of how people with psychiatric problems can get access to psychiatric treatment in the community network (Hall et al., 1978).

The PES in an urban catchment area may at one time or another make decisions regarding the immediate treatment and follow-up of a relatively large proportion of the clientele of the community psychiatry network and thereby contribute to the shaping of policy and the allocation of resources. For example, if the PES transferred all patients with psychiatric disorders to state hospitals, the quality and style of treatment in the state hospital system would be altered, as would the allocation of resources within the state system. If the PES routinely sent marginally violent people into outpatient follow-up rather than admitting them, it would contribute to raising the rate of violence in the community. Thus the philosophy and commitment of the PES to the community and within the health system have major impact on the locus of care of patients and thereby on the functioning of the system as a whole, in both cost and effectiveness.

Social Control and Legal Issues

Society expects psychiatry to treat those who are suffering or cause others to suffer because of mental illness. However, out of concern for the rights of citizens, society also regulates psychiatric practice. The need to balance these concerns is evident in interactions between law enforcement and psychiatry in the PES. Since dangerous behaviors may be prompted not only by psychiatric illness but also by a variety of other motivations, an element of social control has been inserted into the medical practice of psychiatry by government and by society at large (Watson et al., 1993). The PES must not only establish good and mutually supportive working relationships with the police, but also be well versed and expert in the legal requirements for respecting patients' rights and for implementing involuntary treatment formalities when needed (Chapter 13).

Clinical Methods

The process of care in a Psychiatry Emergency Service involves prioritization and medical "clearance," acute management, crisis intervention, and treatment planning. The quality and success of all these enterprises depends on thorough evaluation of the patient. Evaluation must focus on the whole patient and must attend not only to the potential disease process but also to the patient's history, character structure, patterns of behavior, and social context. This process often requires gathering data from outside informants and outside records. A complete evaluation allows the mental health professional to make an accurate provisional diagnosis and, equally important, to formulate the patient's case, to understand the patient's strengths and weaknesses, and thereby to understand both whether treatment is required, and which treatments and plans are likely to be successful.

Prioritization and Medical "Clearance"

Although a patient in a general emergency department may have already been triaged before reaching the psychiatric worker, timely attention to the most urgent problems requires prioritization among the patients waiting to be seen. Several questions should be addressed: Which patient has the most intense crisis? Who must be admitted? Which patient can be diverted to a less intense setting, such as a day hospital or a crisis bed? Who will be able to follow up with an outpatient treatment plan? Who will need in-home services? Who is medically unstable? Answering these questions allows the clinician to decide whom to see first, and on whom to expend the most time (Rosenzweig, 1992; Birch and Martin, 1985).

The question regarding medical instability hinges on the interaction of mental and medical states and is particularly important since the myth of medical "clearance" persists in many emergency departments. In many medical settings, the evaluation process is sequential. First the somatic physician examines the patient and declares him to be "clear." That physician considers that his task is complete and sends the patient to the psychiatrist. The psychiatrist or other psychiatric clinician then examines the patient and assesses his psychiatric mental state. A basic error is made with this arrangement: The patient is not viewed as a whole person but as a series of real or potential health problems. A better approach is for psychiatric and somatic physicians to work cooperatively, collegially and in parallel, to decide to what extent the patient's medical conditions may mask or account for his psychiatric conditions, and to what extent his psychiatric condition may mask or account for his physical condition. In that way the best treatment plan for the whole patient can be developed. Two experts, one focusing on somatic issues, and one on psychiatric issues, can together develop the appropriate order of treatment priorities for the patient.

Acute Management and Crisis Intervention

Once an initial assessment of the patient's medical and psychiatric state has been made, acute management may begin. This may involve definitive treatments in the emergency department (Forster and King, 1994a; Forster and King, 1994b), or it may involve holding measures such as the practice of using neuroleptics as sedatives (Pilowsky et al., 1992; Coffman et al., 1987). In an era of ever shortening lengths of stay, inpatient treatment may, in effect, begin in the Emergency Department. Initial doses of anti-manic agents, for example, may be started while awaiting an inpatient bed. The advent of SSRI antidepressants has made initiation of antidepressant therapy in the PES a possibility, since unlike the tricyclic antidepressants, these drugs may be started at full therapeutic dose and have high therapeutic indexes, low suicide potential, and relatively low rates of side effects. Patients are being discharged home from emergency departments sicker than ever before due to more stringent criteria for inpatient admission and the availability of alternate treatment strategies. The early initiation of antidepressant treatment is one factor in the success of this approach. Patients who are having hallucinations or delusions or are agitated or dangerous for other reasons may need to be sedated in the PES, typically using neuroleptics or benzodiazepines. This sedation serves to keep the environment safe, as well as to relieve in some measure the patient's suffering, and help him to retain his dignity. For some psychotic patients, the structure of the emergency department, by providing structure and control, may itself be therapeutic, when contrasted with the chaotic world from which he comes, and into which his illness thrusts him.

Breaking the patterns of thoughts, behaviors, and feelings that led to the emergency visit may be as important to the success of a subsequent outpatient or inpatient stay as the initiation of medications. Some patients come to the PES because their psychic pain is intense and they have become demoralized and hopeless at the prospect of ever improving. If a caring provider can say with authority that all will be well and that improvement will eventually come, then the patient may be able to go on. This intervention is often more successful if a change in medication is made at the same time. Other patients come to the PES because the difficulties in their interpersonal relationships have grown to what seem to them to be crisis proportions, independent of major mental illness. It is often possible for the health care provider, after completing an evaluation and formulation of the problem, to point out to the patient an element in his log jam of thoughts, feelings, or behaviors that, if removed, would allow resumption of progress or normal living. It may be possible for the health care provider to help the patient de-catastrophize his situation, and see that though it may be bad, it is not horrible, awful, or intolerable. Finally, it may be possible for the health care provider to use the crisis as a catalyst to bring many of the elements of the patient's support network together in the same room, in order to mediate a new accommodation to family or neighborhood stresses which the identified patient may cause or endure. These psychotherapeutic interventions are as important to a successful subsequent inpatient stay as they are to any outpatient disposition. If executed carefully, they may, for some patients, allow an outpatient disposition where an inpatient admission had seemed inevitable.

Treatment Planning

After acute crises are addressed, the emergency psychiatrist or team begins planning subsequent treatment for the patient. For some patients this may involve inpatient admission in a state or a private facility. For others, it may mean arranging admission to a crisis holding bed or to a day hospital. For still others it may mean inpatient or outpatient drug rehabilitation. If definitive treatment or temporizing measures in the emergency department have been effective, the treatment plan may continue with an outpatient clinic referral.

Deciding among these various alternatives involves a series of risk-benefit analyses from the perspective of the patient, the community, and the inpatient milieu. In making the decision to admit, the health care provider must weigh the benefit to the patient of discharge—freedom to act, ability to work, free access to family and friends—with the risk of discharge, for example, violence toward self, continued suffering, exposure to a chaotic life circumstance, and worsening of illness if unmonitored. Similarly, the risk of inpatient admission—dependency, loss of autonomy, restricted access to friends and family—must be balanced against the benefit, including assured compliance with medication treatment, reduction of risk of self-harm, and reduction of suffering (Gordon and Beresin, 1981; Slaby, 1985).

In making the decision where to admit a patient, the clinician must weigh similar risks and benefits for the patient, but must also consider the risks and benefits to the inpatient unit and to the community. On inpatient units and in communities, for example, one must consider the patient's effect on people around him, consider whether the setting is equipped to handle any behavioral disturbances, and consider whether it can provide him the treatment he requires.

Community Connections and Networks

In order to fulfill its roles as point of entry into the community network, back-up for other services, and patient and system advocate, and to perform its functions of triage, management, and treatment planning, the PES must have a community-oriented philosophy. The emergency department must be accessible and must be able to access diverse sources of information. In order to make effective treatment plans, the PES staff must understand the culture both of the people it treats, and of the people who care about them—their families, friends, churches, and other community institutions. The PES must know what financial and physical hardships the patient and his community endure. To know the likelihood of compliance, it is important to understand prevalent community attitudes toward treatment. This knowledge allows the PES to understand just how accessible it must be, based on community need, and allows it to structure itself to meet this need. Knowledge of the community provides opportunity to obtain supplemental information to augment a patient's history and to know how to seek and find outside informants.

For effective treatment planning, the PES must have particularly good connections to the rest of the psychiatric service network. Lists and directories of phone numbers and contact people in the various agencies and disposition sites are invaluable to the PES worker. Even more important is a trusting relationship among all those negotiating the care of the patient, so that transitions between caretakers occurs smoothly and without surprise for patient or staff. This again allows the PES to plan treatments that will work in the community in which it exists. It allows the PES to share the records of previous treatment successes and failures with other components of the community psychiatry program. It allows the emergency psychiatrist to use the patient's existing social network to plan treatment in a way that will be successful in the long term and to make appropriate referrals to agencies interested in caring for the patient (Bachrach, 1991).

Problems in the System

Problems arise in the Psychiatric Emergency Service even when it is operating at its best. They arise due to the kind and quality of complaints and behaviors that psychiatric patients present, the nature of the Community Psychiatric System, and the influence of managed care on the Psychiatric Emergency Service.

Misuse of the PES

Emergency departments are open to everyone who walks in the door, and are thus vulnerable to "misuse" by persons who use the facility to seek some form of help that is not truly within the realm of medical emergencies. Some antisocial patients may have goals relating to comfort or personal gain of some kind rather than treatment. They may be seeking to fulfill basic needs, such as food, shelter, or safety, and may see the Psychiatric Emergency Room as a clearinghouse for such resources. They may feign psychiatric symptoms in order to gain admission. Alternatively, they may not desire admission at all but merely want to have some need met in the middle of the night. Some people may present to the PES with the goal of obtaining psychoactive medications such as benzodiazepines, opiates, or anticholinergics for recreational use. Others may have actual psychiatric symptoms, but have a lower than average threshold for seeking help; their symptoms and distress do not seem, in the eyes of the PES, to constitute an emergency. These patients misuse the availability and easy accessibility of the PES and may, for example, repeatedly spend the night in the PES, gladly accepting discharge the next morning. Since the PES is costly to the health system, the extra load placed by these patients can have economic consequences for providers as well. Sorting them out from the truly disturbed population is costly in time and morale for the PES staff, whose workload may be excessive and who must set priorities among the various people seeking help (Ellison et al., 1986). Identification of "ER abusers" is needed in such cases. Treatment plans for these individuals can be established and kept available to the emergency department staff not only to minimize inappropriate PES use, but also to foster more constructive approaches to meeting their needs.

System Failures

"Inappropriate" patients, those without real emergency needs, may present even though the PES and community system are working at their best. However, the presence of these patients may also reflect deficits in the PES itself or in other aspects of the community system. Inappropriate presentation to the PES may reflect long waits to be seen at outpatient clinics, or a failure to respond to minor crises. It may also reflect poor coordination between multiple care-givers within the community network. It may not be only the patient who is misusing the PES: If the regular clinic therapist sends the patient to the PES without there being a true emergency, she or he is misusing the service as well.

PES Failures

The PES may also fail to perform its role effectively. For example, rather than confronting troublesome patients when they inappropriately present to the service, the clinicians in the PES may admit patients for an unnecessary inpatient stay. They may not seek outside informants to confirm history, or they may fail to confer with the regular treatment team. Failures of these sorts often reflect inadequacy of training, resources, or organization in the PES or elsewhere in the community system.

Mobile Crisis Teams

As the importance of the PES within the community network has become evident, it has also become evident that emergency services can be moved out of the hospital emergency room, and many community networks have had great success with mobile emergency treatment teams or mobile crisis services. Mobile teams can be responsive to persons who cannot or will not come to an emergency department, and they can also take some of the stress off the traditional emergency department. Mobile emergency teams go wherever they are needed in the community, at the request of family members or concerned individuals. Treatment is provided *in situ* or by bringing individuals in to the emergency department or to an outpatient clinic for more formalized care. Such interventions can lead to de-escalation of patients who would otherwise require involuntary transportation to the PES, involvement of police, or inpatient admissions. Evaluations at home can also lead to increased appreciation by the treatment team of the patient's social milieu, adversities, support systems, and other substrates of behavior. Further, once a plan is devised, an in-home team can more easily recruit a support system from the patient's own setting. Mobile interventions may facilitate problem-solving, due to mobility and continuity with the community. In addition to avoiding admission, mobile interventions may avoid the involvement of law enforcement with its attendant stigma (Zealburg et al., 1993; Yu-Chin and Arcuni, 1990).

The crisis team must always be aware of potential danger to staff members. Unlike the hospital-based psychiatric emergency service, a mobile crisis team sees patients without the benefit of seclusion rooms, restraints, or security personnel. Furthermore, like the hospital-based service, a mobile crisis team is seeing both patients who want treatment and those who do not want treatment. The combination of dangerousness and variable willingness to be treated leads to a particular style of intervention. Greater care must be taken to avoid the appearance of being threatening. The threat of dangerousness may, however, be less in a setting familiar to the patient, and diminished by the social conventions of hospitality. Still, the greatest difficulty is in knowing which patients absolutely require to be brought in to the center and which ones may be treated by the mobile team. A high-level triage process is required, therefore, and is best carried out by people with experience in dealing with psychiatric patients in general but with emergency psychiatric patients in particular. Sensitivity to causative or complicating medical problems must be very high.

Summary

Emergency services are a vital component of a community psychiatric service system, acting as a portal of entry into the system for many patients, but also as a back-up to the rest of the system when urgent needs for treatment arise. The PES provides an interface between psychiatry and somatic medicine, and often great skill is needed to clarify the physical and psychological causes of acute states. The PES also interacts with police and other agencies of the society in dealing with the many problems that patients encounter. Increasingly, mobile emergency services are being developed to expand the capacity of emergency services to respond effectively to crises.

References

Bachrach, L. (1991) Planning high-quality services. *Hospital and Community Psychiatry,* 42: 268–269.

Birch, G., and Martin, M. (1985) Emergency mental health triage: A multidisciplinary approach. *Social Work,* 30:364–366.

Coffman, J.A., Nasrallah, H.A., Lyskowski, J., MCalley-Whitters, M., and Dunner, F.J. (1987) Clinical effectiveness of oral and parenteral rapid neuroleptization. *Journal of Clinical Psychiatry,* 48:20–24.

Craig, T.J., Huffine, C.L., and Brookes, M. (1974) Completion of referral to psychiatric services by inner city residents. *Archives of General Psychiatry,* 31:353–357.

Ellison, J.M., and Wharff, E.A. (1985) More than a gateway: the role of the emergency psychiatry service in the community mental health network. *Hospital and Community Psychiatry,* 36:180–184.

Ellison, J.M., Blum, N., and Barsky, A.J. (1986) Repeat visitors in the psychiatric emergency service: a critical review of the data. *Hospital and Community Psychiatry,* 37:37–41.

Forster, P., and King, J. (1994a) Definitive treatment of patients with serious mental disorders in an emergency service, Part I. *Hospital and Community Psychiatry,* 45:867–869.

Forster, P., and King, J. (1994b) Definitive treatment of patients with serious mental disorders in an emergency service, Part II. *Hospital and Community Psychiatry,* 45:1177–1178.

Gillig, P.M., Grubb, P., Kruger, R., Johnson, A., Hillard, J.R., and Tucker, N. (1990) What do psychiatric emergency patients really want and how do they feel about what they get? *Psychiatric Quarterly,* 61:189–196.

Gordon, C.D., and Beresin, E. (1981) Emergency ward management of the borderline patient. *General Hospital Psychiatry,* 3:237–240.

Hall, R.C.W., Popkin, M.K., Devaul, R.A., Faillace, L.A., and Stickney, S.K. (1978) Physical illness presenting as psychiatric disease. *Archives of General Psychiatry,* 35:1315–1320.

Hillard, J.R. (1994) The past and future of psychiatric emergency services in the U.S. *Hospital and Community Psychiatry,* 45:541–542.

Huffine, C.L., and Craig, T.J. (1974) Social factors in the utilization of an urban psychiatric emergency service. *Archives of General Psychiatry,* 30:249–255.

Lazarus, A. (1993a) Improving psychiatric services in managed care programs. *Hospital and Community Psychiatry,* 44:709.

Pilowsky, L.S., Ring, H., Shine, P.J., Battersby, M., and Lader, M. (1992) Rapid tranquilisation. *British Journal of Psychiatry,* 160:831–835.

Public Law 88-164 (1963) CMHC Act of 1963.

Public Law 94-63 (1975) CMHC Act of 1975.

Rosenzweig, L. (1992) Psychiatric triage: a cost effective approach to quality management in mental health. *Journal of Psychosocial Nursing,* 30:5–8.

Slaby, A.E. (1985) Crisis-oriented treatment. In Lipton, F.R., Goldfinger, S.M. (eds.) *Emergency Psychiatry at the Crossroads,* pp. 21–34. San Francisco: Jossey-Bass.

Watson, M.A., Segal, S.P., and Newhill, C.E. (1993) Police referral to psychiatric emergency services and its effect on disposition decisions. *Hospital and Community Psychiatry,* 44: 1085–1090.

Wellin, E., Slesinger, D.P., and Hollistter, C.D. (1987) Psychiatric emergency services: evolution, adaptation and proliferation. *Social Science and Medicine,* 24:475–482.

Yu-Chin, R., and Arcuni, O.J. (1990) Short-term hospitalization for suicidal patients within a crisis intervention service. *General Hospital Psychiatry,* 12:153–158.

Zealburg, J.J., Santos, A.B., and Fisher, R.K. (1993) Benefits of mobile crisis programs. *Hospital and Community Psychiatry,* 44:16–17.

18

Partial Hospitalization

GERALD NESTADT

Compared to the psychiatric hospital, with its long and varied history, partial hospitalization is a relatively recent development in psychiatric care. The first day hospitals were established a half-century ago, but despite its 50-year lifespan, partial hospitalization remains remarkably unfamiliar to many in the psychiatric community. Partial hospital services have had a checkered history and at various times and places have developed in differing incarnations. The principles, philosophies, and methods of care have been affected by competing needs and changing therapeutic strategies reflecting developments in the practice of psychiatry.

Because partial hospitals have remained peripheral to the mainstream of psychiatric practice, they have been influenced more by individual innovators than by traditions encompassing psychiatry in general. This has resulted in the scope and focus of these services remaining relatively broadly defined and often vague in conception. Furthermore, most programmatic developments have occurred locally rather than nationally. Nevertheless, efforts have been made to develop a coherent framework for this treatment approach.

Although partial hospitals, much like psychiatric services in general hospitals, often function as discrete treatment services independent of other service providers, they are more effective when they are incorporated as an integral component of the community service network, taking advantage of those features of the partial hospital which patients and providers find attractive: flexible attendance schedules engendering less stigma, lower cost, and fewer family and social disruptions. Moreover, a permeable interface with other community services permits both intervention and the exchange of information to occur in the community or in the hospital. Despite a number of limitations, utilization of partial hospitals has fluctuated, and in the 1990s growth appears to be exploding and interest expanding so that the American Association of Partial Hospitalization (AAPH, 1991) has developed guidelines and standards for partial hospitals in the United States.

History

The first day hospital was developed by Dzahagrov in the Soviet Union in 1937 to deal with a paucity of psychiatric inpatient beds and additional economic pressures. The concept spread: Cameron in Montreal and Bierer in London opened the first day hospitals in Canada and the United Kingdom. In the United States, the first day hospitals were founded at the Menninger Clinic and Yale University in the 1950s. Vigorous interest emerged in the 1960s and 1970s when the community psychiatry movement gained momentum and the use of alternate treatment facilities to replace the overcrowded psychiatric hospitals was encouraged. This movement sought services in local rather than distant communities, services that would be closer to home and the family.

A landmark study by Wing and Brown (1970) revealed the inadequacies of mental hospitals in the rehabilitation of chronic psychiatric patients, particularly those with schizophrenia. Their work indicated that an active, medically directed, rehabilitative program was necessary to reduce disability. This and parallel work in psychiatry fostered a movement toward the use of day hospitals as an appropriate stage in the treatment and rehabilitation of chronic mental patients discharged from hospitals.

Simultaneously, there was a growth of outpatient services and a keen interest in treating non-chronic patients who did not require hospitalization. Results of epidemiological surveys revealed an abundance of psychological disturbance in the population, undetected and underserved by the existing health service system. Many of these patients had psychiatric syndromes for which outpatient services alone did not suffice, and partial hospitalization services were conceived of as an appropriate way of providing enhanced services. The Joint Commission on Mental Illness and Health in its 1961 report, *Action for Mental Health,* mandated partial hospitals for community mental health centers receiving federal funds. This aligned partial hospitalization services further with the community psychiatry movement during a period of optimism for psychiatry and with an articulated aim of bringing psychiatry to the community.

This optimism, however, was not fully realized. In the 1980s, the development of partial programs stagnated, and most of the existing programs were under-utilized. More recently, trends to curtail escalating health care expenditures by seeking alternative, less costly services to substitute for the more expensive acute hospital episodes of care have led to renewed interest in partial hospitalization. With this trend, the emphasis is on the development of services that substitute for acute hospital care but are provided at lower cost.

Definitions

The nature of any particular partial hospitalization program is dependent on the specific psychiatric service system in which it resides. Programs are often tailored more to their niche in the system than to specific patient goals. Furthermore, the form of the programs does not necessarily reflect the results of empirical research.

The absence of a clear and unambiguous definition is particularly troublesome. *Partial hospitalization* ought to refer to the duration of the daily treatment period rather than the nature of the services offered. As Hoge and colleagues (1988) pointed out, this is not "partial care." Competing interests in the delivery sector and a diversity of programs make any specific definition incapable of satisfying all involved interests. The resultant heterogeneity makes it difficult for patients, families, providers, and insurance companies to decide on the utility of the partial hospital. Programs differ as to the patients they admit, their staffing, the treatments they offer, and the duration of care. One program may be appropriate for a specific patient while another may not. Faced with these differences and a lack of guidance as to how to make choices, consumers often avoid the partial hospital altogether.

The AAPH guidelines published in 1991 address admission and discharge criteria, staffing patterns, and program procedures. Using this set of standards, one can assess the different programs and make decisions about their utility. The guidelines define partial hospitalization as "a time-limited, ambulatory, active treatment program that offers therapeutically intensive, coordinated structured clinical services within a stable therapeutic milieu." This definition does not distinguish programs that offer an acute, intensive, medically oriented alternative to inpatient services from those that offer a rehabilitative perspective on the provision of care.

Rosie (1987) recommends a broad categorization of programs. He suggests that *day hospitals* are an alternative to traditional psychiatric inpatient units that provide diagnostic and therapeutic services for the acutely ill patient; *day treatment programs* provide care for less acute patients, such as those patients transitioning from inpatient treatment or as an alternative to outpatient treatment; and *day care* has the aim of maintenance and habilitation or rehabilitation of chronic patients. These definitions appropriately articulate a hierarchy of patient acuity and treatment goals.

Functions

The partial hospital serves a variety of functions in the delivery of patient care. There is a guiding principle mentioned repeatedly by proponents of partial hospitals that only one function ought to be served in a particular program so as not to dilute the program and confuse its mission. Nevertheless, there appear to be three recurring themes.

First, a partial hospital is recommended as an alternative to full inpatient hospitalization. The implication is that certain patients can be adequately managed in either setting. It is not intended to suggest that this is the case for all patients: It is crucial to recognize the importance of the 24-hour hospital and to identify the specific role it performs for each patient. Nonetheless, empirical research, described later in this chapter, has shown that one-third to one-half of patients currently provided care on an inpatient service can be treated in a partial hospital. Which particular patients are best suited for partial, as opposed to 24-hour care, remains undefined. There is probably no ready formula that will define the needs of a given patient; the decision, like most others in medicine, must be individualized. Experience with both forms of services provides the clinician with a sense of the appropriate patients for each.

A second common and popular use of the partial hospital is the transition of patients from an acute inpatient service back into the community. This functions as a method to aid and assess the discharge readiness of a patient. In this way, it provides a more structured and formal method than the traditional leave of absence from the 24-hour hospital to assess the practicality and the reality of the treatment plan. This is useful from several vantage points. Often symptoms presented by patients are hidden or subdued while under hospital care and emerge once the patient returns to the community. Medication regimens that appear sensible in the hospital may be unworkable once the patient is at home. Decisions about residential placement, while appearing appropriate from the hospital, may prove untenable in real life. This transition can actually be bi-directional; that is, patients can be "guested" briefly on the inpatient services if the need arises because community care plans have turned out to be inadequate for the patient's needs.

Finally, a partial hospital can provide a more intensive form of evaluation and treatment than can be provided on an outpatient basis. Without the availability of a partial hospital patients may have to be hospitalized for further observation and assessment. In other cases outpatient diagnosis and treatment may be prolonged, with deleterious effects on both patient and cost. Partial hospital programs can provide a sufficient period of intense observation, medical investigation, and assessment of response to medication, with the involvement of an active multidisciplinary team in the diagnostic and management process.

Treatment Model

As discussed in the preceding pages, partial hospital programs vary substantially in the patients they serve and the methods they employ. Nevertheless, they have features in common. They generally function daily, providing care 6 to 8 hours during the day. Most programs operate during weekdays, with some exceptions. There are also evening, weekend, and night hospitals which primarily focus on patients who are employed. All modalities of psychiatric treatment are offered in a partial hospital, including individual, group, behavioral and family psychotherapy, medical care, social work interventions, and occupational therapy. Treatment should be individualized to the needs of the patient and provided by a multidisciplinary team of providers including psychiatrists, psychologists, nurses, occupational therapists, and social workers. In most cases, the daily program is structured, with a variety of therapy and educational groups available to the patients. Treatment is time-limited, although there are substantial variations in the length of stay. In the more acute facilities, the average length of stay is usually less than 30 visits.

Partial hospitals are located in a variety of settings including general hospitals, psychiatric hospitals, multi-service mental health organizations, and as free-standing entities. The location often influences the source and diagnostic makeup of the patients and in the organization of community services, it is optimal to have close links between the components of the system. The ability to move patients rapidly between services with the fewest obstacles is optimal. Likewise, psychiatric staff in all the components should communicate with and advise each other frequently.

Therapeutic Issues

The emphasis of an effective program is on providing care in the context of other components of the community service network in a manner that is in keeping with the character of the community served. This requires an appreciation of the assets and limitations of other service agencies and the development of intimate collaborative relationships. To ensure continuity of care and smooth transitions between services, it is helpful to maintain low thresholds for admission and discharge. The degree of outreach to the community, particularly for absent or physically ill patients, varies across programs; the more this is available, the more able the program is to deal with sicker patients. Contact with families and other social supports are actively pursued.

The management of medical problems and the use of psychotropic medications are conducted much as on an inpatient service. In addition, several unique features contribute to the efficacy of partial hospitals in dealing with particular types of patients. Weil (1984) refers to the "half-time in plus half-time out" distribution of treatment—the interplay between active involvement of the patient in the therapeutic setting simultaneous with active involvement in the community, family, social, and domestic affairs. This circumstance promotes an understanding of the patient in the community context and provides the opportunity for observation of behaviors and stressors that affect the individual. In addition, any emotional or psychiatric difficulties that emerge can be dealt with immediately in the day hospital program.

Partial programs permit and encourage autonomy. Rather than being the passive recipient of treatment and care in a 24-hour program, the individual is required to be responsible for treatment and for personal affairs, which discourages dependence and promotes self-reliance. While family intervention can and does occur in various inpatient and outpatient settings, the alliance between the family, patient, and medical staff in the partial hospital is vital. From the first, families are encouraged to be active members of the treatment team, to observe the patient outside partial hospital hours, and to participate with the patient in health-promoting behaviors. Psychiatric illness in a family member becomes an event that is observed and dealt with, not by extruding the person into a institution until he or she is better, but through an active involvement with the patient during periods of substantial psychopathology. This results in a greater understanding of the nature of the psychopathology, the impairment, and the handicap, and ultimately results in a willingness to accept and help the patient during future exacerbations.

Prevocational assessment is in many cases an important early step for patients in the partial hospital, recognizing the importance of appropriate role functioning for the patient. Skills that are crucial for employment or education are actively pursued, such as time management, timeliness, the use of discretion, and how to relate appropriately to peers and supervisors. Close contacts are kept with rehabilitation programs, employers, schools, sheltered work, and sheltered workshops. This naturally leads into another intervention partial hospitals provide that is unavailable in other services: the gradual weaning of the patient back into the community and into his or her social and occupational role. The partial hospital program, with its flexibility, permits a person to work or attend a rehabilitation program while continuing as a patient in the program. In this way, the adjustment that the patient has to make is part of the active treatment process and discussed on a regular basis. Any assistance and supports needed by the patient are provided during the hours when they are participating in the rehabilitation program.

Medication compliance can be dealt with more effectively than in other treatment settings because patients are personally responsible and are active participants in any mediation regimen. In contrast to an inpatient service, where the patient somewhat passively receives medication as ordered, patients in the partial hospital setting are to a much greater extent required to take responsibility for this aspect of their treatment. Difficulties with compliance therefore become evident rather than remaining hidden, and as a consequence, attempts can be made to deal with this more effectively. A good example is the presence of bothersome side effects from medications. These may not appear as troublesome when in a confined environment; however, when the patient is actively involved in the community, problems may emerge, resulting in discontinuation of medications. In the partial hospital, discussion and modification of medication regimens can occur in the natural setting.

Finally, daily or near daily attendance in a program is in itself a substantial therapeutic intervention. The "coming-and-going" requires an active decision on a daily basis by patients that treatment is appropriate and necessary and that they are making an effort to obtain it. There is a sense of autonomy and owning one's treatment which one does not necessarily have on an inpatient setting. There is also the behavioral aspect of motivating and activating oneself on a regular basis to obtain a goal that one has selected. This certainly provides a foundation, together with involvement of the family, for dealing with issues of insight into the nature of the illness, or as often is the case, the actual recognition of the presence of psychopathology. On a daily basis, this issue is reexplored by patients, their families, and the therapeutic team, which leads to an ultimate acceptance of the nature of the disorder being treated.

A variety of additional therapeutic factors are discussed by Hoge and colleagues (1988). Patients report deriving benefit from factors that stem from the therapeutic milieu. These include perceiving the environment as accepting and fostering altruism and providing a sense of companionship and belonging. There are educational opportunities in the therapeutic setting. Successful completion of the program itself fosters growth in self-esteem.

Utilization Trends

With the contemporary concerns over health care costs, partial hospitalization is under greater scrutiny than at any other time in its history. Insurance providers, administrators, and prospective patients have now turned their attention to this resource as a means of cost containment. There remains a sense of caution on the part of payors, with the recognition that new services do not necessarily replace the old but may merely augment them, at added cost. Nevertheless, since the late 1980s there has been a dramatic increase in the number of programs. According to Leibenluft and Leibenluft (1988), the increase in programs in the 1980s occurred in the private sector, with a coincident decline in the public sector. Still, partial hospital admissions remain a relatively small proportion of total patient care episodes in the United States; the number of patients admitted to partial hospitals is 2 percent of those admitted to outpatient services and 7.6 percent of those admitted to inpatient services.

Empirical Studies of Partial Hospitalization

Empirical evidence of effectiveness provides the best justification for treatment recommendations. Studies that evaluate the effectiveness of partial hospital programs are difficult to conduct and fraught with limitations and flaws (Guy and Gross, 1967), but a number of studies have been conducted since the 1960s, and there have been several comprehensive reviews of this research (Green and De La Cruz, 1981; Rosie, 1987; Creed et al., 1989b). Partial hospitalization research can be categorized according to the specific functions of these programs or the populations studied. The first category evaluates partial hospitals as an alternative to inpatient hospitalization, as a transition from the hospital, and as an alternative to outpatient treatment.

Two relatively early studies compared patients randomly assigned to a day hospital or to an inpatient service. The first, at the Bronx Municipal Hospital, revealed that 66 percent of subjects could be randomized into either a day hospital or inpatient group. Several patients in the day hospital group, however, did require brief inpatient stays. There was no difference between the two randomized groups at follow-up with respect to clinical and social variables (Zwerling and Wilder, 1964). A second study, by Herz and colleagues (1971), was remarkable in that it used the same treatment setting for both groups. This study revealed that 22 percent of patients could be treated effectively in the day hospital mode. In addition to those considered too ill for randomization, others were not randomized because they were "too well" or refused for one of several reasons. There was an equivalent clinical outcome in both groups; however, social outcome was better in the day hospital group, and the inpatients required a longer hospital stay.

More recently, Creed and colleagues (1990) conducted a prospective, randomized controlled trial, comparing day hospital and inpatient services with follow-up at 3 and 12 months. Although 185 patients were eligible for participation, only 175 patients consented to randomization. Of these, 102 (58 percent) could be randomly allocated to either condition, whereas 42 percent could not be allocated. At one-year follow-up, there was no difference between the two groups on clinical, social role, or behavioral measures.

A landmark study was conducted at the Massachusetts Mental Health Center (Gudeman et al., 1983). In 1981, the traditional inpatient services were rearranged in such a way that all patients were admitted directly to one of two day hospitals which replaced the inpatient services. A room-and-board "inn," providing accommodation but no treatment, was available for those patients who needed it, and an intensive care unit provided 24-hour inpatient care if this was essential. The outcome, comparing the periods 19 months before and after the change, revealed no substantial utilization differences except for reductions in length of stay, patient-related staff accidents, elopement, and the use of seclusion or restraint. The remarkable finding was that all patients could be managed in this system, based on the partial hospital.

In summary, research comparing the use of the day hospital as an alternative to 24-hour hospitalization suggests that from one-third to one-half of patients served by the inpatient service can be successfully managed in a partial hospital.

The use of partial hospital programs as transitional facilities from inpatient services is frequently discussed. However, this function has only rarely been studied. Glick and colleagues (1986) compared referral to a day hospital and to routine outpatient services for a group of hospitalized patients. They found a substantially lower dropout rate among the day hospital patients (14 percent) compared to those referred to the outpatient condition (43 percent). However, outcome, based on a variety of indicators including clinical variables and continued medication compliance, did not distinguish the two groups. Patients with affective disorders tended to do better in the day hospital than in outpatient care. These investigators admit that certain factors may have biased the results. For instance, inpatient clinicians may have been reluctant to allow randomization of certain patients, for whom they felt day hospitals would be more appropriate.

An additional body of research examines the third role of day hospitals as alternatives to outpatient services. Tyrer and colleagues (1987) randomized a group of patients with neurotic conditions to either a day hospital or outpatient program. They found no clinical differences between the two groups at follow-up. Given the additional expense of day hospital over outpatient treatment, this mitigates against the use of day hospital services as a routine treatment site for all patients with neurotic conditions. Dick and colleagues (1991) extended the study of this population by studying patients with persistent anxiety or depression who had been referred for day hospital treatment. For this presumably more impaired group, clinical outcomes were significantly superior for the patients treated in the day hospital. Furthermore, the day hospital group fared better on several other outcome measures including structuring of time, socialization, self-rated coping ability, and a preference for the treatment modality.

In the United States, Piper and colleagues (1993) studied patients with affective disorders and anxiety disorders with or without personality disorders, using a different study design. The control population in this case had treatment delayed. The authors found, at 8-month follow-up, significantly better outcome of day hospital treatment.

They reported that the average day hospital patient's clinical improvement exceeded that of the control group by 76 percent.

The other population for whom day hospitals have traditionally provided service are the chronically mentally ill. Ferber and colleagues (1985) studied a day hospital in New York in which the day hospital was the "entry point to a long flexible network of long-term services." Eighty-two percent of patients who completed day hospital treatment were receiving psychiatric services 6 months or more after discharge, a treatment continuity rate twice that for those who did not complete day hospital treatment. Factors that influenced successful completion of treatment included older age, prior hospitalization, family involvement, and the absence of a criminal record. Younger males who were new to the mental health service system were at greater risk for dropping out of treatment, suggesting that a more intensive "treatment indoctrination" is necessary for this group.

Several of the studies cited above evaluated the utility of partial hospital programs for specific patient populations. Two studies by Creed's group (1990; 1989a) suggest which patients are amenable to management in a partial hospital: The majority of patients with neurotic and personality disorders and approximately half of their patients with schizophrenia could be managed in this setting. Patients with manic disorders more frequently had inpatient care recommended. The patients who could not be treated in the day hospital were either involuntary patients or were considered "too ill." A small proportion of individuals could not be managed in the day hospital due to a social factor such as the absence of an adequate living situation. Two clinical features discriminated day hospital patients from inpatients: overactivity and self-neglect.

Cost-Effectiveness

That partial hospitals are more economic than inpatient hospitals should be self-evident; only one shift of staffing is required, compared to three on an inpatient unit. However, this saving in per diem cost is offset by additional costs resulting from greater length of stay, use of emergency facilities, differential post-discharge treatment, and cost to the family, such as loss of employment. Studies by Fink (1979) and Washburn (1976) and their colleagues have compared partial hospital and inpatient treatments with respect to cost. Both studies showed evidence of fiscal advantage to the day hospital. The Massachusetts Mental Health Center program discussed previously revealed that the transition to a day hospital–based service resulted in a 13.5 percent savings with equivalent patient outcomes. In another study, 75 patients were identified as high-frequency psychiatric hospital users. Partial hospital care was substituted for inpatient care for this group with a consequent $400,000 saving over a 4-month period (Leibenluft and Leibenluft, 1988).

Advantages of Partial Hospitalization

Lower cost is the most obvious advantage of partial hospitalization. This is crucial where there are fiscal limits to the quantity of service available for a given population.

Because of lack of understanding of partial hospital services, incentives provided by payers are often perverse, however, and for an individual there may be a cost disadvantage. This occurs where reimbursement is poorer or where co-payment is greater for partial hospitalization relative to 24-hour inpatient care. In this case it is advantageous for the patient to choose 24-hour hospitalization. These circumstances often result in unnecessary 24-hour hospitalization and additional cost to the system.

The second great advantage for partial hospitalization is that it diminishes the disruption of patients' ties to their families and to the community. Care providers (parents, case-managers, etc.) continue in their role, which reduces a sense of isolation and fosters a sense of remaining part of the family and community.

A third important advantage is a lessening of the stigma that is still associated with psychiatric disorders. Attending a partial hospital on a regular basis during daytime hours and returning in the evening is a more normal behavior pattern, one that reduces the impression, for both patient and neighbor, that there is a problem that requires isolation and one that needs to be taken care of behind locked doors beyond the scrutiny of others.

Limitations

Difficulties in obtaining reimbursement for partial hospital care is a major problem in the United States (Leibenluft and Leibenluft, 1988). Reimbursement varies considerably between health insurance providers and between states, where regulations differ as to mandated requirements for mental health insurance benefits. Overwhelmingly, it is more difficult to obtain reimbursement for partial hospital care compared to inpatient care. There is no general agreement in the health insurance industry regarding the utility of the partial hospital as an alternative to inpatient care. Suggestions have been made, and in some instances accepted, to provide equivalent reimbursement for partial and 24-hour hospitalization on a ratio basis where payment for two or three partial hospital days can be substituted for one inpatient day. In some instances, particularly in those cases where managed care organizations are influencing the utilization of services, there is a trend to actively encourage partial hospital treatment rather than inpatient care.

Safety is a major concern with acutely disturbed patients. Careful initial evaluation and preadmission screening are vital to ensure that patients will be safe in the partial hospital program and will not act dangerously toward themselves or others. Given these precautions, as well as daily vigilance with respect to any potentially deleterious behavior, and the willingness to admit patients to 24-hour care when dangerousness is a concern, patients in partial hospitals do not appear to have an increased risk of harm to themselves or to others.

The treatment of the severely disturbed patient in a partial hospital setting requires consideration of the burden on the family. There is no doubt that for some patients, clearly those excluded from randomization in the research trials described earlier, full inpatient hospitalization is necessary because the disorganization of the patient would be overly distressing and burdensome to the family. Because this form of care is still considered novel and patients have often previously experienced 24-hour hospitalization, there is a reflex response by the family that it would be too burdensome to manage the patient while he or she attends a partial hospital. These views are often unwarranted. No studies have revealed evidence of greater burden on the family of patients admitted to a partial hospital. In fact, in many cases, families have reported greater satisfaction with the partial hospital treatment.

Second only to the limited reimbursement, and probably related to it, professional attitudes toward partial hospitals contribute substantially to their under-utilization. There continues to be a reluctance on the part of many psychiatrists to refer patients for partial hospital care. One study found that of patients referred to partial hospitals, by far the majority are referred by psychiatrists who have had substantial experience with this method of care (Fink et al., 1978). This has also been the experience of many other investigators in the field. Clearly, a concern about adequate reimbursement influences the decision of some professionals, but there also is an impression that it is safer to manage a person in a 24-hour hospital than in the partial hospital, though no evidence to this effect exists. It is less anxiety-provoking for many professionals to manage a patient in a 24-hour hospital where the patients are captive, decisions can be deferred, and where contact with a patient can occur over a longer span of time during the day. Unfortunately, it is the exception for professionals to be trained in partial hospitals and, until this situation reverses, there will probably be a continued reluctance to utilize this approach.

The Future of Partial Hospitalization

There are three distinct domains in which partial hospitalization programs should thrive. First, this method provides an excellent cost-containing alternative to general inpatient care. This persists as the predominant factor encouraging the growth of partial hospital programs and therefore is likely to be accompanied by more stringent utilization review. In the future, partial programs will be integrated into an array of different services within systems, thus providing continuity for the delivery of patient care. In the same way, specialty services will increasingly include partial hospital programs as part of their delivery systems. Such specialty programs include geriatric, child and adolescent, pain-treatment, eating disorder, and chemical dependence programs. Increasingly, special partial hospital programs will be specifically geared to addressing the needs of these patient groups.

References

AAPH (1991) *Guidelines and standards for partial hospitalization.* Washington, D.C.

Creed, F., Anthony, P., Godbert, K., and Huxley, P. (1989a) Treatment of severe psychiatric illness in a day hospital. *British Journal of Psychiatry,* 154:341–347.

Creed, F., Black, D., and Anthony, P. (1989b) Day-hospital and community treatment for acute psychiatric illness: a critical appraisal. *British Journal of Psychiatry,* 154:300–310.

Creed, F., Black, D., Anthony, P., Osborn, M., Thomas, P., and Tomenson, B. (1990) Random-ised controlled trial of day patient versus inpatient psychiatric treatment. *BMJ,* 300: 1033–1037.

Dick, P., Sweeney, L., and Crombie, I. (1991) Controlled comparison of day-patient and out-patient treatment for persistent anxiety and depression. *British Journal of Psychiatry,* 158:24–27.

Ferber, J.S., Oswald, M., Rubin, M., Ungemack, J., and Schane, M. (1985) The day hospital as entry point to a network of long-term services: a program evaluation. *Hospital and Community Psychiatry,* 36:1297–1301.

Fink, E.B., Heckerman, C.L., and McNeill, D. (1979) An examination of clinician bias in patient referrals to partial hospital settings. *Hospital and Community Psychiatry,* 30:631–632.

Fink, E.B., Longabaugh, R., and Stout, R. (1978) The paradoxial underutilization of partial hospitalization. *American Journal of Psychiatry,* 135:713–716.

Glick, I.D., Fleming, L., DeChillo, N., Meyerkopf, N., Jackson, C., Muscara, D., and Good-Ellis, M. (1986) A controlled study of transitional day care for non-chronically-ill pa-tients. *American Journal of Psychiatry,* 143(12):1551–1556.

Greene, L.R., and De La Cruz, A. (1981) Psychiatric day treatment as alternative to an transition from full time hospitalization. *Community Mental Health Journal,* 17:191–202.

Gudeman, J.E., Shore, M.F., and Dickey, B. (1983) Day hospitalization and an inn instead of inpatient care for psychiatric patients. *New England Journal of Medicine,* 308:749–753.

Guy, W., and Gross, G.W. (1967) Problems in the evaluation of day hospitals. *Community Mental Health Journal,* 3:111–118.

Herz, M.I., Endicott, J., Spitzer, R.L., and Mesnikoff, A. (1971) Day versus inpatient hospital-ization, a controlled study. *American Journal of Psychiatry,* 127:1371–1382.

Hoge, M.A., Farrel, S.P., Munchel, M.E., and Strauss, J.S. (1988) Therapeutic factors in partial hospitalization. *Psychiatry,* 51:199–210.

Leibenluft, E., and Leibenluft, R.F. (1988) Reimbursement for partial hospitalization: a survey and policy implications. *American Journal of Psychiatry,* 145(12):1514–1520.

Piper, W., Rosie, J., Azim, H., and Joyce, A. (1993) A randomized trial of psychiatric day treatment for patients with affective and personality disorders. *Hospital and Community Psychiatry,* 44:757–763.

Rosie, J.S. (1987) Partial hospitalization: a review of recent literature. *Hospital and Community Psychiatry,* 38:1291–1299.

Tyrer, P., Remington, M., and Alexander, J. (1987) The outcome of neurotic disorders after outpatient and day hospital care. *British Journal of Psychiatry,* 151:57–62.

Washburn, S., Vannicelli, M., and Scheff, B.J. (1976) A controlled comparison of psychiatric day treatment and inpatient hospitalization. *Journal of Consulting and Clinical Psy-chology,* 44:665–675.

Weil, F. (1984) Day hospitalization is a therapeutic tool. *Psychiatric Journal of the University of Ottawa,* 9:165–169.

Wing, J., and Brown, G. (1970) *Institutionalism and Schizophrenia: A Comparative Study of Three Mental Hospitals 1960–1968.* Cambridge: Cambridge University Press.

Zwerling, I., and Wilder, J.F. (1964) An evaluation of the applicability of the day hospital in treatment of acutely disturbed patients. *Israel Annals of Psychiatry,* 2:162–185.

19

Inpatient Services

WILLIAM R. BREAKEY

The practice of psychiatry requires ready access to high-quality inpatient care when needed. Community-oriented inpatient services are thus a vital component of a responsive service system. Community psychiatry developed in the context of dein-stitutionalization. The diminishing emphasis on inpatient care in favor of community-based ambulatory services and the transfer of resources to the community sector are fundamental to the field, so that the success of integrated service systems is often judged on their ability to keep people out of hospital. In this context it must be all the more strongly emphasized that avoiding inpatient admission is not *per se* an in-dicator of good outcome for a person who may be distressed by severe symptoms and experiencing poor quality of life. Nonetheless, time spent in hospital is often used as an outcome measure for evaluating the effectiveness of mental health programs be-cause it is important from a policy perspective, but also because it is relatively easily recorded and often available from existing data sets—a major attraction to program evaluators. The ready availability of this measure, and the lack of more direct or definitve outcome measures, should not, however, tempt clinicians or policy makers into believing that programs that reduce inpatient utilization are necessarily providing good care.

In recent years, inpatient services have seen several major changes: the phasing out or downsizing of large state-run institutions, the development of units in general hospitals, and reduction in length of stay. American state and county hospital censuses peaked in 1955, at which time there were 560,000 resident patients; by 1990, however, the number had reduced to 91,000 (Redlick et al., 1994). In Britain in 1954 there were 148,000 patients in psychiatric hospitals, but the number had reduced to 64,800 by 1985 (Audit Commission, 1986). This loss of mental hospital beds was offset to some extent, however, by an increase in use of general hospital psychiatric units over the same period. In Europe, these units were developed as a matter of public policy (Barbato et al., 1992), while in the United States their growth has reponded more to marketplace opportunity. In 1970 there were 22,000 psychiatric beds in general hospitals in the United States; by 1990, the number had increased to 53,000 (Redlick et al., 1994). As inpatient care is restricted more and more to the sickest patients, general hospital psychiatric units have the advantage that they are well positioned to handle cases who have general medical as well as psychiatric needs, but they may have the disadvantage that they are small and cannot offer the range of milieus and treatments available in larger psychiatric facilities (Summergrad, 1991). Overall, there are fewer psychiatric beds available in the 1990s, but with widespread access to health insurance for employed people and support from Medicaid and Medicare for the poor, the disabled, and the elderly, admissions have continued to to increase. In the United States in 1969, the admission rate was 650 per 100,000 civilian population, but by 1986 it had risen to 750 per 100,000; this has only been possible because of the marked reduction in length of stay that has occurred with changes in treatment philosophy and practice. Parallel with these changes in inpatient utilization, there has been a very large increase in outpatient and partial hospital care. Whereas in 1955, 77 percent of all episodes of psychiatric care were in inpatient settings and 63 percent of these were in state hospitals, by 1990 only 26 percent of episodes were inpatient episodes and only 16 percent of these were in state hospitals (Redlick et al., 1994).

Reducing Use of Inpatient Services

There are a number of theoretical and practical reasons why psychiatrists accept more and more widely that inpatient admission should be used only when ambulatory treatment methods have failed, or appear doomed to failure and that, in general, patients should be treated in the "least restrictive" setting. One is the desirability of causing as little upheaval as possible for the patient; admission to hospital disrupts the life of the patient and his or her family and removes him or her from social and family support systems. Another is to reduce the stigma that still attaches to psychiatric inpatient care, particularly when it is prolonged, which is very painful for both patients and their families. A third reason concerns involuntary admission, which interferes with the civil rights of the patient, and therefore should be avoided if at all possible, both because of respect for those rights, and also because of the intrusion of the legal system into the clinical interaction which necessarily follows. However, the predominant reasons for reducing use of inpatient care have been economic and practical. With the continuing reliance on inpatient care, the increase in inpatient admissions, the shift in the main locus of inpatient care out of the major mental hospitals into the general hospitals, and escalating costs resulting from these factors, a drive for greater cost efficiency has been pursued energetically.

The norm, now, is for psychiatric disorders to be treated in ambulatory settings. Inpatient admission may be necessary, even life-saving on occasion, but it represents a failure of psychiatric management, either because the illness was too severe to be controlled by currently available methods, or because the treatment team was not sufficiently skillful or did not have access to adequate resources to maintain the patient outside hospital, or because for some reason the ill person could not be persuaded to accept proffered help.

Controlling Utilization

Economists, purchasers of care, and planners of public systems all look to reduction in inpatient utilization as a major way of reducing the rate of inflation of health care budgets and of freeing up health service resources to be applied to other, more cost-efficient approaches. This has prompted the search for alternatives to inpatient care and methods to provide incentives and controls to direct patients elsewhere. In ideal circumstances reduction in patient utilization is obtained by improvement in the quality of outpatient care so that admission is avoided. In practice, administrative measures have proved necessary to bring about changes. Two strategies are employed: reduction of availability of beds and control of admission and discharge decisions.

The most direct method is the reduction in availability of beds. Planners constantly confront the issue of how many beds are needed to serve a given population, but there is no agreed-upon measure. Although it has been shown that bed utilization correlates with social deprivation (Jarman et al., 1992; Thornicroft et al., 1992), utilization is not the same as need. Estimates of need have, indeed, generally been based on prior utilization experience, but this reflects the practices in a particular time and place—practices that are constantly changing. Many people who would have been considered definitely in need of inpatient care only a decade ago are now treated as outpatients or in other ambulatory services. Many patients who two decades ago would have spent weeks in hospital are now discharged in a matter of days. Geographic variations are also significant: Lengths of stay for psychiatric care on the West coast of the United States are consistently shorter than on the East coast. In spite of a lack of professional consensus as to what is needed, planners attempt to make rational decisions about closure of hospitals or opening of new units in order to ensure that resources are distributed as efficiently and equitably as possible. Many cities have too many expensive hospitals competing with each other in a narrow geographic area, while smaller cities or rural areas are underserved. Mechanisms are therefore established by governments to develop estimates based on variables such as previous utilization history, known information about prevalence, and the socioeconomic characteristics of the population served (Hirsch, 1988). For example, in 1975 the British government suggested targets of 50 general hospital beds per 100,000 population, with 35 for the elderly and 17 for new long-stay patients. Ten years later, the Royal College of Psychiatrists recommended 44 beds per 100,000 population (Thornicroft and Bebbington, 1989). Such estimates can be integrated into regional or district planning processes. Permission to develop new inpatient facilities can be witheld if sufficient beds are available, or hospitals can be compelled to close beds, close wards, or close down altogether.

Where hospitals are under the management control of government, as in the case of American state hospitals or British National Health Service hospitals, run-down or closure of inpatient facilities can be accomplished by administrative fiat, always subject to political priorities and pressures. This has been the basic strategy for deinstitutionalization. Where hospitals are under other management, other regulatory methods must be used to control bed availability. This is important because of the well-known phenomenon that supply creates demand—if beds are available, they will be used—and increased use leads to increased cost to the system.

Closing beds requires reduction of admissions, and in the public sector this is generally accomplished through preadmission screening procedures that require a referring physician to obtain clearance from the screening agency before a patient can be admitted. Preadmission screening is in general performed by agencies other than the hospital staff themselves, who have a vested interest in filling beds. As beds are emptied and then closed, admission criteria become increasingly restrictive, so that dangerousness or very severe disability become the principal or only criteria for inpatient treatment.

One of the systemic problems in many areas is the separation between community services and hospital administrations, which may operate under different incentive structures and are likely to have difficulty in developing joint strategies with agreed-upon objectives. Hospital managers in some circumstances want to keep their beds full by encouraging admissions, while community service providers and funding agencies would prefer to avoid inpatient treatment where possible. When the two sectors can be integrated with an agreed-upon set of service objectives, use of inpatient care can be reduced considerably without sacrificing quality of outcome.

Utilization review is the other method widely used to control cost by third-party payers in the United States. Utilization review has two components, preadmission screening and concurrent review. Preadmission screening requires the clinician who wishes to arrange an admission to consult a screener who must give approval before the patient can be admitted, or, in the case of some insurance plans, before the insurance company will accept responsibility for paying for the admission. The intent is to deflect "inappropriate" or "unnecessary" admissions into alternative treatment settings. Concurrent review requires the clinician to continue to justify to the reviewer the patient's continuing treatment in the hospital. If continuing approval is not given, the hospital will not be reimbursed. Clinicians find these procedures objectionable and not generally in the patients' best interests (Melnick and Lyter, 1987). They often find themselves in a struggle with screeners on the telephone who may or may not have a good understanding of what constitutes good treatment and whose aim is to avoid cost for the payer rather than necessarily to provide the best care for an individual patient. Utilization review is effective in reducing inpatient utilization, but it has not been established whether it leads to a superior or inferior quality of psychiatric care overall, or whether in the long run there is a cost reduction.

Length of Stay

Possibly the most striking change that has occurred in psychiatric care is a dramatic reduction in length of inpatient stay. This has resulted from advances in psychiatric practice but also from the reduced availability of beds and the effects of utilization review. For example, in the St. Louis County Insane Asylum at the end of the nineteenth century, the mean length of stay was 683 days. By 1980, it had reduced to 34 days (Evenson et al., 1994). By 1985 the mean length of stay across state and county hospitals in the United States was 28 days (Manderscheid and Sonnenschein, 1990). In hospitals that deal only with treatment of acute episodes of illness, average lengths of stay are now often less than two weeks, and many patients are discharged in less than one week.

Psychiatric hospitals before deinstitutionalization served both chronic patients, whose stay in hospital was indefinite, and acute patients, who were expected to be discharged when their mental state became stabilized or their problems resolved. Even acute patients, however, until relatively recently, would often spend long periods in hospital. Although obviously long-term inpatient care may be necessary in certain clinical situations, research has demonstrated in a variety of ways that briefer episodes of inpatient care are generally as effective as longer episodes (Gordon and Breakey, 1983). Whereas the intent of inpatient psychiatrists had once been to return a person to as normal a state as possible before discharging him or her to home, the aim now is to stabilize the situation to the extent that the patient can be safely transferred to another less costly and less restrictive treatment setting. As pressures from third-party payers and administrative authorities result in ever-shorter hospital stays, coordination between inpatient and ambulatory services becomes increasingly important for continuity of care.

Indications for Inpatient Care

Inpatient treatment is generally indicated because it provides the best setting for thorough evaluation and expeditious treatment for the relief of distress. There is a public expectation that psychiatrists will provide care and protection (asylum) to those who are disabled by mental illness and not able to care for or protect themselves, that they will protect patients who are at risk of harming themselves, and that they will protect the public from persons who, by reason of mental illness, are liable to harm others. Meeting these expectations may require the structure and control provided by an inpatient facility. Thus the general indications for inpatient care are (1) risk of self-injury, (2) dangerousness to others, (3) severely distressing affects or behaviors, and (4) the need for intensive observation for diagnostic evaluation and stabilization.

The Risk of Self-Injury

Suicidal acts or impulses indicate the need for close supervision of a psychiatric patient that can only be provided in a controlled setting. In some cases this control can be provided by a family or in some type of highly structured community residential facility, but in general the supervision of skilled nursing staff is needed to protect the person until the suicidal impulses have been brought under control. Self-injury can also take other forms. Patients, because of the symptoms of their illnesses, can place themselves at risk of accidental injury by failing to take normal precautions, for example when crossing the street or operating machinery, or by engaging in risky sexual behaviors. They may be so disabled that they are unable to take care of their basic survival needs and impose risk to their health or their life. They may risk social harm by acting imprudently in a manic episode to an extent that will cause great embarrassment to themselves or their family. Admission to hospital may be indicated in such a situation.

Dangerousness to Others

Assaultive behavior occurring as a symptom of psychiatric illness is an indication for admission, although it is much less common in reality than in the popular imagination. All criminal acts committed by a mentally ill person are not necessarily the result of insanity, and some violent acts or threats should be an indication for police involvement rather than hospital admission. Traditionally, very violent patients have been cared for or treated in special forensic hospitals, staffed both by clinical staff and by security staff. These hospitals have been government-run and closely linked with courts and correctional systems. Increasingly, forensic psychiatrists also are experimenting with alternatives to traditional models such as community supervision strategies for the criminally insane and secure units in general psychiatric hospitals.

Acutely Disturbed Affects or Behaviors

The major role for any physcian is the alleviation of suffering, and sometimes this can be accomplished most effectively by admitting the sufferer to hospital where the intensive efforts of a highly skilled professional team can be brought to bear to provide the variety of supports and treatments that will help the person recover most rapidly. It is probably true that most psychiatric illness, even though quite severe, can be treated in an ambulatory setting, but an inpatient setting can provide a level of support, observation, and rapid intervention when needed that is difficult to provide elsewhere. Hospital admission is often a great kindness to patients and their families, relieving them of the tremendous burden of coping with severe illness in the home environment.

Evaluation and Observation

The formulation of a diagnosis in some cases requires more detailed and continuous observation than is feasible in an outpatient or day hospital environment. This type of careful evaluation requires repeated skilled examinations of mental status, careful elicitation of history, gathering of data from a wide variety of sources, and the combined skills of a multidisciplinary team. In some cases, a complex series of laboratory, radiological, and psychometric evaluations may be needed; these can be accomplished much more expeditiously if the patient is admitted.

Stabilization

Certain patients are referred into the mental health service system at a point of crisis. Not only is the patient's life in crisis, but the family is in uproar, the clinical picture confusing, mobilization of resources impossible, and the situation possibly dangerous. In other cases, patients may have established patterns of noncompliance with treatment recommendations, frequent failures to cope with everyday matters, and resulting chronic chaos. In circumstances such as these an admission may be extremely useful to impose structure on the person's daily life, to reevaluate the clinical problems, to initiate a rational treatment plan, to permit the family or social support system to regain its equilibrium, and then to return the patient to a more stable situation in which a coherent long-term treatment plan can be pursued.

Alternatives to Inpatient Care

The above listing of indications for inpatient care underscores the fact that, in current practice, inpatient treatment is resorted to much less frequently than formerly, and only where there is a very good reason why the patient cannot be evaluated and treated at home or in a setting that provides less intensive supervision. The drive to reduce use of inpatient care has led to the development of a number of alternative ways of addressing the needs of patients and their families.

Assertive Community Treatment

The Program for Assertive Community Treatment (PACT), originated by Stein and Test (1985), was seminal in demonstrating that quite ill people could be managed without recourse to inpatient admission if a community team were available to provide intensive services in the home environment or wherever services were needed (Chapter 21). The model has been tested in different settings in different countries (Hoult and Reynolds, 1984; Marks et al., 1994) and has been found to be effective. The principles underlying this approach have been used in many places to establish programs which resemble the original model to greater or lesser degrees (Bond, 1991; Burns et al., 1993). For example, intensive case management teams have been adopted as a central component of community care systems in the United Kingdom to provide support and treatment for chronically disabled individuals in community settings and to minimize utilization of inpatient services.

Respite Care

Formerly it was not unusual to admit a person to hospital to ease the burden on the caring family, for example by permitting them to take a vacation or simply to get a break from the burden of caring for their family member. In some cases respite is needed because the usual care provider is ill. Various models of respite care facilities have been developed to care for the ill person for a short time. A usual way of doing this is to provide a house staffed by people familiar with mental illness and the needs of mentally ill people who can provide the necessary support and supervision for several weeks.

Crisis Services

Many admissions to hospital have been occasioned by a crisis for which no other response could be mustered. Such crises can include acute depression or anxiety, excerbations of schizophrenic symptoms, acute manic episodes, or responses to traumas or disasters. Alternative methods of dealing with crises can avert some admissions to hospital (Bengelsdorf and Alden, 1987). Crisis services in communities may have several different components, including crisis counseling services, hot lines, crisis teams, community crisis beds, and ultra-short-stay inpatient crisis units. Crisis counseling services, provided through telephone services or face-to-face in emergency departments or by mobile teams, provide a patient with an opportunity to ventilate and process the anxiety-producing situation in such a way that the acute emotional reaction is attenuated and the risk of harm diminished. Where a severely mentally ill person is confronting a crisis, problem solving and adjustment of medication dosage can on occasion bring symptoms under control quite rapidly.

When additional support over a longer period is needed to avoid hospital admission, crisis beds can be used. This is most appropriate where a person's symptoms or behavior are such that the usual care provider can no longer cope or, if the person lives alone, he or she can not manage alone. If the problems are not severe enough to need the full panoply of hospital nursing and medical care, a less intensive, less costly, more home-like setting can be used for a few days to help the person through the crisis. Generally a facility of this sort is an ordinary house in an ordinary neighborhood, staffed around the clock with mental health professionals who may or may not have nursing credentials. It is important, however, that they have access to on-call psychiatric services as needed to address any acute treatment needs that may arise at any hour of day or night. In-home supporters provide an alternative to crisis beds. These supporters have mental health knowledge and training and can stay in a patient's own home overnight to provide support and supervision over a crisis period.

Brief stay units or "overnight" beds in a hospital, providing care and treatment for a few days, are often linked closely with emergency departments for those patients who pose greater risk and who need a brief period of inpatient treatment in a crisis. A staff that is specially geared to dealing rapidly with acute crises can accomplish this better than is possible in a setting where patients normally stay for longer periods. The specific knowledge and skills of the staff are important in ensuring rapid discharge, but equally important is the level of expectation of patients and staff alike that the stay will only be for a matter of days. If it is assumed that more time is available to address the problems, they will be tackled with less energy, but if staff, patients, and their families all appreciate the need for urgency, issues will be addressed and problems solved more quickly.

Partial Hospitalization

In many cases admitting a person to a day hospital can be a very effective way of addressing his or her psychiatric needs and avoiding 24-hour inpatient care. It is necessary that the person have a means of traveling to and from the day hospital, that there be adequate support and supervision at night, and that the risks of self-injury or harm to others be minimal (Chapter 17).

Practice Issues

Continuity of Care

Within a service network, where a patient may move from one component to another, continuity of care becomes a major issue (Bachrach, 1981). This is particularly so in the transitions to and from inpatient care, because of the demonstrated risk of relapse at this stage of treatment (Goldacre et al., 1993) and because inpatient treatment teams may have a poor appreciation of what is involved in the provision of community services. Frequently an inpatient team may go to work in evaluating a case without taking advantage of the knowledge base possessed by the outpatient therapist. In some cases it may be beneficial for another team to take a fresh look at a case, but more often the inpatient care will proceed more smoothly if the inpatient psychiatrist is fully informed about what has gone before. Similarly, as a patient is discharged, the transition back to the community should go as smoothly as possible, with maximum sharing of relevant information. A longitudinal perspective is essential when confronting a chronic illness. Many patients have gone from care provider to care provider, and their treatment histories come to resemble a smorgasbord of medications and interventions. Instead, under ideal circumstances, the primary treatment provider should have a longitudinal perspective of the individual and the evolution of the illness in the person over time. Any one exacerbation or crisis should be understood in the light of this history and its treatment designed in a way that is mindful of the longer term view.

Continuity of care has been defined as continuity of provider, continuity of treatment, or continuity of planning. Continuity of provider may sometimes be possible when a person moves into an inpatient treatment unit where the same physician can continue to supervise the treatment. More often, however, for practical reasons this is not possible, and the focus is on ensuring continuity of treatment and planning. Continuity of treatment requires that the patient not lose contact with the treatment providers during the transition from inpatient to outpatient care. Setting up appointments, face-to-face meetings with outpatient staff prior to discharge, short waiting periods before first appointment, and mail or telephone reminders will all increase the likeli-hood of smooth follow-through (Chen, 1991).

Continuity of care requires good communication channels between the elements of the treatment system. Unfortunately, these channels are often inadequate, and in some cases the smooth flow of shared information is impeded by confidentiality con-cerns between agencies—a problem that requires an administrative solution. Written discharge plans or treatment plans can be useful, but may often be completed more with a view to complying with regulations than as a meaningful communication. Face-to-face contact between treatment providers is more likely to enable effective com-munication and to provide opportunity for ensuring continuity of care as the patient makes the transition.

Voluntary and Involuntary Admission

For many reasons, where a patient has to be admitted to hospital, voluntary admission is greatly to be preferred. It is normalizing and destigmatizing for a psychiatric ad-mission to be as little different from any other medical admission as possible, and when a patient is admitted by mutual agreement with the treatment provider, a ther-apeutic alliance occurs more naturally than where the admission has been the result of a struggle of wills in which the patient's wishes have been overruled. When an involuntary admission occurs, with the legal and procedural processes involved, the legal system by necessity intrudes upon the medical interaction. This introduces dy-namics that are undesirable at best and can be quite harmful in the therapeutic rela-tionships that the treatment team seeks to establish. Consumer advocacy organizations that represent the interests of patients are often critical of the concept and implemen-tation of involuntary admission practices; the most extreme viewpoint is that invol-untary hospital admission is never justifiable. Psychiatrists in general support the need for involuntary admission mechanisms but agree that they should only be used where admission is vital and consent cannot be obtained, even after great effort has been made to obtain it. In some instances the process has been corrupted by the circum-stances where beds are so scarce relative to demand that a policy is established that only the most severely ill patients—or those who are the most dangerous—can be admitted, which translates into a policy to admit only those who are involuntary. In this circumstance desperate physicians are tempted to certify patients as involuntary to gain their admission.

Indications for Long-Term Hospitalization

It is now comparatively rare for a person to be admitted to a psychiatric hospital for more than a few weeks. The development of intensive case management, assertive treatment teams, and supervised community residential alternatives permit people to be treated and cared for in the community in almost every instance.

The first exception is where an individual is too dangerous or antisocial to be safely maintained in a community setting. This includes those individuals who are repeatedly assaultive, but also, for example, those who have intractable paraphilic or pedophilic disorders. The second group of patients who need long-term hospitalization, less clearly defined, comprises those patients who are so severely disabled that they cannot be adequately supported in a community setting. These are individuals who repeatedly escape from even the most diligent supervision, who fail to take medication and frequently relapse, requiring emergency treatment and rehospitalization, as well as others who have complex medical needs or physical disability complicating their psychiatric disorder that can only be addressed satisfactorily in an institutional setting. A third category includes those patients with complex disorders that resolve only slowly. These people have histories of frequent readmissions because in a brief period in hospital it is not possible to fully address all the factors that lead to relapse or, in some cases, to persuade the person of the need for continuing treatment. A patient like this may appear fit for discharge relatively quickly, but after returning home relapses rapidly and requires readmission. A longer period of inpatient support in certain of these cases would end the revolving door cycles and be cost-effective as well as humanely preferable.

These individuals constitute a very small minority of patients in any community. The numbers of beds required to provide care for these special categories are small compared to what was considered neccessary only a few years ago, and as community treatment methods improve, these estimates are constantly being revised downward.

References

Audit Commission (1986) *Making a Reality of Community Care.* London: HMSO

Bachrach, L. (1981) Continuity of care for chronic mental patients: a conceptual analysis. *American Journal of Psychiatry,* 138:1449–1456.

Barbato, A., Terzian, E., Sraceno, B., Barquero, F.M., and Tognoni, G. (1992) Patterns of aftercare for psychiatric patients discharged after short inpatient treatment. *Social Psychiatry and Psychiatric Epidemiology,* 27:46–52.

Bengelsdorf, H., and Alden, D.C. (1987) A mobile crisis unit in the psychiatric emergency room. *Hospital and Community Psychiatry,* 38:662–665.

Bond, G.R. (1991) Variations in an assertive outreach model. *New Directions in Mental Health Services,* 52:65–80.

Burns, T., Beadsmoore, A., Bhat, A.V., Oliver, A., and Mathers, C. (1993) A controlled trial of home-based acute psychiatric services. I: Clinical and social outcome. II: Treatment patterns and costs. *British Journal of Psychiatry,* 163:49–61.

Chen, A. (1991) Noncompliance in community psychiatry: a review of clinical interventions. *Hospital and Community Psychiatry,* 42:282–287.

Evenson, R.C., Holland, R.A., and Cho, D.W. (1994) A psychiatric hospital 100 years ago: I. A comparative study of treatment outcomes then and now. *Hospital and Community Psychiatry,* 45:1021–1025.

Goldacre, M., Seagroatt, V., and Hawton, K. (1993) Suicide after discharge from psychiatric inpatient care. *Lancet,* 342:283–286.

Gordon, T., and Breakey, W.R. (1983) A comparison of the outcomes of short- and standard-stay patients at one year follow-up. *Hospital and Community Psychiatry,* 34:1054–1056.

Hirsch, S. (1988) *Psychiatric Beds and Resources: Factors Influencing Bed Use and Service Planning.* London: Gaskell.

Hoult, J., and Reynolds, I. (1984) Schizophrenia: A comparative trial of community oriented and hospital oriented psychiatric care. *Acta Psychiatrica Scandinavica,* 69:359–372.

Jarman, B., Hirsch, S., White, P., and Driscoll, R. (1992) Predicting psychiatric admissions. *British Medical Journal,* 304:1146–1151.

Manderscheid, R.W., and Sonnenschein M.A. (eds.) (1990) *Mental Health, United States, 1990.* DHHS Publication No. (ADM)90-1708. Rockville, Maryland: U.S. Department of Health and Human Services.

Marks, I.M., Connolly, J., Muijen, M., Audini, B., McNamee, G., and Lawrence, R.E. (1994) Home-based versus hospital-based care for people with serious mental illness. *British Journal of Psychiatry,* 165:179–194.

Melnick, S.D., and Lyter, L.L. (1987) The negative impacts of increased concurrent review of psychiatric inpatient care. *Hospital and Community Psychiatry,* 38:300–303.

Redlick, R.W., Witkin, M.J., Atay, J.E., and Manderscheid, R.W. (1994) Highlights of organized mental health services in 1990 and major national and state trends. In Mandersheid, R. W., Sonnenschein, M.A. (eds.) *Mental Health, United States, 1994.* DHHS Publication No. (SMA)94-3000. Rockville, Maryland: U.S. Department of Health and Human Services.

Stein, L., and Test, M.A. (1985) *The Training in Community Living Model: A Decade of Experience.* San Francisco: Jossey-Bass.

Summergrad, P. (1991) General hospital inpatient psychiatry in the 1990s: problems and possibilities. *General Hospital Psychiatry,* 13:79–82.

Thornicroft, G., and Bebbington, P. (1989) Deinstitutionalization—from hospital closure to service development. *British Journal of Psychiatry,* 155:739–753.

Thornicroft, G., Margolius, O., and Jones, D. (1992) The TAPS Project. 6: New long-stay psychiatric patients and service deprivation. *British Journal of Psychiatry,* 161:621–624.

20

General Health Care

GERARD GALLUCCI
BRUNO R. LIMA

Health-care providers are challenged with understanding and treating patients who present with overlapping psychiatric and somatic symptoms. Primary-care practitioners encounter many psychiatric problems in general practice, and over the years community psychiatrists have struggled with the need to ensure that patients with psychiatric illness receive appropriate general medical care in addition to treatment for their psychiatric illness.

As a medical discipline, psychiatry has developed a specialty approach to the treatment of psychiatric conditions, encouraged by the growing knowledge of psychopathology and the greater sophistication of psychiatric diagnosis and treatment. At odds with this specialization is the view of psychiatry as a primary-care discipline, alongside family practice, pediatrics, and general internal medicine. Establishing the point of authority for coordinating the general medical care of psychiatric patients is necessary for providing comprehensive treatment. Unfortunately, that point of authority is often undefined and care remains fragmented. In the United States, health maintenance organizations have continued to grow and have established the primary medical care providers as the gatekeepers for access to specialty services, including psychiatry. Conversely, in community mental health programs, it is generally the psychiatrist who is reponsible for ensuring that the general health needs of patients are attended to.

Historically, patients with psychiatric illness have been treated in settings that promote isolation from patients with other medical conditions. Patients with mental disorders traditionally received care in the large, state-run psychiatric facilities. These institutions were designed to be self-sufficient centers where the medical as well as the psychiatric needs of patients could be addressed. Patients in the better run state hospitals were provided with general medical care including regular physical exams, dental care, and hearing and speech assessments. Surveillance for infectious diseases including tuberculosis and syphilis became routine, and chronic diseases such as diabetes and hypertension were managed by the medical staff.

At the inception of the federal Community Mental Health Center initiative in 1963, President Kennedy proposed that the CMHCs would "return mental health to the mainstream of American medicine." By 1981 there were 761 federally funded Community Mental Health Centers in operation, developed under the auspices of the National Institute of Mental Health which since its establishment after World War II had been administratively and financially independent from the National Institutes of Health that sponsor research on other aspects of health. There were thus separate federal budgets for mental health research, service, and training programs, guaranteeing separation from the "mainstream of American medicine." CMHCs, as they developed into the 1970s, were thus separate from their counterparts in general health, the neighborhood health centers and primary health care clinics (PHCs). These were sponsored by the Bureau of Community Health Services, and by 1983 there were 1,000 such centers in operation. These competing trends, as well as separate funding sources and different administrative controls, quite apart from the professional boundaries that always tend to exist between psychiatry and general medicine, helped to create a schism between the CMHCs and the general health care system that continues to exist today.

The coordination of services between CMHCs and PHCs has always been minimal, and insufficient funds have been assigned to develop adequate linkage programs. In 1978, a linkage initiative was implemented that was to be expanded under the Mental Health Systems Act of 1980. This act, however, was subsequently repealed by Congress as part of the Reagan administration's budget cuts.

When this historical perspective on the development of community psychiatry and primary health care in the United States is compared with the main trends modeling the development of general psychiatry in the same period of time, an interesting contrast emerges. As psychiatry was returning to the mainstream of medicine, the biological understanding of major mental illnesses was gaining acceptance and psychopharmacology was becoming increasingly more effective and better accepted as a legitimate intervention for certain disorders. And as psychiatric units were established in general hospitals, CMHCs were created with a specific mission that set them apart from this mainstream movement. They replicated in the community some aspects of the isolation state hospitals had faced, and they perpetuated the historical separation of mental health and general health care delivery they were supposed to have bridged.

Community Psychiatry Clinics and General Health Care

In some areas, the mental health centers have seen it as their role to be primary-care providers for patients with severe mental illness. This is as much a practical position as a philosophical one. Patients attending the center often fail to pursue somatic care but continue a relationship with the mental health center that spans a period of years.

Since psychiatric visits are usually no less frequent than monthly and visits to the family doctor or medical clinic are generally much less frequent, it becomes a *de facto* responsibility of the mental health center to monitor its patients' physical problems and to develop effective community treatment plans that include management of their medical needs. Long-term health maintenance issues can be addressed since patients have ongoing contact with their mental health care providers over many years.

Some CMHCs have learned to interface with both the social services agencies and the general health care sector in order to provide comprehensive care to the severely disabled, multiply handicapped chronic patient. A mental health program can establish linkages with general medical clinics or primary-care providers that improve communication between the various disciplines. Mental health program staff can provide consultation to assess patients attending general medical clinics who present with psychiatric symptoms. They can provide follow-up psychiatric care in that setting or facilitate entry into the CMHC for those patients requiring more intensive treatment. A number of different approaches have been described to foster such links between the mental health and general health care systems, and different models need to be considered to meet the specific needs of a given situation (Pincus, 1980). Differences in patient populations, geographic settings, management and financing issues, and overall philosophy of care may influence the type of relationship that is most effective.

Within mental health centers, some have utilized "physician extenders" such as nurse practitioners in the assessment of the medical needs of their patients. The psychiatrist may be unavailable or overwhelmed by the increasing demands on his or her time for clinical supervision of psychiatric treatment, and non-medical therapists may lack the necessary training to identify, refer, and coordinate patients' medical treatment. The nurse practitioner, on the other hand, can perform physical exams, draw blood, administer medications, coordinate consultation and follow-up of patients, and interface with medical and surgical specialists. Coordinated activities between the nurse practitioner and physician staff help to minimize the likelihood of fragmented care. Others have expanded the role of the nurse practitioner to include education and prevention, direct health maintenance, and quality assurance as pertains to the overall medical needs of patients attending the CMHC (McConnell et al., 1992).

Comorbid Conditions and Differential Diagnosis

Attention to the medical care of patients with psychiatric illness becomes even more important when the special needs of this population are considered. As early as 1937, Phillips had described the medical problems seen in psychiatric patients. A number of other investigators also noted the association between psychiatric illness and medical disorders in both the inpatient and outpatient settings. Hall and colleagues (1981) found a very high prevalence of physical illness in 100 consecutive admissions to a state hospital. Forty-six percent of patients had a previously unrecognized medical condition that either caused or worsened their psychiatric illness, and 80 percent had a medical condition that required treatment. These findings supported earlier work that indicated high rates of physical illness in patients attending a psychiatric outpatient clinic. A study by Koranyi in 1972 showed that 49 percent of a sample of consecutive outpatients suffered from a significant physical condition.

More recently, Bartsch and colleagues (1990) found that when physical exams and diagnostic tests were performed on a group of outpatients attending two community mental health centers, a substantial number had medical conditions or abnormal laboratory studies that warranted further diagnostic work-up. In addition, nearly one-fifth had a previously undetected health condition and 16 percent had medical conditions that could either cause or exacerbate their psychiatric condition.

Explanations for the high rates of physical illness in patients with mental disorders include theories of somatization and the effect of stress on physical and mental health. The severely and persistently ill patient with psychiatric disease may have poor coping skills, be liable to suffer increased stress and anxiety, and thus be vulnerable to both physical and psychiatric symptoms. Hypertension, cardiovascular disease, gastrointestinal problems, and a variety of neurological symptoms are associated with stress and stressful life events.

The co-occurrence of psychiatric disorders, including major affective illness and anxiety disorders, with cardiovascular disease has been well-described (Chignon et al., 1993; Dalack and Roose, 1990). One study that examined the course of depression in patients with a history of heart disease found that depression was more complicated and severe in patients with a previous history of myocardial infarction (Wells et al., 1993). It has been suggested that the cardiac condition may result in limitations in functioning and vocational ability, and in various psychosocial changes that impact on an individual's sense of well-being. Conversely, the depressive illness itself may adversely affect the course of the cardiac disease, resulting in a poorer prognosis (Roose and Dalack, 1992). Treatment strategies for patients with comorbid affective illness and cardiovascular disease must also acknowledge the possibility of adverse drug effects as well as drug-drug interactions that can worsen both psychiatric and cardiac symptoms (Lane et al., 1994).

Panic disorder and anxiety symptoms have been associated with functional cardiac symptoms as well as with organically based cardiac or thyroid disease. Katon (1990) found that in a sample of patients referred to primary care because of chest pain or tachycardia, 40 percent met DSM-III criteria for panic disorder. Other studies have shown high rates of panic disorder in patients with atypical chest pain who had normal coronary arteries by angiography and normal treadmill studies (Beitman et al., 1987). Clignon and associates (1993) suggest that 15 percent of patients who were assessed for possible cardiac arrhythmia had panic disorder. Other research has highlighted the direct association between anxiety symptoms and various gastrointestinal conditions (Fossey and Lydiard, 1990).

In recent years, more attention has been given to the psychiatric conditions associated with HIV infection (Katz, 1994). Central nervous system involvement from HIV infection leads to the development of psychiatric symptoms, including cognitive difficulties such as delirium and dementia, paranoid delusions and hallucinations, mood disorders, anxiety symptoms, and other behavioral problems. The primary-care physician and psychiatrist must be able to discern the etiology of neuropsychiatric symptoms in patients infected with HIV, intervene when there is an organic basis for the symptomatology, and treat or refer patients for more intensive psychiatric care when symptoms are a result of a primary psychiatric disorder (Chapter 29).

These examples serve to emphasize that psychiatrists working in community settings must be skilled in differentiating the pathological processes driving such symptoms in order to effectively and safely intervene and treat their patients. Treatment plans are often complex and include somatic medications, psychotropic agents, psychotherapy, or a combination of all of these.

A number of factors may contribute to the increased prevalence of medical disorders in patients with psychiatric illness. Lima and Pai (1987) have pointed out that patients with psychiatric illness receiving care in the community are often from lower socioeconomic groups and consequently are at greater risk for developing a number of medical problems at higher rates than are found in the general population. Another factor in these higher prevalence rates may be that people with severe mental illnesses are frequently noncompliant with treatment recommendations for medical follow-up and are poorly compliant with both prescribed psychiatric and medical regimens (Lima and Pai, 1987). They often have difficulty maneuvering through the complex maze of social and medical services as a consequence of cognitive limitations, active psychiatric symptomatology such as paranoid ideation, and mistrust of medical interventions. General physicians may also have difficulty in responding to the medical needs of psychiatric patients. In a medical clinic patients with psychiatric illness may have an odd appearance, display poor personal hygiene and manneristic behavior, have difficulty understanding and complying with follow-up treatment, relate poorly to the staff, and provide an ''unrewarding experience'' to the clinician. Emergency room personnel may limit their medical evaluation when a patient with a known diagnosis of psychiatric illness presents complaining of pain or discomfort; they may hasten the physical exam in order to ready the patient for a psychiatric evaluation. Laboratory and other diagnostic studies are sometimes neglected and organic illness overlooked. Patients may be prematurely discharged from the emergency room or admitted to a psychiatric ward without full evaluation of an underlying medical problem. Barriers to treatment of this sort obstruct access to treatment and serve to increase prevalence.

Medical Complications of Psychiatric Treatments

Psychiatrists must be alert to the many actions of the medications they use and be ready to intervene quickly if patients develop medical problems. A number of medical problems seen in psychiatric patients can be side effects of psychotropic medication. For example, hypothyroidism or nephrogenic diabetes insipidus may result from chronic lithium use in patients with bipolar disorder. Carbamazepine as a treatment for mood disorders has the small but definite risk of agranulocytosis and requires hematological monitoring. The anticholinergic properties of the tricyclic antidepressants and other psychotropic medication may result in a number of medical problems including cardiac, genitourinary, and gastrointestinal difficulties. Clozepine carries the risk of agranulocytosis, and patients are required to have a complete physical examination and a series of laboratory studies before treatment can be initiated. Some community mental health centers have attempted to respond to the medical issues associated with specific pharmacotherapies by establishing special clinics. Patients who are treated with clozepine, for example, participate in standardized protocols including preliminary medical evaluation and routine assessments that include review of systems, weight monitoring, and orthostatic blood pressure and pulse checks.

Mortality Risk of Patients with Psychiatric Illness

A number of studies have pointed to the higher mortality of patients with psychiatric illness. For example, Martin found that the mortality of psychiatric outpatients was approximately twice that of reference population rates (Martin et al., 1985). Other investigators have found increased mortality rates for patients with various psychiatric diagnoses, including a two-fold increase in mortality in patients with schizophrenia (Allebeck and Wistedt, 1986) and similar rates in patients with affective illness. Murphy and her associates (1987, 1988) demonstrated that elderly depressed patients tended to have more physical ailments and higher mortality rates. It was noted that mortality rates were higher in this group even if physical illness was controlled for, suggesting a possible direct effect of depression on physical health. Other studies have demonstrated the higher mortality risk associated with alcohol dependence and other substance abuse (Fossey and Lydiard, 1990).

Bruce and colleagues (1994) looked at follow-up data on the vital status of older adults who participated in the New Haven ECA study and found that 33.5 percent had died during a 9-year period. A greater risk of mortality was associated with recent and past episodes of psychiatric illness as assessed by the NIMH Diagnostic Interview Schedule. Major depression, schizophrenia, and alcohol disorders were all associated with increased mortality.

Psychiatric Treatment in General Health Care Settings

Several surveys of general health services utilization suggest that patients with psychiatric diagnoses use general health services 1.5 to 2 times as frequently as persons without a psychiatric diagnosis. Burns and colleagues (1979) pointed out that for health economics and policy planning reasons it is important to know the extent to which the primary-care sector can contribute to mental health services. In part, this means it is essential that there be an accurate assessment of the burden of mental illness in the primary-care sector.

The groundbreaking work of Michael Shepherd and his colleagues, outlined in *Psychiatric Illness in General Practice* (1966), helped to lay the foundation for future studies. Responding to trends in Great Britain and the United States that supported identification and management of psychiatric illness in the community, Shepherd and his collaborators sought to describe the extent of psychiatric illness in general practice and then to ascertain the role and effectiveness of the general practitioner in treating psychiatric conditions. In a carefully designed survey, Shepherd found a total prevalence rate of 140 per 1,000 persons for all psychiatric disorders combined. Earlier rates of 60.5 and 93.4 had been reported by Lemkau (Lemkau et al., 1941) and Pasamanick (1959), respectively, in the United States. Shepherd noted that there were significant variations in the reported morbidity rates between various practice settings and suggested that these differences might reflect the different interest and capacity of general practitioners to diagnose psychiatric illness. It should be pointed out that while 64 percent of patients identified by the survey as having a psychiatric disorder suffered from a "neurotic" illness, only 4 percent were diagnosed with a psychosis.

Despite the fact that most psychiatric illness seen by the general practitioners were relatively minor, Shepherd was able to show that the GPs surveyed were inadequately prepared to diagnose and treat them. The conclusion of this important study was that psychiatric illness was widespread in general practice and that the general practitioner had an important role to play in providing mental health services in the community. However, it was apparent that the primary care practitioners would require additional training in psychiatric illness before they could do so effectively.

Subsequent epidemiological surveys confirmed Shepherd's findings. For example, Hankin and Oktay (1979) were able to estimate prevalence rates of mental disorders in the range of 15 to 50 percent. More recently, broad-based population surveys have found prevalence rates for psychiatric illness and substance abuse to be in the range of 20 to 30 percent, including the multi-site NIMH Epidemiologic Catchment Area Program that found the annual prevalence rate of mental and addiction disorders to be 28.1 percent (Regier et al., 1993).

By the early 1970s in the United States, the already overburdened and inadequate mental health system was unable to meet the demand for services by large numbers of patients with psychiatric illness and, consequently, the idea was advanced that the primary-care sector would provide the most likely setting for the bulk of mental health services. In 1977, a NIMH workgroup helped to clarify U.S. health policy on the issue of integrating mental health and primary care services (Regier, 1977). The workgroup supported efforts to strengthen the training of primary-care practitioners to better enable these practitioners to respond appropriately to the mental health needs of their patients. It highlighted the importance of training general practitioners to develop the skills to prevent, diagnose, and treat mental illness in the primary-care setting. The non-psychiatrist physician would therefore require comprehensive mental health training in order to effectively deal with the wide variety of psychiatric conditions seen in their practice.

The National Institute of Mental Health in the United States and the National Health Service in Britain have provided the administrative structures that have encouraged an integrated approach to mental health and primary care services. The 1978 President's Commission on Mental Health noted the important role of the general health care sector and further encouraged an integrated system of mental health and primary care services in the community.

These efforts were more successful in Britain than in America. In the United Kingdom, the well-organized national cadre of general practitioners has a major role, in concert with community psychiatrists, in meeting the mental health needs of the community. In the United States, however, in the absence of such a system, despite national policy statements, integration between primary-care services and mental health services is haphazard and often nonexistent.

The importance of establishing more accurate data on the extent of psychiatric disorder in the primary-care setting has become more apparent as treatments for both the minor and major psychiatric disorders have become more rational and specific. A number of tools have been developed for this purpose. Perhaps the best known of these instruments, still widely used in services research, is the General Health Questionnaire (GHQ) developed by Goldberg in 1972. The GHQ has been valuable for detecting psychiatric illness in various clinic populations. Prevalence studies in the United States and elsewhere that have employed the GHQ for assessment of mental disorders have found high rates of psychiatric illness in both urban and rural primary-care settings. However, the usefulness of the GHQ may depend, in part, on other concurrent diagnostic assessments. For example, Benjamin and colleagues (1992), using the GHQ, reported psychiatric "caseness" approaching 69 percent in patients attending primary-care clinics in Israel. He found that when the Schedule for Affective Disorders and Schizophrenia, Lifetime Version (SADS-L) was administered to a sample of the clinic population and used to estimate prevalence, the rate dropped to 15 percent. The general practitioners' estimate was 31 percent. This study shows how detection rates for psychiatric illness in the general health care setting vary depending on the instrument or interview schedule used as well as the training and beliefs of the person making the diagnosis. In this study the GHQ was a suitable tool for detecting psychiatric illness after the threshold score was raised. Thus, the specificity and positive predictive value of the GHQ were improved when used in conjunction with other interviews and methods for identification of psychiatric disorders.

Spitzer and colleagues (1994) developed a screening procedure for detecting and diagnosing mental disorders in the primary-care setting. The PRIME-MD is a 2-stage assessment tool consisting of a 26-item patient checklist that can be followed by a 12-page structured interview administered by a primary-care physician. Patients who respond positively to various symptoms on the initial patient questionnaire are assessed further by the clinician, using five diagnostic modules that may result in 18 possible psychiatric diagnoses. The usefulness and validity of the PRIME-MD has been established by data collected in various primary-care settings. In one study, 1,000 patients were assessed by the PRIME-MD and 26 percent met criteria for a DSM-III-R diagnosis. This finding resulted in treatment or referral in 62 percent of the patients diagnosed with a mental disorder by the PRIME-MD who had not previously been in treatment. Prevalence rates compared favorably with results obtained using other schedules, and construct validity was determined by findings that showed greater impairment in functioning as well as increased health care utilization of services in patients diagnosed with the PRIME-MD. The structured physician interview took less than 9 minutes to administer.

Summary

Patients with psychiatric illness have unique medical needs that may be directly or indirectly related to their primary psychiatric condition and treatment. Identifying and treating the medical problems of these patients has been a challenge both for the community psychiatrist and the general medical practitioner. Access to general medical care has frequently been a problem for these patients because of financial, motivational, or other boundaries that limit contact with the general health care setting. Consequently, community psychiatrists have assumed greater responsibility for assuring that patients with severe and persistent mental illness receive adequate medical care by providing general health maintenance at the CMHC or acting as liaison between the patient and the primary-care providers. Attempts have also been made to train general practitioners to recognize and treat the more common psychiatric illness seen in the primary-care setting and to refer individuals with more complicated psychiatric conditions to the psychiatric specialist.

References

Allebeck, P., and Wistedt, B. (1986) Mortality in schizophrenia. *Archives of General Psychiatry,* 43:650–653.

Bartsch, D.A., Shern, D.L., and Feinberg, L.E. (1990) Screening CMHC outpatients for physical illness. *Hospital and Community Psychiatry,* 41:786–790.

Beitman, B.P., Basha, I., Flaker, G., et al. (1987) Atypical or nonanginal chest pain: panic disorders or coronary artery disease? *Archives of Internal Medicine,* 147:1548–1552.

Benjamin, J., Maoz, B., Shiber, A., et al (1992). Prevalence of psychiatric disorders in three primary-care clinics in Beersheba, Israel. Concurrent assessment by the General Health Questionnaire, General Practitioners, and Research Diagnostic Criteria. *General Hospital Psychiatry,* 14:293–295.

Bruce, M.S., Leaf, P.J., Rozal, G.P., et al. (1994) Psychiatric status and 9-year mortality data in the New Haven Epidemiologic Catchment Area Study. *American Journal of Psychiatry,* 151:716–721.

Burns, B.B., Regier, D.A., Goldberg, I.D., et al. (1979) Future directions in primary care/mental health research. *International Journal of Mental Health,* 8:130–140.

Chignon, J., Lepine, J., and Ades, J. (1993) Panic disorder in cardiac outpatients. *American Journal of Psychiatry,* 150:780–785.

Dalack, G.W., and Roose, S.P. (1990) Perspectives on the relationship between cardiovascular disease and affective disorder. *Journal of Clinical Psychiatry,* 51 Suppl:4–9; discussion 10–11.

Fossey, M.D., and Lydiard, R.B. (1990) Anxiety and the gastrointestinal system. *Psychiatric Medicine* 8:175–186.

Goldberg, D.P. (1972). *The Detection of Psychiatric Illness by Questionnaire.* London: Oxford University Press.

Hall, R.C., Gardner, E.R., and Popkin, M.I. (1981) Unrecognized physical illness prompting psychiatric admission: A prospective study. *American Journal of Psychiatry*, 138:629–634.

Hankin, J., and Oktay, J.S. (1979) *Mental Disorder and Primary Medical Care: An Analytical Review.* Rockville, MD: National Institute of Mental Health.

Katon, W.J. (1990) Chest pain, cardiac disease, and panic disorders. *Journal of Clinical Psychiatry*, 51:27–30.

Katz, M.H. (1994) Effect of HIV treatment on cognition, behavior, and emotion. *Psychiatric Clinics of North America*, 17:227–230.

Koranyi, E.K. (1972) Physical health and illness in a psychiatric outpatient department population. *Canadian Psychiatric Association Journal*, 17:SS109–SS116.

Lane, R.M., Sweeney, M., and Henry, J.A. (1994) Pharmacotherapy of the depressed patient with cardiovascular and/or cerebrovascular illness. *British Journal of Clinical Practice*, 48:256–262.

Lemkau, P., Tietze, C., and Cooper, M. (1941) Mental hygiene problems in an urban district. *Mental Hygiene*, 25:624–630.

Lima, B.R., and Pai, S. (1987) Concurrent medical and psychiatric disorders among schizophrenia and neurotic outpatients. *Community Mental Health Journal*, 23:30–39.

Martin, R.L., Cloninger, C.R., Guze, S.B., and Clayton, P.J. (1985) Mortality in a follow-up of 500 psychiatric outpatients. *Archives of General Psychiatry*, 42:47–54.

McConnell, S.D., Inderbitzin, L.B., and Pollard, W.E. (1992) Primary health care in the CMHC: A role for the nurse practitioner. *Hospital and Community Psychiatry*, 43:724–727.

Murphy, E., Smith, R., Lindesag, J., and Slattery, J. (1988) Increased mortality rates in late-life depression. *British Journal of Psychiatry*, 52:347–353.

Murphy, J.M., Monson, R.R., Olivier, D.C., Sobol, A.M., and Leighton, A.H. (1987) *Archives of General Psychiatry*, 44:473–480.

Pasamanick, B. (ed.) (1959) *Epidemiology of Mental Disorder.* Washington, D.C.: American Association for the Advancement of Science.

Phillips, R.J. (1937) Physical disorders in 164 consecutive admissions to a mental hospital: the incidence and significance. *British Medical Journal* 2, 363–366.

Pincus, H.A. (1980) Linking general health and mental health systems of care: conceptual models of implementation. *American Journal of Psychiatry*, 13:315–320.

Regier, D.A., Narrow, W.E., Rae, D.S., Manderscheid, R.W., Locke, B.Z., and Goodwin, F.K. (1993) The defacto U.S. mental and addictive disorders services system. Epidemiologic catchment area prospective-year prevalence rates of disorders and services. *Archives of General Psychiatry*, 50:85–94.

Regier, D.A. (1977) *The Report of the NIMH Workgroup on Mental Health Training of Primary Care Providers.* Rockville, MD: National Institute of Mental Health.

Roose, S.P., and Dalack, G.W. (1992) Treating the depressed patient with cardiovascular problems. *Journal of Clinical Psychiatry*, 53 Suppl:25–31.

Shepherd, M., Cooper, B., Brown, A., and Kalton, G. (1966) *Psychiatric Illness in General Practice.* London: Oxford University Press.

Spitzer, R.L., Williams, J.B., Kroenke, K., Linzer, J., deGruy, F.V., Hahn, S.R., Brody, D., and Johnson, J.G. (1994) Utility of a new procedure for diagnosing mental disorders in primary care. The Prime-MD 1000 study. *JAMA*, 272:1749–1756.

Wells, K.B., Rogers, W., and Burnam, M.A. (1993) Course of depression in patients with hypertension, myocardial infarction, or insulin-dependent diabetes. *American Journal of Psychiatry*, 150:632–638.

21

Psychiatric Rehabilitation

RUTH A. HUGHES
ANTHONY F. LEHMAN
THOMAS E. ARTHUR

Patients being discharged to the community in the 1960s and 1970s found that the supports and services necessary for community adjustment were not in place. Such needs as a home, income, easily accessible health and mental health care, skills to cope with community living, support during crises, friends, and meaningful work were all too often unmet, and outpatient clinic services had limited impact in these crucial areas. The field of psychiatric (or psychosocial) rehabilitation grew from the need to meet this challenge.

Early programs grew from the recognition that medical interventions were not sufficient for persons with serious mental illnesses, and these programs sought to develop nonclinical approaches. There was a strong emphasis, still apparent in the field today, on practical, commonsense interventions in a normal social environment. The names of agencies such as Fountain House, Horizon House, and Thresholds reflect the informal, nonhierarchical nature of the programs. Participants are often called members, not patients or clients, to emphasize the contributions and responsibilities of every participant to the running of the program. Functioning in every-day life is the focus, with an emphasis on personal strengths rather than clinical symptoms.

The field of psychiatric rehabilitation has grown from its beginnings in a few isolated programs to be a major and integral part of mental health systems across the United States and Canada. Similar programs can now be found throughout the world. The field has been enriched by a number of different models of service delivery, including clubhouse programs, Fairweather lodges, consumer-run alternatives, high-expectancy programs, assertive community treatment, and rehabilitation case management services. The number of U.S. agencies describing themselves as providing psychiatric rehabilitation services for persons with psychiatric disabilities had grown to more than 1,600 in 1990, and over 3,000 in 1995 (IAPSRS, 1991), as mental health service systems became aware of the need and mobilized their responses.

The Psychiatric Rehabilitation Movement

The psychiatric rehabilitation movement began in the late 1940s and early 1950s with a handful of programs dedicated to providing services to people with chronic mental illnesses. These programs sought alternatives to long-term institutionalization and to the pattern of repeated hospitalizations so frequently experienced by persons with mental illness. Much of the early program design and practice was developed from common sense, practical intervention, and trial and error. Exciting and innovative programs were established, but there was little replication or growth in the field until it became apparent in the 1970s that deinstitutionalization was creating a new set of problems.

In 1977, the U.S. Government Accounting Office issued a report that decried the large number of patients being discharged from state hospitals and returning to communities ill prepared to provide support. Shortly thereafter, the National Institute of Mental Health launched its Community Support Program, which encouraged states to develop systems of care in the community for persons with psychiatric disabilities. As community treatment and rehabilitation slowly became priorities, interest in psychiatric rehabilitation grew. It was only in the 1980s and 1990s that psychiatric rehabilitation became an accepted and integral part of the mental health delivery system.

There is enormous diversity in the field. There are a number of different program models with a growing assortment of services. Typically, a psychiatric rehabilitation program can be identified because it provides services to persons with serious psychiatric disabilities, subscribes to the philosophical principles of psychiatric rehabilitation (see below), and provides an array of services designed to help a person cope successfully with life in the community. Those services include training in community living skills, vocational rehabilitation, social rehabilitation, housing, and case management. Irving Rutman, one of the early pioneers in the field, gave the following definition:

> Psychosocial rehabilitation refers to a spectrum of programs for persons with long term mental illness. The programs are designed to strengthen an individual's abilities and skills necessary to meet their needs for housing, employment, socialization, and personal growth. The goal of psychiatric rehabilitation is to improve the quality of life of psychiatrically disabled individuals by assisting them to assume as much responsibility over their lives and to function as actively and independently in society as possible.
>
> Major psychosocial rehabilitation services, which are offered on a continuum, include socialization, recreational services, vocational services, residential services, training in the skills of daily community living, and case management. In addition, psychosocial rehabilitation facilities may also provide client assessment and goal planning activities, educational programs, advocacy training and personal and family support.
>
> The individual may need to use these programs on a short term basis or indefinitely. The programs are offered in the context of a supportive, non-stigmatizing environment in the community, and in a manner that emphasizes the "personhood" rather than the "patienthood" of the individual, maximizes the individual's feelings of responsibility and self

worth, and encourages ownership in the rehabilitation process. The services are coordinated with those offered by other mental health and human service agencies.

(Rutman, 1989)

Structure, practices, location, staffing, funding and resources, and the role of clients/members may vary dramatically from one agency to another, or from one model to another. This variety has contributed to a rich and productive range of ideas in psychiatric rehabilitation.

Psychiatric Rehabilitation Principles

At its very core, psychiatric rehabilitation focuses on the functioning of each person, rather than on the illness. The goal is to assist each person to compensate for deficits related to the illness, through coping skills and a supportive environment. Often an individual needs to develop and practice community living skills. These skills may include personal hygiene, housekeeping, street survival, use of public transportation, social skills, problem solving, prevocational skills, and any area of a person's life affected by the psychiatric disability. Developing competency in these community activities is best achieved in the "real" community. The more activities are integrated into the normal life of the participants, the more effective the interventions will be.

Another core concept of rehabilitation is the empowerment of the person with mental illness. Much of the experience of a patient with mental illness has been disempowering. A sense of hopelessness and helplessness is a common outcome of years of being labeled mentally ill. In rehabilitation, the individual must begin to make decisions, accept responsibility for behavior, take risks, and even make mistakes. Through the process of empowerment, the individual begins to rebuild a more normal life.

As the field has matured, a number of authors have attempted to clarify the principles of psychiatric rehabilitation (Anthony et al., 1982; Anthony et al., 1983; Anthony and Liberman, 1986; Beard, 1978; Beard et al., 1982; Cnaan et al., 1988; Dincin, 1975; Dincin and Pernell-Arnold, 1985; Farkas and Anthony, 1989; Fairweather, 1980; Lanoil, 1982; McRae et al., 1990; Olfson, 1990; Hughes, 1994; Propst, 1990; Rapp and Wintersteen, 1989; Rutman, 1989; Rutman, 1981; Spaniol et al., 1991; Tanaka, 1983). They include:

- A belief in the potential for growth and change in the most severely disabled person. Hope is an essential ingredient in psychiatric rehabilitation.
- The whole person, not the illness, is the focus of psychiatric rehabilitation. "Personhood, rather than patienthood."
- Behavior and functioning, not symptoms, are the focus of interventions. "Health induction rather than symptom reduction."
- The distance between practitioners and clients/members is minimized in order to strengthen the working partnership between them.

- Psychiatric rehabilitation services are oriented toward the practical, day-to-day needs of each person.
- All interventions are based on the principle of client self-determination. Efforts are made to involve the client/member as an active participant in all areas of the program.
- Psychiatric rehabilitation services provide opportunities for people to participate as fully as possible in normal roles and relationships in the community.
- Unnecessary hospitalizations are avoided.
- Activities are *experiential.*
- Interventions are designed to meet the individual needs of each person.
- Psychiatric rehabilitation programs strive to develop supportive communities and/or networks of support.
- The development of coping skills is a major goal.

This is not an exhaustive listing, but there is general agreement about many of these basic principles. While most of the proponents of a particular model or approach would agree with them, there are differences in the priority or weight given to a particular principle. For instance, all models support the concept of self-determination. In a Fairweather Lodge program, self-determination is interpreted as fostering autonomy in the running of the residence and business, with the staff only having a facilitative role. In the intensive case management model, self-determination may mean asking the client his preferences for services, but still fostering dependency on the case manager. A consumer-run alternative program might encourage no reliance at all on mental health professionals or the mental health system. The meaning of self-determination is quite different in each model.

The Practice of Psychiatric Rehabilitation

The goal of psychiatric rehabilitation is to enable individuals to compensate for or eliminate the functional deficits, interpersonal barriers, and environmental barriers created by the disability, and to restore ability for independent living, socialization, and effective life management. Interventions help the individual learn to compensate for the effects of symptoms of the illness through the development of new skills and coping techniques and through creation of a supportive environment. Psychiatric rehabilitation practices also counteract the effects of the secondary symptoms by restoring a sense of confidence and building on the strengths of each person, emphasizing wellness rather than illness.

The activities in a rehabilitation program designed for learning and practicing new coping skills are sometimes confused with vocational, educational, and social interventions. An example may help to clarify the rehabilitation process: A young woman with schizophrenia participates in the food preparation unit each day making lunch. The effects of the mental illness are evident in her slow movements and disinterest in the activities around her (apathy), in her withdrawal from interactions with others (isolation and withdrawal), and in the difficulty she has understanding and communicating with others (cognitive deficits). The intent of the rehabilitation process is not to teach her to cook or to find a job in food preparation. Rather she is learning to follow directions, to ask for clarification when she does not understand, to complete tasks, to relate to others appropriately, to control bizarre behavior, etc. Most important, she is learning to manage the symptoms of her illness in a normal setting. Such activities also raise self-esteem, combat hopelessness, and provide a testing ground for new coping skills in a supportive and caring environment. Through such real-life and normal activities, the rehabilitation process takes place.

Program and Practice Models

One of most replicated models of psychiatric rehabilitation is the *clubhouse*. First developed at Fountain House in New York City in the late 1940s, clubhouse programs strive to develop an intentional community in which members have the opportunity to take on productive and essential roles in the management of the clubhouse, with the support and encouragement of peers and staff. Participants are called members (as in any social club) and may not be excluded from any activity of the organization, including staff meetings. Within the club, each member takes on responsibility. Any person interested in working, no matter what level of functioning he or she is currently exhibiting, is placed in a part-time job in competitive employment, a *transitional employment placement.* Staff and other members provide on-the-job support and training. Members needing a home are assisted in finding an apartment with other members of the clubhouse. At Fountain House, members who participated in the program regularly have been shown to have a lower rate of rehospitalization, with fewer days spent in the hospital and a higher level of functioning while in the community, than a control group (Beard, 1976; Beard et al., 1982).

The National Clubhouse Expansion Program, a Robert Wood Johnson Foundation project, developed standards for clubhouse programs (Propst, 1990). These standards highlight some of the unique elements of the model. Members, not staff, determine their level of involvement in the program. There are no staff offices that could be seen as placing barriers between staff and members. The staff have generalist roles and are involved in all aspects of the program with their members. For instance, a staff member may help a member obtain Social Security benefits, provide on-the-job support to a working member, and be responsible for programming within the club. Staff/member ratios are kept intentionally high to ensure the major involvement of members in running the program. Fountain House has trained thousands of colleagues from all over the world in the clubhouse model. There are approximately 250 such programs in the United States today, with a much larger number of agencies replicating aspects of this approach.

There are a number of early psychiatric rehabilitation agencies that could be characterized as ascribing to a *high-expectancy* model. These programs are more structured than the clubhouse model and set up expectations with each client regarding goals and progress. Often the program is designed with a series of sequential steps for clients to move through as they become more independent, skilled, and employed. If clubhouse programs provide a surrogate family, then high-expectancy programs are similar to going to school. Clients may attend classes and are assisted in developing new skills and competencies. Examples of high-expectancy programs are Thresholds in Chicago, Portals in Los Angeles, Horizon House in Philadelphia, and Stairways in Erie, Pennsylvania. There is no formal system to encourage replication of this model, nor any network of high-expectancy programs, but a large number of agencies have adopted an educational approach that utilizes segments of this model (Rutman, 1989; Dincin, 1975, 1981).

The *assertive community treatment* model has been described as psychiatric rehabilitation without walls. Rather than having a client come into a facility, a team takes the clinical and rehabilitative services to the client in the community (Chapter 16). Originally developed as a way to provide services to those clients who had high rates of rehospitalization and were less than cooperative with existing services, the model was designed to use the community as the training ground. Stein and Test first developed this approach in Madison, Wisconsin (Stein and Test, 1975, 1983; Thompson et al., 1990). Members of a treatment team would visit a person in their home or on the job, go grocery shopping together, or meet at the local coffee shop. By utilizing a team approach, the client is always assured of being able to contact someone he knows. The amount of contact varies depending on the client's needs at any point in time. The Program for Assertive Community Treatment (PACT) has been shown to be a cost-effective alternative to hospitalization (Weisbrod et al., 1980) and to be effective in helping clients maintain a stable adjustment to the community (Taube et al., 1990).

In the *strengths* model of case management, each client has an individual case manager. It tends to be a less clinically oriented approach than PACT and focuses more on the personal and social needs of each client. Again, the natural resources of the community are used to meet the client's needs. A study of 12 programs using this approach found significantly lower rehospitalization rates than with clients of other community support services (Rapp and Wintersteen, 1989; Wintersteen and Rapp, 1986).

A growing consumer movement has led to the development of *consumer run alternatives* to the more traditional mental health services. These programs are based on the premise that a person who has experienced the anguish of mental illness, and also experienced the system of mental health services as a patient, is in the best position to assist other people with psychiatric disabilities. Frequently, consumer-run programs are designed as drop-in centers or social clubs that are a place for the participants to develop a network of caring and supportive friends. There is usually a strong advocacy component to consumer-run programs, as the participants discover they can influence the mental health system more effectively by banding together. Because few of the consumers have mental health degrees, treatment is usually received elsewhere, though some consumer-run programs hire their own clinical staff.

There is enormous diversity among consumer-run alternatives; some examples are Project Share in Philadelphia, On Our Own in Baltimore, Project Stay in Michigan, and the Mental Patients' Liberation Front in Boston (Rutman, 1989; Chapter 12).

Another model that strongly emphasizes consumer autonomy is the *Fairweather Lodge*. George Fairweather originally developed this approach to help move people from the hospital to the community. In a typical lodge program, a group of persons with psychiatric disabilities live together, setting their own rules and expectations of one another. The group will frequently launch a small business venture, which is owned and operated by the residents. The more heterogeneous the group, the more likely they will succeed in their endeavors. The staff role in this approach is as a facilitator or consultant. The responsibility is on the group to tackle problems and set goals. Lodge programs tend to form highly cohesive, task-oriented groups, which function well in the community (Fairweather et al., 1969). Lodge programs have been shown to significantly reduce hospitalization and significantly increase employment among participants (Fairweather and Fergus, 1988).

While others were developing program models, Robert Liberman and William Anthony have used behavioral theory and social learning theory to develop effective practices in rehabilitation. There is a strong emphasis on assessment, planning, skill development, and resource development to support and strengthen the individual's level of functioning. Anthony and his colleagues have developed training curricula in the methods of assessment, planning, skill development, and resource development. Utilizing role play and behavioral exercises, Liberman has developed training packages to be used with clients to teach specific sets of skills such as medication management and social skills (Anthony and Liberman, 1986; Liberman, 1988). The techniques can be used in any setting and in combination with other program models. Dion and Anthony (1987) reviewed 35 experimental and quasi-experimental studies and found that psychiatric rehabilitation interventions positively affect recidivism, time spent in the community, employment, skill development, and client satisfaction.

In addition to the models described, there is a growing number of new approaches to specific services, such as supported employment, transitional employment, supported housing, and supported education. Underlying each of these approaches is a strong commitment to help the individual fully integrate into the community by providing the necessary supports in the community environment. For example, in *supported employment* a person with a serious mental illness is placed in a competitive job, usually part-time. A job coach may work side-by-side with the client at the work place until the client has mastered both the job skills and the social behaviors needed in the work environment. Once the client is stable in the job position, the job coach will begin to withdraw, only making periodic visits to the job site. If necessary, the job coach will intensify the amount of support and on-the-job supervision during periods of change (e.g., a new supervisor) or if symptoms intensify. The job coach is also responsible, with the client, for ensuring that other support services such as mental health treatment, medication, transportation, stress management, and social skill training are available as necessary.

Outcome Research

While there is general agreement that psychiatric rehabilitation is effective in reducing hospitalizations and in increasing the level of functioning in the community, little is known about which interventions or practices make the difference for a client. There is no method to predict which clients will most benefit from which interventions or strategies of rehabilitation. The relative recency of the development of this field, the complexity of psychiatric rehabilitation interventions (and of the outcomes they address), as well as problems in designing research on services that may not be readily conducive to standard research methodologies, such as randomized clinical trials, have posed major barriers to the development of definitive outcome research. Nonetheless, there is currently a much-expanded agenda of rehabilitation research underway.

Social Skills Training (SST)

Considerable research effort has been devoted to the assessment of the efficacy of this approach. Several observations and conclusions can be derived from these studies. First, SST can successfully modify specifically targeted behavioral skills, such as eye contact, voice volume, active listening skills, and problem-solving strategies (Liberman et al., 1986). This is an important finding in itself because it demonstrates that the social skill deficits of persons with serious mental illnesses are modifiable. Second, intensive SST can enhance clinical outcomes, such as symptoms and relapse rates, as well as improve social skills (Wallace and Liberman, 1985; Bellack et al., 1984). Finally, the evidence on the generalization and enduring nature of the immediate effects of SST are mixed. Some studies have found that the effects of SST generalize to other situations in the patient's life and endure over a period of time (Liberman et al., 1984; Wallace and Liberman, 1985); others have questioned this and reported failure to generalize or rapid deterioration in social skill gains after discontinuation of SST (Dion and Anthony, 1987; Mattson and Stephens, 1978). Generalization and durability may be enhanced through use of behavioral homework assignments, involvement of significant others in the SST program, and supervised practice of the social skills in real-life situations.

Vocational Rehabilitation (VR)

Assessment of the efficacy of vocational rehabilitation interventions is complicated because of the wide variety of these programs and the rapid evolution underway from sheltered programs to transitional and supported work models. In general, the employment rates among persons with serious mental illness are low, typically in the range of 25 percent (Anthony et al., 1978). This has not improved over the past decade. Bond and Boyer (1988) reviewed the existing controlled evaluations of vocational rehabilitation programs for persons with serious mental illness and found rather discouraging results. Among 31 studies, 11 found enhanced occupational outcomes among VR clients compared to control cases, 19 found no advantage for the VR cases, and one found negative effects of a VR program. In this review VR programs appeared to have the most benefit on sheltered vocational outcomes, that is, VR patients were more likely than control cases to be employed, but in sheltered settings. Only 1 of 13 studies that examined competitive employment found advantages to VR programs, and of the 9 studies that examined employment after the VR program, only 3 found advantages for VR. In considering these somewhat discouraging results, it is important to keep in mind that models of VR are currently in flux, and not enough is known as yet about the efficacy of such innovative VR models as supported employment and transitional employment. Work remains such an important outcome for persons with serious mental illness that developing the optimal VR strategy for the individual patient who wants to work is an important priority (Tashjian et al., 1989).

Residential Services

Appropriate housing constitutes an essential component of community care for persons with serious mental illness (Chapter 22), yet little is known about the efficacy of various housing options for enhancing outcomes. The research that does exist has focused on consumer preferences and has shown consistently that most patients would prefer to live in their own homes or apartments with flexible supports (Carling, 1988). One study found that the quality of life experience of persons with serious mental illness living in private apartments or small group homes were superior to the experience of persons in large board-and-care homes or long-term hospitals (Lehman et al., 1991). However, there is still no adequate research data base upon which to base any firm conclusions about housing for persons with serious mental illness. It is probably safe to say that a continuum of housing options is needed, that every attempt should be made to allow persons with serious mental illnesses to live in the least restrictive settings of their choice, and that more effective models need to be developed for linking services with housing.

Linking Clinical Treatments with Rehabilitation

Perhaps one of the most important general findings in the rehabilitation research literature is that combining effective clinical treatment with psychiatric rehabilitation is more effective than providing either service alone. The best example of this is a study by Hogarty and colleagues (1991). In a randomized study they compared four treatment conditions for schizophrenia: (1) depot fluphenazine (FPZ) alone; (2) FPZ plus social skills training (SST); (3) FPZ plus family training (FT); and (4) FPZ plus SST plus FT. The most striking result is that combining medication with family training appeared to substantially reduce relapse rates throughout the 2-year follow-up period. An even more intriguing finding was that among the patients who did not relapse, those who received family training had considerably better *employment* outcomes compared to non-relapsed patients who did not receive family training. Fifty percent of those receiving family training were competitively employed at follow-up compared to 27 percent of those not receiving family assistance. While this finding is in need of replication, it suggests that a supportive and positive environment itself (in this case a family environment) can enhance the rehabilitation outcome in unexpected ways.

In summary, the research on outcomes of rehabilitation strategies for persons with serious mental illness indicates that psychiatric interventions in general are an essential component of treatment; we do not yet know exactly what rehabilitation interventions work for which patients; and combining clinical treatment with psychiatric rehabilitation will likely yield the best results.

Role of the Psychiatrist

We are only now discovering the complexity and range of community services needed to adequately serve people with serious mental illness (Bachrach, 1991; Breakey, 1990; Hogg et al., 1990; Lamb, 1991). Those initially targeted for deinstitutionalization are now being joined by emerging populations requiring specialized services, such as young adults, the elderly with mental illness, and individuals with dual diagnosis of mental illness and substance abuse. In addition, the advances in understanding biomedical theories of mental illness and the development of new medications add to the complexity of providing adequate community-based services to this population. While treatment focuses on stress relief, symptom alleviation, and curing diseases, and rehabilitation emphasizes increasing functioning levels, neither outpatient treatment nor community rehabilitation can stand alone (Bachrach, 1991; Breakey, 1990; Hazel et al., 1991; and Wintersteen and Rapp, 1986).

In the past, primary care of people with serious mental illness was left to mental health providers with the least amount of training and experience. The complexities of the community-based system require a wide range of expertise from mental health professionals and psychiatric rehabilitation practitioners alike. In the past, psychiatric rehabilitation services and clinical treatment have often been separated. More and more frequently, clinical agencies such as community mental health centers are now developing psychiatric rehabilitation components, and free-standing psychiatric rehabilitation agencies are developing clinical components and hiring psychiatrists. Psychiatrists can play an essential role in this system of care. Several roles emerge as primary for the psychiatrist: clinician, clinical supervisor, teacher, consultant, and liaison for other mental health and health services.

As clinician, the psychiatrist provides diagnostic evaluation, treatment planning, prescribing, psychiatric counseling, rehabilitation referral, and overall treatment monitoring. It is critically important for the psychiatrist to assess not only the symptoms but the level of functioning of the patient. Medication side effects may interfere with functioning and the rehabilitation process. On the other hand, rehabilitation may induce stress and lead to an increase in symptoms. The psychiatrist, psychiatric rehabilitation practitioners, and client must continually monitor and balance the various interventions to enhance the highest level of functioning. The psychiatrist has a key role in helping the client and rehabilitation staff develop a plan of intervention in case of relapse. Such a plan, which identifies early prodromal symptoms and the most effective early interventions for the client, can be essential as a person with serious mental illness becomes more independent or moves away from the sheltered environment in a rehabilitation program.

In the environment of a psychiatric rehabilitation program, a psychiatrist is a teacher and consultant for psychiatric rehabilitation staff, for the clients in the program, and for family members. The more everyone understands about mental illness, treatment, and rehabilitation, the more effective these interventions will be. Clients, families, and staff all benefit from being educated about the nature of mental illness, medication, and coping mechanisms (Dincin, 1990; Hazel et al., 1991; Streicker et al., 1986). As teachers, psychiatrists also serve as role models for psychiatric students entering the field and can have a significant impact on these future psychiatrists serving people with serious mental illness (H&CP Gold Award, 1989; Weintraub et al., 1991).

A seldom mentioned benefit for psychiatrists involved with psychiatric rehabilitation programs is the opportunity to see clients functioning at a much higher level than they often do in clinical settings. When contact with patients occurs in inpatient units, emergency rooms, and even clinics, the focus is on the client's illness and the severity of the symptoms. In a rehabilitation program the focus is on the client's wellness and ability to function. Mental health professionals who work in both clinical and rehabilitation settings often express amazement at the difference observed in the same clients in different settings.

In the consultant role, the psychiatrist can provide programmatic consultation to community rehabilitation programs on a variety of issues ranging from staff inservice to effective communications with others in the medical profession. At times the psychiatrist can serve as a liaison or bridge between the psychiatric rehabilitation program and other physicians. This role can be essential to ensuring good relationships between providers and continuity of services for members.

Summary

Psychiatric rehabilitation services are an integral and crucial component of the system of community care for persons with serious mental illness. A wide variety of psychiatric rehabilitation models and interventions has emerged in the last 15 years. All emphasize providing supports to help an individual improve the quality of life and to function as actively and independently in society as possible. Based on the current research evidence, it may be concluded that psychiatric interventions in general are an essential component of treatment, but it is not yet known exactly which rehabilitation interventions work for which patients. The role of psychiatrists in psychiatric rehabilitation programs has been relatively undefined but is now emerging as greater integration between clinical and rehabilitative interventions occurs.

References

Anthony, W., Cohen, M., and Cohen, B. (1983) Philosophy, treatment process, and principles of the psychiatric rehabilitation approach. In *New Directions for Mental Health Services.* (ed. L. Bachrach) San Francisco: Jossey-Bass.

Anthony, W., Cohen, M., and Farkas, M. (1982) A psychiatric rehabilitation treatment program: Can I recognize one when I see one?'' *Community Mental Health Journal,* 18:83–96.

Anthony, W., Cohen, M., and Vitalo, R. (1978) The measurement of rehabilitation outcome. *Schizophrenia Bulletin,* 4:365–383.

Anthony, W., and Liberman, R. (1986) The practice of psychiatric rehabilitation: historical, conceptual and research base. *Schizophrenia Bulletin,* 12:542–559.

Bachrach, L. (1991) Planning high quality services. *Hospital and Community Psychiatry,* 42: 268–269.

Beard, J. (1978) The rehabilitation services of Fountain House. In Stein, L., Test, M. (eds.), *Alternatives to Mental Hospital Treatment.* (eds. L. Stein and M. Test). New York: Plenum Press

Beard, J. (1976) Psychiatric rehabilitation at Fountain House. In Meislin, J. (ed.), *Rehabilitation Medicine and Psychiatry.* Springfield, Ill.: Charles C. Thomas.

Beard, J., Propst, R., and Malamud, T. (1982) The Fountain House model of psychiatric rehabilitation. *Psychosocial Rehabilitation Journal,* 5:47–59.

Bellack, A., Herson, M., and Luber, R. (1984) An examination of the efficacy of social skills training for chronic schizophrenic patients. *Hospital and Community Psychiatry,* 35: 1023–1028.

Bond, G., and Boyer, S. (1988) The evaluation of vocational programming for the mentally ill: A review. In Ciardiello, J., Bell, M., (eds.), *Vocational Rehabilitation of Persons with Long Term Mental Illness.* Baltimore: Johns Hopkins University Press.

Breakey, W.R. (1990) Networks of services for seriously mentally ill in the community. In Cohen, M. (ed.), *Psychiatry Takes to the Streets.* New York: Guilford Press.

Carling, P.J. (1988) Review of research on housing and community integration for people with psychiatric disabilities. *NARIC Quarterly,* Vol. 1, No. 3.

Cnaan, R., Blankertz, L., Messinger, K., and Gardner, J. (1988) Psychosocial rehabilitation: toward a definition. *Psychosocial Rehabilitation Journal,* 11:61–78.

Dincin, J. (1990) Speaking out. *Psychosocial Rehabilitation Journal,* 14:83–85.

Dincin, J. (1981) A community agency model. In Talbott, J. (ed.), *The Chronically Mentally Ill: Treatment, Programs and Systems.* New York: Human Sciences Press.

Dincin, J. (1975) Psychiatric Rehabilitation. *Schizophrenia Bulletin,* 13:131–147.

Dincin, J., and Pernell-Arnold, A. (1985) *Psychosocial Rehabilitation: Definition, Principles and Description.* Columbia MD: International Association of Psychosocial Rehabilitation Services.

Dion, G., and Anthony, W. (1987) Research in psychiatric rehabilitation: A review of experimental and quasi-experimental studies. *Rehabilitation Counseling Bulletin,* 30:177–203.

Fairweather, G. (ed.) (1980) *The Fairweather Lodge: A Twenty-Five Year Retrospective.* San Francisco: Jossey-Bass.

Fairweather, G., and Fergus, E. (1988) The Lodge Society: A look at community tenure as a measure of cost savings. Michigan Lodge Dissemination Project, Michigan State University.

Fairweather, G., Sanders, D., Cressler, D., and Maynard, H. (1969) *Community Life for the Mentally Ill.* Chicago: Aldine.

Farkas, M., and Anthony, W. (eds.) (1989) *Psychiatric Rehabilitation Programs: Putting Theory into Practice.* Baltimore: Johns Hopkins University Press.

H&CP Gold Award (1989) Integrating training and research with clinical services in a community setting. *Hospital and Community Psychiatry, 40:1175–1179.*

Hazel, K., Herman, S., and Maubray, C. (1991) Characteristics of seriously mentally ill adults in a public mental health system. *Hospital and Community Psychiatry, 42:518–525.*

Hogarty, G.E., Anderson, C., Reiss, D., Kornblith, S., Greenwald, D., Jauna, C., and Madonia, M. (1991) Family psychoeducation, social skills training, and maintenance chemotherapy in the aftercare treatment of schizophrenia. *Archives of General Psychiatry, 48:340–347.*

Hogg, L., Hall, J., and Marshall, M. (1990) Assessing people who are chronically mentally ill: new methods for new settings. *Psychosocial Rehabilitation Journal, 13(3):117.*

Hughes, R. (1994) *Psychiatric Rehabilitation Is an Essential Health Service for Persons with Serious and Persistant Mental Illness.* Columbia, MD: IAPSRS.

International Association of Psychosocial Rehabilitation Services (1991) *Organizations Providing Psychosocial Rehabilitation and Related Community Support Services in the United States.* Columbia MD: IAPSRS

Lamb, R. (1991) Community treatment for the chronically mentally ill. *Hospital and Community Psychiatry, 42:117.*

Lanoil, J. (1982) An analysis of the psychiatric psychosocial rehabilitation center. *Psychosocial Rehabilitation Journal, 5(1):55–59.*

Lehman, A.F., Slaughter, J.C., and Myers, C.P. (1991) Quality of life in alternative residential settings. *Psychiatric Quarterly, 62:37–51.*

Liberman, R. (ed.) (1988) *Psychiatric Rehabilitation of Chronic Mental Patients.* Washington, DC: American Psychiatric Press.

Liberman, R., Mueser, K., and Wallace, C. (1986) Social skills training for schizophrenic individuals at risk for relapse. *American Journal of Psychiatry, 143:523–526.*

Liberman, R., Mueser, K.T., Wallace, C.J. (1984) Social skills training for relapsing schizophrenics. *Behavior Modification, 8:155–179.*

Mattson, J., and Stephens, R. (1978) Increasing appropriate behavior of explosive chronic psychiatric patients with a social skills training package. *Behavior Modification, 2:61–77.*

McRae, J., Higgins, M., Lycan, C., and Sherman, W. (1990) What happens after five years of intensive case management stops? *Hospital and Community Psychiatry, 41:927–928.*

Olfson, M. (1990) Assertive community treatment: an evaluation of the experimental evidence. *Hospital and Community Psychiatry, 41:634–641.*

Propst, R. (1990) *Standards for Clubhouse Programs.* New York: Fountain House/National Clubhouse Expansion Program.

Rapp, C., and Wintersteen, R. (1989) The strengths model of case management: results from twelve demonstrations. *Psychosocial Rehabilitation Journal, 13:23–32.*

Rutman, I. (1981) Community based services: characteristics, principles and program models. In Rutman, I. (ed.), *Planning for Deinstitutionalization.* Rockville, MD: Department of Health and Human Services.

Rutman, I. (1989) The psychosocial rehabilitation movement in the United States. In Meyerson,

A., Fine, T. (eds.), *Psychiatric Disability: Clinical, Legal and Administrative Dimensions.* Washington DC: American Psychiatric Press.

Spaniol, L., Zipple, A., and Cohen, B. (1991) Managing innovation and change in psychosocial rehabilitation: key principles and guidelines. *Psychosocial Rehabilitation Journal,* 14: 27–38.

Stein, L., and Test, M. (1983) The community as the treatment arena in caring for the chronic psychiatric patient. In Barofsky, I., Budson, R. (eds.), *The Chronic Psychiatric Patient in the Community.* New York: SP Medical and Scientific Books.

Stein, L., and Test, M. (1975) Training in community living: research design and results. In Stein, L., Test, M. (eds.), *Alternatives to Mental Hospital Treatment.* New York: Plenum Press.

Streicker, S., Kaluzny, S., Andur, M., and Dincin, J. (1986) Educating patients about psychiatric medications: failure to enhance compliance. *Psychosocial Rehabilitation Journal,* 9:16–23.

Tanaka, H. (1983) Psychosocial rehabilitation: future trends and directions. *Psychosocial Rehabilitation Journal,* 6(4), 7–12.

Tashjian, M., Hayard, B., Stoddard, S., and Kraus, L. (1989) *Best Practice Study of Vocational Rehabilitation Services to Severely Mentally Ill Persons.* Washington, D.C.: Rehabilitation Services Administration, U.S. Dept of Education.

Taube, C., Morlock, L., Burns, B., and Santos, A. (1990) New directions in research on assertive community treatment. *Hospital and Community Psychiatry,* 41:642–646.

Thompson, K., Griffith, E., and Leaf, P. (1990) A historical review of the Madison Model of Community Care. *Hospital and Community Psychiatry,* 41:625–633.

Wallace, C., and Liberman, R. (1985) Social skills training for patients with schizophrenia: a controlled clinical trial. *Psychiatry Research,* 15:239–247.

Weintraub, W., Nyman, G., and Harbin, H. (1991) The Maryland Plan: the best of the story. *Hospital and Community Psychiatry,* 42:52–55.

Weisbrod, B.A., Test, M.A., and Stein, L.I. (1980) Alternative to mental hospital treatment II: economic benefit-cost analysis. *Archives of General Psychiatry,* 37:400–405.

Wintersteen, R., and Rapp, C. (1986) The young adult chronic patient: a dissenting view of an emerging concept. *Psychosocial Rehabilitation Journal,* 9:3–13.

22

Housing

ANTHONY F. LEHMAN
SANDRA J. NEWMAN

Liberty like charity must begin at home.

(Conant, 1942)

Everyone needs to know there is a place in society for them, that there's a place where they can belong.

(Harp, 1988)

The essence of the major transition in the care afforded persons with severe mental illnesses in the United States over the past 40 years has been the change in where they live. For the first half of the twentieth century the majority of these persons lived predominantly in large public hospitals. Since then there has been a steady effort, largely successful, to shift the residences of these persons from long-term care hospitals to community-based settings. Today persons with severe mental illnesses live in a wide variety of housing settings in the community, ranging from such community institutions as nursing homes and locked care facilities to "mainstream" settings including independent housing and the homes of their families.

There is little that is more basic to the practice of community psychiatry than understanding and dealing with the issues related to where our patients live. This chapter reviews national policies relating to housing for persons with severe mental illnesses, describes the various types of housing programs that have been developed and what is known about their effectiveness, and discusses the functions of the community psychiatrist relevant to housing.

Background and Policy Issues

Housing Programs for Persons with Severe Mental Illnesses

Ridgway and Zipple (1990) identified two major paradigm shifts in housing for persons with severe mental illnesses during the past 40 years. The first was the shift from housing large numbers of persons in mental hospitals to living in the community; the second is the shift from the provision of structured housing programs to the concept of supporting individuals who live in ordinary housing arrangements, the "supported housing" concept. These conceptual shifts on the part of housing experts have been mirrored by shifts in public policy from "supply side" to "demand side" funding mechanisms.

The first paradigm shift began in the early 1950s and peaked in the 1970s. Ridgway and Zipple refer to this first wave of community-based residential care as the "paradigm of the linear continuum." Central to this paradigm was the development of a graduated continuum of residential *treatment* programs in the community through which a person progresses toward higher functioning and less restrictive settings.

Considerable variety characterizes the community residential care settings offered to persons with severe mental illnesses under the "linear continuum," and the literature is replete with various terminologies for referring to these settings. Budson (1990) identifies eight basic types: transitional halfway houses, long-term group residences, cooperative apartments, intensive care community residences, total rural environments, foster care, board and care homes, and nursing homes. These types of residential care differ according to the length of time a person is allowed to stay, the intensity of on-site staff supervision, the degree to which they emphasize clinical or rehabilitation services versus simple housing, and the level of aggregation of patients in the living space. The most common programs are transitional halfway houses, long-term group residences, and cooperative apartments (also referred to as "satellite housing," "landlord supervised apartments," and "post halfway house accommodations") (Budson, 1990).

Transitional halfway houses provide 24-hour daily supervision, a planned program, and the expectation that the patient will move on to more permanent housing in the community. They are conceived as a bridge between the hospital and the community. These programs are often closely linked administratively and functionally to psychiatric hospitals and clinics. In contrast, *long-term group residences* are designed to offer 24-hour daily supervision on a longer term basis, and may be the sequel setting for a transitional halfway house resident who is unable to move on to more independent living. These residences typically have less clinical input and expertise than transitional halfway houses. *Cooperative apartments* typically have no on-site supervision, but provide regular staff oversight and supervision for a small number of residents living together in an apartment. *Intensive care or "crisis" residences* offer an acute, short-term alternative to hospitalization and are staffed by clinicians. *Nursing homes* offer a longer term version of clinically supervised residential care for those persons needing ongoing intensive nursing care and supervision. Under the *foster care* model, a private family or citizen in the community takes a mentally disabled person into their home. These homes are analogous to foster care for children. The family assumes responsibility for meeting the needs of the disabled person with oversight and supervision from a social case worker. *Board and care homes* are proprietary homes that provide room, board, and some minimal but ongoing supervision. Typically they are converted apartment buildings, hotels, or motels. Their staffing and programming typically are minimal, providing meals and a bed. One staff member may be on-site at all times to supervise up to 150 residents. Finally, total *rural environments,* a rare version of residential care, are residential farms, supervised by staff, that emphasize rehabilitation through working and living together.

The goals, administration, and funding for these residential alternatives vary. Transitional halfway houses, intensive care or "crisis" residences, nursing homes, and rural environments have treatment and/or rehabilitation as explicit goals. They may be independently operated or be components of a larger health care network, and funding mixes third-party health payors (i.e., health insurance or government support) with payments by patients and families. Oversight and licensing by public health departments is typical. Foster care rests within the social welfare system. The goal of foster care is primarily support and shelter for persons who are unable to live independently and who are essentially "wards of the state." Funding for foster care may come directly from a government agency with case worker oversight and monitoring, although "private pay" foster care is also available. Cooperative apartments are often affiliated with more intensive residential programs (e.g., halfway houses or clinical programs) and are viewed as a step toward greater independence. Their funding relies more on patient and family self-pay (rent), but they may be subsidized by government programs. In contrast, board and care homes have the more modest goal of food and shelter. Patients pay rent to stay in these homes; the rent is typically geared to the amount of funds that patients receive under government disabilities programs.

The research on these alternative residential settings is limited and leaves many unanswered questions, in particular their relative efficacy for various patient subgroups. However, in general the research indicates that many of these settings offer viable and preferable alternatives to long-term hospitalization (Braun et al., 1981), and that some patients benefit from higher expectations setting (e.g., transitional halfway houses), whereas others adapt better to low-expectation situations (e.g., board and care homes or foster care) (Budson, 1990).

It can be argued correctly that the "linear continuum" is a misnomer. Although its name derives from the notion that a patient leaving an institution ideally may progress along a continuum from greater to lesser restrictive housing (e.g., from hospital to halfway house to cooperative apartment to independent living), the fact is that this is not what usually occurs. Typically patients move from the hospital to one of these settings and remain there for an extended period of time.

Patient dissatisfaction with this linear continuum paradigm is illustrated by the following comment.

I could get out [of the hospital] under the condition that I went to live in what was called a group home. . . . In a group home, I was [sic] . . . little more than community institutionalized, I was told when I could get up, when I could go to bed, when I could eat, and when I could go to the bathroom, and I was highly resentful of it. Every time I would attempt to go out on my own, I would be told, "You need to continue to live in the group home, it's part of your therapy, and, if you leave, we'll have to re-commit you."

(Crafts, 1988).

Due to a variety of problems with this linear continuum paradigm, Ridgway and Zipple denote a second major shift in housing for persons with severe mental illnesses that is now underway. This they refer to as the "paradigm of supported housing." "In the new paradigm of supported housing there is, first and foremost, a conceptual and real shift away from the exclusive reliance on residential treatment settings as the sole model of delivery and a new emphasis on the development of normal housing options as a person's own home" (pp. 16–17).

The differences between these two paradigms as conceptualized by Ridgway and Zipple are summarized in Table 22–1 (from Ridgway and Zipple, 1990).

It is evident from the terminology in the table that the conceptual shift from the "linear continuum" to "supported housing" is substantial and to an extent political. Central to the conceptual shift is a greater emphasis on normalization of housing and client choice. The terminology in the table probably exaggerates the actual shift and may be unfairly pejorative with regard to residential services other than supported housing. The conceptual shift to promoting more normalized housing and client choice is essential, but the fact remains that a range of housing options, with varying capacities for support depending upon the patients' needs and preferences, is both necessary and desirable. Clearly the more options available, the greater the opportunity for appropriate choices.

In practice, supported housing allows the client to chose an appropriate place to live and supportive services are provided to enable the client to succeed. Supportive case management is an essential component of supported housing. The case manager provides periodic supervision and is available to provide clients with support and training in community living. The case manager also provides rehabilitation training in such daily living areas as money management, cooking, grocery shopping, and household cleaning.

Table 22–1   Comparison of Supported Housing and Linear Continuum

Supported Housing	Linear Continuum
A home	Residential treatment settings
Choice	Placement
Normal roles	Client role
Client control of home	Staff conrol
Social integration	Grouping by disability
Real-world learning in permanent settings	Transitional preparatory settings
Individualized flexible services and supports	Standardized levels of service
Most facilitative environment, long-term supports	Least restrictive environment, independence

Housing Policies for Persons with Severe Mental Illnesses

Public policies in the United States aimed at providing housing services for persons with severe mental illnesses also reflect the evolving nature of these housing paradigms. Traditionally housing policies at the federal and state level have emphasized the linear paradigm, providing funding to residential care providers, so-called "supply-side" housing interventions (Goldman and Newman, 1990; Newman and Struyk, 1988). These supply-side interventions take the form of tax incentives to developers of low-income housing, supplements to Supplemental Security Income (SSI) programs to cover the additional cost of special housing programs, and direct state funding of housing for persons with severe mental illnesses (e.g., state hospital–operated residences and state grants to private residential care providers). This supply-side approach reinforces the linear continuum paradigm under which treatment and housing providers make the key decisions about the type of housing offered.

In contrast, government housing programs have more recently added "demandside" interventions, that is, subsidies provided directly to housing consumers, who in turn make their own choices about their housing. Examples of these interventions include the Section 8 Housing Certificate Program and the Housing Voucher Program (Goldman and Newman, 1990). Section 8 vouchers are rent subsidy vouchers that are issued by the government to income eligible individuals, including the disabled. They may be used to rent any housing that meets basic federal housing quality criteria, thus maximizing recipient choice. This demand-side approach encourages the paradigm shift to supported housing.

The Role of the Community Psychiatrist in Housing

As we have discussed, the array of housing alternatives for persons with severe mental illness is quite varied, and the housing options that are available to these persons change as concepts and policies evolve. What then are the roles of the community psychiatrist with regard to housing?

Case Example: A 50-year-old woman with chronic paranoid schizophrenia was readmitted to the hospital for an acute exacerbation of her illness following noncompliance with her antipsychotic medication. The intake assessment ascertained that she had been living at a large board and care home in an impoverished area of the city, and it was the staff's opinion that this home paid little attention to medication compliance. While the patient was being restabilized on medication, the staff arranged for the patient to move to a nicer board and care home in a residential neighborhood near the ocean where the care provider would supervise her taking of medication. Arrangements for this move, including time to convince the patient that she should move, extended the hospital stay by at least two weeks. At the time of discharge, the patient was given bus tokens and directions to her new home. She left the hospital and returned instead to her previous board and care residence. When asked why, she indicated that she liked the board and care provider, had friends in the home, and felt more comfortable in the inner-city neighborhood, despite its poverty.

This case illustrates the common failure of clinicians to take into account patients' housing preferences in arranging "placements." In this woman's case, a housing situation that provided better medication supervision would have been preferable from a clinical perspective, but the manner in which the discharge planning occurred was insensitive to other highly relevant factors in her choice of housing. The clinicians failed to make an adequate assessment of the patient's housing situation, especially her preferences, and to use this assessment in planning for the patient's needs.

What else could the clinicians have done? While housing decisions are often difficult, there is actually a great deal that a community psychiatrist can do to facilitate suitable housing for patients. This involvement begins with a thorough assessment to understand that patient's clinical and housing needs.

Assessment

Assessment seems an obvious starting point, but all too often clinicians fail to pay more than perfunctory attention to the patient's living circumstances. The assessment should begin with information about how patients feel about their current living arrangements. Is the arrangement satisfactory? If yes, why does the patient feel this way? If not, why not? Also important are the perceptions of significant others in the patients' life. How does the patient's family feel about the housing arrangement? If the patient is living in a supervised setting, how do the staff perceive the patient's situation?

An adequate assessment also should include information about where the patient lives, the type of housing, its neighborhood, and the availability of local services, such as public transportation, grocery stores, coffee shops, and the like. With whom does the patient live? How many others live there? What are their characteristics (age, gender, race, disability status), and what are their relationships to the patient—relatives, friends, support staff?

Is the housing situation time-limited? Many existing housing services for persons with severe mental illnesses incorporate the linear continuum model of housing and therefore place time limits on the patient's stay. For example, in a survey of 2,538 state-affiliated community residential programs for persons with severe mental illness, half imposed length of stay limits, including 20 percent with a length of stay restricted to less than 12 months (Randolph et al., 1991). It is important to know if this is the case.

What are the house rules and expectations? Housing rules may vary from only the most basic expectations about safety and common decency (such as in single room occupancy hotels) to high-expectation housing programs in which patients are expected to participate actively in a residential milieu and to attend goal-directed activities (such as rehabilitation programs, day hospital, school, or a job).

Planning

This information about the patient's living situation becomes extremely important in planning for the patient's needs. Decisions about housing are made in conjunction with the treatment team, the patient, and often someone else associated with the patient's housing circumstances. This other person may be a family member, if the patient is living at the family home, a staff member of a supervised housing program, or a friend or significant other, if the patient is living unsupervised in the community. The point is to have input from all relevant persons in the decision about housing. Goals and concerns need to be laid out, discussed, and addressed.

Usually the psychiatrist is asked about how the patient's clinical condition bears on the choice of housing. How independently can the patient function? What clinical problems need to be anticipated? How likely is relapse, and if it occurs, how should the housing provider (including the patient's family, if they are providing housing) respond? How should the provider respond to other problems, not necessarily as extreme as relapse? These are all questions with which the community psychiatrist can be extremely helpful.

Supportive Consultation

In assisting with the development of an optimal housing situation for a patient, there is no substitute for a home visit by the psychiatrist. This emphasizes to both the patient and the housing provider the importance of appropriate housing. Typically, both the patient and the care provider are grateful for this interest. It should be noted that patients have a right to decide whom to welcome into their home, but this usually is not a problem if a good clinical relationship has been established. At times housing providers may feel threatened by the prospect of the psychiatrist coming to visit, but usually this anxiety can be allayed with a clear explanation that the purpose of the visit is to gain a better understanding about the patient's life outside the clinic and to be helpful. Indeed, one of the major functions of a home visit is to establish a good working relationship with both the patient and the housing provider so that the psychiatrist can be more responsive to their questions and needs.

Beyond just visiting the home, a community psychiatrist can help in other ways. Perhaps the best information for guiding housing-related interventions derives from the development of psychoeducational interventions for families of persons with schizophrenia (Anderson et al., 1986; Bernheim and Lehman, 1985; Falloon et al., 1982; McFarlane, 1983). While they vary in their details, these interventions have the common goals of educating families and patients about the signs and symptoms of mental illness, the efficacy of available treatments and interventions, techniques for effective problem solving, and communication skills aimed at reducing hostility and criticism and enhancing positive interactions. The efficacy of these interventions for reducing relapse among persons with schizophrenia who live with their families in a stressful climate has been demonstrated repeatedly (Falloon et al., 1982; Berkowitz et al., 1981; Hogarty et al., 1991).

Although research data are still lacking, these techniques most likely can be applied to non-family residential settings as well. Non-family residential supervision of persons with severe mental illnesses is often provided by persons highly motivated by humanistic concern, but with minimal education about mental illnesses and treatment. In their survey of 24,663 staff in state-affiliated residential care programs, Randolph and colleagues (1991) found that 52 percent of the staff were paraprofessionals or had no formal training and that only 22 percent had more than a bachelor's degree. This is analogous to the situation that families face in caring for an ill relative. The interpersonal styles and the reactions of non-family care providers to mental illness probably show the same wide variability as those of family members, and therefore there is good reason to believe that they also would benefit from psychoeducational interventions. Drake and Osher (1987) have described the anecdotal success of a psychoeducational program for residential care staff, and Ranz and associates (1991) more recently reported on a large controlled clinical trial of a psychoeducational program for residential care staff currently underway in residential facilities operated in New York State.

Some of the most common concerns raised by residential care providers focus on symptoms, problematic behaviors, negotiating mutually acceptable solutions, dealing with the variability in a patient's condition, and accessing support services when needed. The psychiatrist can utilize the principles of psychoeducation to help with these concerns. The psychiatrist can meet with the patient and the residential care provider to discuss the patient's illness—not simply the abstract notion of the diagnosis, but how the illness manifests itself for that particular patient. What signs and symptoms does the patients experience? What helps? What doesn't? In this context the importance of medication compliance, monitoring signs and symptoms to provide feedback to the psychiatrist, and environmental interventions to modulate stress in the home can be discussed. Housing providers often have only a vague notion of the signs and symptoms of mental illness, and this provides an opportunity to help them understand the patient's disorder. Other conflicting belief systems held by the housing provider regarding mental illness and psychiatric treatment may emerge, and these should be discussed because they will likely affect the patient's situation in the home.

The dysfunctional behaviors associated with severe mental illnesses, more than such symptoms as hallucinations and delusions, are the most common sources of complaints by housing providers. These include poor personal hygiene; behaviors inconsiderate of the privacy of others (leaving clothes lying around the house, walking into bathrooms without knocking, borrowing others' possessions); unsafe behaviors (leaving the oven on, not locking the front door at night); substance use and abuse; and crisis behaviors, especially suicidality and violence. Patients may have the same complaints about other residents in the home. Conversely, patients may complain about the rules of the house relating to these behaviors and feel that their autonomy and privacy are being threatened. The psychiatrist can assist greatly in the resolution of these conflicts about behaviors. The goal is not necessarily to simply reenforce the housing provider's rules and expectations with the patient, although this may be necessary at times. Rather, the psychiatrist can assist the patient and care provider in resolving their differences regarding behavioral expectations. Sometimes this can be as simple as clarifying the rules of the house for the patient. Other times it may be necessary to assist the patient in renegotiating the house rules or helping the care provider understand that a different approach for behavioral change may be indicated. For example, some of the guidelines included in the New York State residential psychoeducational program (Ranz et al., 1991) include: "Go slow," "Give people space," "Ignore what you can't change," and "Solve problems step by step."

The psychiatrist may feel conflicting loyalties toward the patient and care provider in this supportive, mediating role. The physician's ultimate loyalty is to the patient, and residential care providers may change. However, it is important that the providers feel supported in their roles. With support they can more often respond effectively to the patient's needs. By establishing a helpful relationship with the provider, the psychiatrist is better able to advocate for the patient.

Beyond these interventions with the residential provider in the care for an individual patient, the community psychiatrist can function as a general consultant and source of support for residential care staff. One of the most common complaints from housing providers is that psychiatrists are unresponsive to them, do not listen to their concerns, do not respond when needed, and in general view the housing staff as irrelevant. This may at times be a misconception on the part of the housing staff, but more often than not their complaints are well founded.

Some simple interventions will greatly improve the relationship between psychiatrists and housing care providers. First, community psychiatrists can act as educational consultants. Informal, relatively brief in-service seminars at the housing program can be offered to answer such staff questions as: What is mental illness? What do diagnoses mean? Why are medications prescribed? What other treatments and rehabilitation services are helpful? What should residential providers expect of other service providers (clinics, emergency rooms, etc.)? What do other providers expect of them? How can they establish better rapport with treating psychiatrists? Similar seminars for patients living together in the residence can be offered as well.

Second, there is no substitute for a mutually supportive relationship between the psychiatrist and the residential care staff. Being available to discuss individual patients, providing more general educational consultations, and conducting support groups for the staff are all possible roles for the psychiatrist and engender a tremendous sense of collaboration and trust.

Regardless of where a patient lives, the psychiatrist can visit the patient's home, meet those with whom the patient lives, assess the patient's needs within the housing context, provide education and consultation to the patient and others in the home to promote a supportive environment, and be available to assist with problems and crises. A collaborative relationship with the patient, those with whom the patient lives, and other service personnel providing support to the patient is a critical role for the community psychiatrist.

References

Anderson, C.M., Reiss, D.J., and Hogarty, G.E. (1986) *Schizophrenia and the Family.* New York: Guilford Press.

Berkowitz, R., Kuipers, L., Eberlein-Frief, R., and Leff, J. (1981) Lowering expressed emotion in relatives of schizophrenics. In Goldstein, M.J. (ed.), *New Developments in Interventions with Families of Schizophrenics.* San Francisco: Jossey-Bass.

Bernheim, K.F., and Lehman, A.F. (1985) *Working with Families of the Mentally Ill.* New York: Norton and Co.

Braun, P., Kochansky, G.K., Shapiro, R., Greenberg, S., Gudeman, J.E., Johnson, S., and Shore, M.F. (1981) Overview: deinstitutionalization of psychiatric patients, a critical review of outcome studies. *American Journal of Psychiatry, 138:*736–749.

Budson, R.D. (1990) Models of supportive living: community residential care. In Herz, M.I., Keith, S.J., Docherty, J.P. (eds.), *Psychosocial Treatment of Schizophrenia; Handbook of Schizophrenia, Vol. 4.* New York: Elsevier.

Conant, J.B. (1942) Address at Harvard College, June 30.

Crafts, J. (1988) in *Ex-Patients View Housing Options and Needs.* (ed. P. Ridgway) Burlington, Vt.: Center for Community Change Through Housing and Support.

Drake, R.E., and Osher, F.C. (1987) Family psychoeducation when there is no family. *Hospital and Community Psychiatry, 38:*274–277.

Goldman, H.H. and Newman, S. (1990) Financing and reimburement issues. In Morrissey, J.D. and Dennis, D.L. (eds.) *Homelessness and Mental Illness: Toward the Next Generation of Research Studies.* Rockville, MD: National Institute for Mental Health.

Falloon, I.R.H., Boyd, J.L., McGill, C.W., Razani, J., Moss, M.B., and Gilderman, A.M. (1982) Family management in the prevention of exacerbations of schizophrenia. *New England Journal of Medicine, 306:*1437–1440.

Harp, H.T. (1988) in *Ex-Patients View Housing Options and Needs.* (ed. P. Ridgway) Burlington, Vt.: Center for Community Change Through Housing and Support.

Hogarty, E.G., Anderson, C.M., Reiss, D.J., Kornblith, S.J., Greenwald, D.P., Ulrich, R.F., and Carter, M. (1991) Family psychoeducation, social skills training, and maintenance chemotherapy in the aftercare treatment of schizophrenics (II). *Archives of General Psychiatry, 48:*340–347.

McFarlane, W.R. (ed.) (1983). *Family Therapy in Schizophrenia.* New York: Guilford Press.

Newman, S., and Struyk, R. (1990) Housing and supportive services: federal policy for the frail elderly and the chronically mentally ill. In Di Pasquale, D., Keyes, L. (eds.), *Building Foundations.* Philadelphia: University of Pennsylvania Press.

Randolph, F.L., Ridgway, P., and Carling, P.J. (1991) Residential programs for persons with severe mental illness: a nationwide survey of state-affiliated agencies. *Hospital and Community Psychiatry, 42:*1111–1115.

Ranz, J.M., Horen, B.T., McFarlane, W.R., and Zito, J.M. (1991) Creating a supportive environment using staff psychoeducation in a supervised residence. *Hospital and Community Psychiatry, 42:*1154–1159.

Ridgway, P., and Zipple, A.M. (1990) The paradigm shift in residential services: from the linear continuum to support housing approaches. *Psychosocial Rehabilitation Journal, 13:*11–31.

23

Case Management

PAULA N. GOERING
DONALD WASYLENKI

Mental health case management developed in response to the need for coordinating complex services for mentally ill people living in communities. This chapter provides a brief overview of the historical and conceptual underpinnings of case management; defines this approach to service delivery; addresses administrative issues; describes the nature of the clinical practice, identifying some of the key issues; and summarizes the findings from selected descriptive and evaluative research studies.

Historical and Conceptual Underpinnings

The shift from inpatient to community care resulted in a number of serious problems. A major issue was that the several functions once served by institutions were not adequately provided for by community programs. The nature of the problems that result from inadequate and fragmented service systems can be illustrated with findings from a study of aftercare in metropolitan Toronto in the late 1970s.

Discharge plans, patterns of service use, and client outcomes of 747 patients from 10 inpatient units in provincial, general, and research hospital settings were examined at 6 months and 2 years after discharge (Goering et al., 1984; Wasylenki et al., 1985). Only 13 percent had complete discharge plans. There was overreliance on medical therapeutic services and neglect of housing, vocational, and social recreational needs. Even when needs were identified in clinical areas, referrals to services often were not made. Dropping out was common for all types of services, and considerable client dissatisfaction was expressed. One-third of the 505 subjects assessed at the 6-month follow-up had been readmitted at least once. Two years after discharge the readmission rate had risen to 70 percent. Other indicators of inadequate care were high symptom levels, transiency, inadequate housing conditions, and poor social functioning.

Similar kinds of problems were documented over and over again in the United States, Canada, and Europe. The revolving door syndrome, and the growing numbers of severely mentally ill individuals who were homeless or occupied detention centers and jails, provided evidence of the disorganized, fragmented, and inadequate provision of services to this most needy population.

There are a number of different issues that must be addressed in order to improve services for the severely ill (Wasylenki et al., 1992). Chief among them are the lack of community support services and the absence of mechanisms to organize the various components of treatment and care into a coherent, accessible system. Case management was developed as the principal process, at the client level, to achieve continuity of care.

Bachrach (1981) has defined continuity of care as the need to ensure the orderly, uninterrupted movement of clients among the diverse elements of the service system. She identifies a number of important conditions that must be realized in order to achieve continuity: Care must be available over a long period of time; clients must be treated individually; care must be comprehensive and flexible; the characteristic of relationship must exist; obstacles to accessibility must be overcome; and there must be communication between client and service provider and among the various service providers involved in his or her care. Each of these conditions is incorporated into the principles of practice of case management.

Generic case management had its origins in social casework with the poor and indigent populations in settlement houses (Friday, 1986). It had been used in inner cities in the 1960s (Levine, 1979) and has been applied to various other specific populations including the elderly, children, and the developmentally and physically disabled (Weil et al., 1985). After case management was identified as one of the ten essential components of a community support system by the National Institute of Mental Health (Turner and TenHoor, 1978), a number of writers began to describe more fully the application of case management to mental health (Lamb, 1980; Intagliata, 1982; Schwartz et al., 1982).

Legislation and official government policy now often mandate the provision of case management for the severely mentally ill. Robinson, Bergman, and Scallet (1989) trace how Medicaid and Public Law 99-660 have supported the implementation of case management for the mentally ill in the United States. Thornicroft (1991) describes the development of policy with regard to case management in Great Britain. Most of the new provincial policies in Canada (Goering et al., 1992) also include case management as an essential service. A National Association of Case Management was formed in the United States in 1990 to further define and promote the professional role (Community Support Network News, 1991). Case management is increasingly being applied to other populations including persons with alcohol dependence, victims of child abuse, homeless people, and paroled criminal offenders.

The mental health professions of social work (Johnson and Rubin, 1983; Kanter, 1987) and nursing (Krauss, 1989; Mound et al., 1991) have generally been quicker to incorporate case management into their educational and practice domains than has psychiatry. This is regrettable since psychiatrists definitely need to be knowledgable about this approach. If they work directly with individuals with severe mental illness, acting as case manager will enhance their own understanding of rehabilitation and recovery and will increase their ability to use the service system to the best advantage of their clients. Even if one accepts the argument that psychiatrists should remain specialists and it is not cost efficient for them to assume a primary care role, it is still imperative that there be sufficient knowledge of the practice of case management in order to work as a colleague or to be involved in the supervision and training of other team members who do assume this role. Given the centrality of the approach in both hospital and community settings, psychiatrists should also be prepared to play a major role in the administration, planning, and evaluation of case management at program and system levels.

Defining Case Management

There has been widespread implementation of case management but no standardized definition of the approach. Some mental health programs have defined case management exclusively as a brokerage function that requires no direct contact or therapy with the client. There is now general agreement, however, that both coordination and direct service provision are required for meeting the needs of the severely mentally ill (Bachrach, 1989). Private insurers and managed care organizations continue to use the term *case management* to describe brokerage and fiscal control programs that differ dramatically in their operation and intent. In order to maintain a distinction, increasingly case management for persons with psychiatric disability, which focuses on client needs and explicitly employs a therapeutic relationship, is referred to as *clinical case management* (Harris and Bergman, 1987; Kanter, 1989; Lamb, 1980).

There is some consensus about the goals and basic functions of clinical case management. The goals from a client perspective are described by Furlong-Norman (1991) as "to assist individuals to live in the most supportive community environment possible and advocate the creation of supports and environments suitable to a person's personal goals and needs where these resources do not exist" (p.2). From a systems perspective, the goal is to provide whatever services consumers need in a coordinated, effective, and efficient manner through the enhancement of continuity, accessibility, and accountability (Intagliata, 1982).

There is also considerable agreement that the basic functions of case management include assessment, planning, linking, monitoring, and evaluation (Intagliata, 1982; Thornicroft, 1991). Outreach, direct service provision, meeting special needs, and advocacy are frequent additions in more comprehensive services (Intagliata, 1982; Levine and Fleming, 1985). There may be considerable variation in the relative emphasis given to these functions and the method of carrying them out from program to program, but the essence of case management is the provision of these functions to meet client goals. The main support functions are described by Desisto, Ridgway and Erikson (1986). Table 23–1 provides a listing of activities originally among those categorized as integrating services. In our opinion they comprise a comprehensive listing of clinical case management components.

Table 23–1   Case management functions

Goal: To ensure continuity of care within the system. It is a process of case finding, needs assessment, planning, coordination, direct service provision, monitoring, and evaluating continuing needs in the most efficient and effective way possible. It is a principal supportive function within the entire network of care.

I. Outreach and Case Finding

a. Reaching out to psychiatrically disabled persons and bringing them into contact with the service system,
b. informing family members and other service providers about the availability of case management,
c. assertively maintaining contact so that services are not inappropriately terminated, and
d. providing long-term continuity of helping relationships.

II. Comprehensive Individualized Assessment and Planning

a. Undertaking for each psychiatrically disabled person a comprehensive, individualized assessment of his or her needs that takes into account basic needs and treatment needs and aids each person to set overall rehabilitation goals.
b. Developing with each psychiatrically disabled person a comprehensive individualized plan that fills basic needs, specifies needed treatment, and provides rehabilitation-oriented services and supports.

III. Service Coordination

a. Linking patients/clients to multiple services, supports, and resources,
b. advocating to ensure access and to modify and adapt existing resources to meet individual needs, and
c. maintaining active, ongoing linkages with agencies in the area as a key player in interagency coordination efforts.

IV. Direct Service Provision

a. When there are gaps in existing services and resources, provides assistance with managing problems of daily living, teaching community living skills, and develops natural support systems.

V. Monitoring and Evaluation

a. Monitoring the implementation of each psychiatrically disabled person's service plan,
b. evaluating the achievement of goals and client satisfaction,
c. revising plans and programs of treatment, support, and rehabilitation to ensure appropriate, effective, and timely services.

VI. Meeting Special Needs

a. Ensure access to specialized services for psychiatrically disabled persons with multiple problems traditionally met by separate services sectors, i.e., psychogeriatric, mental retardation, substance abuse, etc.

Under the rubric of clinical case management, there are varying ways of defining and operationalizing this approach to care. Clinical case management programs are usually considered to be intensive if they maintain low staff-client ratios (less than 1:25) and see clients frequently (daily to once a week). Four models have been proposed to distinguish among the various types of clinical case management programs (Robinson et al., 1989). The four models differ along various dimensions. The key distinction is underlying focus. *Expanded broker* stresses the linkage function, *personal strengths* a mentor approach and systems advocacy; *rehabilitation,* improving living skills, and *full support* the reduction and management of symptoms. The full support model, also known as assertive community treatment (Stein and Test, 1980), is the most widely replicated and evaluated model (Solomon, 1992; Deci et al., 1995).

In Ontario, the rehabilitation model, employing the theory and practice of psychiatric rehabilitation (Anthony et al., 1993) has been predominant. Case managers assume individual caseloads and emphasize functional assessments, rehabilitation plans, and skill teaching.

Administrative Matters

Administrators and planners concerned with how to organize clinical case management programs have a number of choices to make. The amount of variation that is possible in program definition can create confusion, especially when the term *case management* is used without specifying its particular attributes. But there are also advantages to having choice and freedom with regard to implementation. The challenge is to develop program models that suit local circumstances and particular client populations while remaining consistent with the basic goals and functions of case management. The following questions must be answered: What is the target population? How comprehensive will the program be? Where will it be situated? Who will staff the program? How will it be structured? What authority will the case managers have in the system? How will they be trained and supervised?

There are a number of options for each of these questions, and a growing body of experience and literature which can inform the decision-making process. Case management for the severely mentally ill has been defined in terms of 12 axes of practice (Thornicroft, 1991). The pros and cons of various organizational models have been examined (Reinke and Greenley, 1986). Common features of case management programs for the homeless mentally ill have been defined (Rog et al., 1987). Training needs have been outlined (Anthony et al., 1988; Cochrane et al., 1991) and the process of planning has been described (Levine and Fleming, 1985). The prevention of staff burnout is an issue of considerable importance (Goering et al., 1989). Team approaches share the responsibility for individual clients among a team of professionals, reducing occupational stress and increasing long-term effectiveness (Bond et al., 1991).

Bachrach (1992) lists several techniques to increase the therapeutic potential of the case manager and stretch case management resources. Team case management, matching case managers and patients, mixing caseloads, clustering case management activities, and supporting people who act as case management extenders are all potential options. The valuable role that family members and consumers can play in the delivery of case management services should not be ignored (Intagliata et al., 1986; Sherman and Porter, 1991).

Because there are great differences in how case management services are delivered and in who delivers them, training needs differ considerably from program to program. The knowledge and skills that are needed for case managers to perform effectively can be described. They include such areas as assertive outreach and identification, forming therapeutic relationships, crisis prevention and intervention, symptom management, and family education. Approaches to training case managers on a wide-scale basis have been implemented by organizations such as the Centre for Research and Training at Boston University, Community Connections Training Institute in Washington, D.C., and the state mental health departments in Colorado and Ohio. These all use practices that allow them to adapt their training programs to the wide diversity in the case management field. Among them are an initial consultation to learn about the agency and its needs, preparation of a variety of teaching modules, practical experiential training methods, and a training-of-trainers component.

Practice Issues

Kanter (1989) has outlined five principles of clinical case management. The first is *continuity of care*. This is a response to the client's need for an ongoing, personal relationship with a case manager, often for an extended period of time. The second principle is use of the case management *relationship*. This suggests that relationships among the case manager, the client, and others in the client's social network are important determinants of outcomes. The third principle is *titration of support* and structure. This requires case managers to avoid providing either excessive or inadequate amounts of support. The fourth principle is *flexibility,* which suggests that case manager qualities, such as firmness, must be employed in relation to ever changing client needs. The final principle is *facilitating patient resourcefulness,* which focuses attention on the need to enhance clients' strengths as well as to bolster deficits.

Although Kanter's outline is comprehensive, it should be noted that it is prescriptive rather than descriptive. There are few empirical accounts of what case managers actually do in clinical programs and, most disappointingly, attempts to correlate what case managers do with client characteristics have reported very little relationship between client needs and type of case manager activity. A study by Clark and Landis (1990), for example, involving 2,152 clients served by case managers at 16 sites found that clients' overall functional levels bore very little relation to the amount of service time provided by case managers. In particular, regardless of client needs, case managers spent a great deal of time providing intake assessment and monitoring client functioning and transportation services and very little time providing advocacy and linkage referral services. The authors conclude that factors such as unavailability of resources, inadequacies in case manager training, and geographic inaccessibility are likely explanations for their findings.

Insofar as case managers attempt to help clients deal with their experiences of the environment, their activities will share some of the attributes of supportive psychotherapy (Wasylenki, 1992). For example, it is essential that clinical case managers master techniques of therapeutic listening. Anthony and colleagues (1990) identify attending, observing, listening, and responding skills as essential for client engagement. A systematic approach to communication not only promotes engagement and self-exploration, but also draws the case manager into an important attending-observing-listening mode in relation to the client. Without this, attempts to build relationships and to understand and explain are bound to produce frustration. In order fully to understand clients' subjective states, it is necessary to move beyond cognitive-observational approaches to an approach that relies more upon empathic listening. Empathy requires the case manager to draw out of himself or herself a state of experience that approximates that of the client. Listening empathically is a subjective mode of perceiving—of placing oneself inside the client's experience (Schwaber, 1981). This subjective perspective sharpens attunement to clients' internal states. Understanding these fluctuating internal states may help to explain many processes that influence the course and outcome of a chronic mental illness.

Goering and Stylianos (1988) have examined the concept of therapeutic alliance as a means of understanding the mechanisms underlying rehabilitation. According to these authors, the ability to form a working relationship depends on the ability and willingness of a client to meet the demands of a given therapeutic environment. Thus "progress" in rehabilitation is seen as due to a combination of practitioner empathy, warmth, and genuineness, along with sufficiently specified goals and tasks. Experiences of success with regard to specified goals, shared by case manager and client, contribute to a strengthening of the clinical relationship which enhances the working alliance. Harris and Bergman (1987) also explain the efficacy of rehabilitation partially as a function of interpersonal processes.

Finally, clinical case management strives to provide clients with some degree of insight. However, as Lamb (1982) suggests, insight must be redefined for working with severely ill people. He proposes that insight should mean a realization that symptoms such as delusions and hallucinations are understandable. They mean that the client is under stress. Having identified the stressor, case manager and client should move to determine what actions need to be taken. Herz (1984) has shown that people with schizophrenia, for example, can learn to recognize early subjective indicators of relapse onset and to restabilize themselves quickly.

Clinical case management is thus seen as a mode of therapy as well as a vehicle to provide coordination of care. Aspects of the case management process are available to clients for modeling and identification in the context of a close working relationship. Through a process involving imitation, identification, and internalization, a client can achieve insight, growth, and development. The case manager counteracts negative aspects of the client's subjective experience by providing a model of healthy functioning with which the client can identify.

In the Continuing Care Division at the Clarke Institute of Psychiatry in Toronto, clinical case management services are provided to approximately 400 severely ill clients by four continuous treatment teams. In evaluating the clinical case management model, which has been largely successful, a number of problems have emerged. The first is the issue of titrating support, which has been discussed by Kanter (1989). It has been observed that case managers often provide a great deal of support for clients who are able to cooperate in identifying and working toward rehabilitation goals, regardless of their capacity to proceed independently. They provide less support to clients who are not able to participate in the rehabilitation process. At times, there is insufficient recognition of clients having progressed to the point of requiring less support, or of clients' inabilities to tolerate active interventions.

A second difficult issue involves the tension between a client-focused, rehabilitation-oriented approach, in which the client has a major role in setting priorities, and a more assertive approach in which the case manager determines what is in the best interests of the client. As the Continuing Care Division program espouses principles of psychiatric rehabilitation, case managers sometimes are confused over the extent to which they should assist severely ill clients to continue to direct the rehabilitation process.

A third issue has to do with relationships between case managers and psychiatrists. As case managers become more knowledgeable about clients' circumstances, tensions sometimes arise with regard to where the primary responsibility rests for decision making about treatment. This is often manifest in disagreements about such things as needs for medication, frequency of contact, and degree of disability.

Caseload size is another difficult issue in clinical case management. Case managers often are caught in having to decide whether to do more for fewer clients or less for more. Caseload size also must be balanced with competing demands for other activities such as education, research, administration, and group therapy.

Finally, personality-related issues are often problematic in a program that targets severely ill clients. Invariably, when case managers feel they have reached an impasse with a difficult client, consultation reveals that transference-countertransference difficulties arising not from the mental illness but rather from a severe personality dysfunction are at the core of the problem.

Harris (1988) has recently identified a number of new directions for clinical case management. The first involves more careful attention to case manager behavior. She identifies a number of different dysfunctional styles of case manager behavior that have implications for effectiveness, and suggests that more attention be paid to training and supervision in the development of clinical skills and approaches. Harris also focuses on the need to become clearer about client needs as determined by such things as chronological age, course of illness, and intra-psychic growth. She also emphasizes the importance of being aware of changes in case management technology. These include ''cluster case management,'' which combines principles of group psychotherapy and case management as a potential substitute for more traditional clinical practice. Finally, Harris recommends guidelines for applying the case management model to persons suffering from character disorders. These include clarity with respect to expectations, limits, and consequences; diffusion of the intensity of the clinical relationship; avoidance of excessive dependency and regression; and monitoring of countertransference reactions.

Research and Evaluation

As case management has emerged as a central element in the provision of community support to severely ill clients, studies to describe the process and to measure outcomes have begun to proliferate. In 1985, Modrcin, Rapp, and Chamberlain reviewed case management research and identified findings in six major areas. Case managers tended to be female, well-educated, and located primarily in community mental health centers.

Although there were indications that case managers are oriented to reality situations and spend most time in direct service activities, other data indicated that case managers in community mental health centers in particular may focus excessively on counseling activities and neglect linking clients to community resources. Most clients served by case managers were chronically mentally ill, were likely to have a diagnosis of schizophrenia, complained of loneliness, and experienced difficulties in performing activities of daily living. Studies of caseload size revealed ratios ranging from 1:15 to 1:35, and case managers reported that an increase from 15 clients to 30 to 50 clients had a significant negative impact on practice. Although few data are reported, team approaches were described as a way of providing support for case managers and helping to avoid occupational stress and burnout. Finally, the authors reviewed seven studies concerned with the impact of case management services. Unfortunately, none of the studies utilized a random control group design, so results are inconclusive. However, the studies suggested that case management services reduce rehospitalization, decrease levels of symptomatology, assist clients in achieving identified goals, increase employment and social activities, and maintain or improve client quality of life.

Chamberlain and Rapp (1991) have commented on "the paucity of rigorously designed outcome research." They could identify only six studies that met defined criteria for methodological rigor. Although the studies differed in a number of important ways, the authors were able to draw tentative conclusions with regard to the current state of outcome research. All of the case management programs studied offered more than service brokerage. The most commonly accepted mode of practice could best be described as clinical case management. Effects of the programs appeared to be discernable after one year, but not before. According to the authors, it is possible to conclude that regardless of the principal focus of the case management programs, the desired effect, if defined clearly, will be achieved. Finally, in measuring outcome it is sometimes unclear if the case management program itself is responsible for change or if those services to which the client is linked by the program have produced the effects. Since 1990, eight more randomized trials of assertive community treatment models of case management have been published (Burns and Santos, 1995). These studies have found strong positive effects on hospital days and on family satisfaction.

Thornicroft (1991) has also reviewed evaluation research and concludes that results from case management demonstration programs have been optimistic, with improvements noted in client social integration, use of hospital services, and overall satisfaction. He also notes that cost outcome studies have reached divergent conclusions, but that when clients' earnings are taken into consideration, case management is cost effective.

A case management program utilizing principles of psychiatric rehabilitation was developed at the Clarke Institute of Psychiatry in Toronto. The outcomes of 82 clients in the program were compared with those of 82 matched controls (Goering et al., 1988). At 2-year follow-up, clients in the case management program were significantly more likely to have better occupational functioning, to live in a more adequate residence, and to be less socially isolated. However, the two groups did not differ in number of hospitalizations.

This research contributed to the development and evaluation of an outreach case management program for homeless mentally ill clients (Goering et al., 1992). This program is operated by two community agencies using a psychiatric rehabilitation model that locates case managers in the shelter system. Eight case managers provide intensive services to small caseloads of 8 to 10 clients. Comparisons of baseline and 9-month post-intervention assessments for a sample of 59 clients have demonstrated significant improvements in housing stability, social networks, psychiatric symptoms, and disability. In this group with severe and persistent mental illness, there was a 66 percent reduction in time spent living in hostels, a 78 percent increase in size of social networks, and substantial reductions in psychotic and non-psychotic symptoms. Gains were also made in various aspects of social functioning.

Several very important research questions remain unanswered. The issue of optimal caseload size is one. This will continue to be a function of the program model, but approaches to caseload weighting that focus on the individual client's need for service await development. Studies also will need to isolate case management functions in relation to client outcomes so that the impact of the entire service delivery system is not being assessed. The indications for assertive case management should be clarified, as this is a more labor-intensive modality and one that should target populations most in need. The relationship between case manager activities and client outcomes should become an important area of research so as to inform case managers and administrators of how time should best be allocated. Studies also should define important characteristics of clients. These should include standardized diagnosis, severity of illness, degree of disability, and presence or absence of personality disorder. As much as possible, agreement should be reached on appropriate outcome measures. Increasingly, these should include sensitive measures of social functioning and quality of life in order to understand the clinical effects of case management programs. Finally, proponents of case management must confront the emerging forces of consumerism and empowerment in the mental health field. Many consumer groups reject notions of "cases" and "management" (Everett and Nelson, 1992) and strongly argue for enveloping service delivery networks that are accessible so that even severely disabled clients can manage their own support. Others have implemented approaches that use consumers as staff in case management programs (Sherman and Porter, 1991). It thus behooves us to demonstrate how these important themes can be integrated into a model of case management that respects client autonomy to the fullest and operates as a true partnership between consumer and provider. This may turn out to be the most important empirical challenge to case management in the 1990s.

References

Anthony, W.A., Cohen, M., and Farkas, M. (1990) *Psychiatric Rehabilitation.* Boston: Boston University, Sargent College of Allied Health Professions.

Anthony, W.A., Cohen, M., Farkas, M., and Cohen, B.F. (1988) Clinical care update: The chronically mentally ill. Case management—more than a response to a dysfunctional system. *Community Mental Health Journal,* 24(3):219–228.

Anthony, W.A., Forbess, R., and Cohen, M.R. (1993) Rehabilitation-oriented case management. In Harris, M., Bergman, H.C. (eds.), *Case Management for Mentally Ill Patients: Theory and Practice.* Langhorne, PA: Harwood Academic Publishers.

Bachrach, L.L. (1981) Continuity of care for chronic mental patients: a conceptual analysis. *American Journal of Psychiatry,* 138:1449–1456.

Bachrach, L.L. (1989) Case management: toward a shared definition. *Hospital and Community Psychiatry,* 40(9):883–884.

Bachrach, L.L. (1992) Case management revisited. *Hospital and Community Psychiatry,* 43(3), 209–210.

Bond, G.R., Pensec, M., Dietzen, L., McCafferty, D., Giezma, R., and Sipple, H.W. (1991) Intensive case management for frequent users of psychiatric hospitals in a large city: a comparison of team and individual caseloads. *Psychosocial Rehabilitation Journal,* 15(1):90–98.

Burns, B.J. and Santos, A.B. (1995) Assertive community treatment: An update of randomized trials. *Psychiatric Services,* 46:669–675.

Chamberlain, R., and Rapp C.A. (1991) A decade of case management: a methodological review of outcome research. *Community Mental Health Journal,* 27:171–188.

Clark, K.A., and Landis, D. (1990) The relationship of client characteristics to case management service provision. *Evaluation and Program Planning.* 13:221–229.

Cochrane, J., Butterill, D., and Durbin, J. (1991) *Psychosocial case management training: Needs assessment and service delivery models.* Final report to Community Resources Consultants of Toronto: Clarke Institute of Psychiatry Consulting Group.

Community Support Network News (1991) National survey of case management programs. *Community Support Network News,* 7(3):8.

Deci, A., Santos, A.B., Hiott, W., Schoenwald, S. and Dias, J.K. (1995) Dissemination of assertive community treatment programs. *Psychiatric Services,* 46:676–678.

DeSisto, M.J., Ridgway, P., and Erikson, G. (1986) *Meeting the needs of psychiatrically disabled persons for treatment, support, and rehabilitation.* Bureau of Mental Health, Maine Department of Mental Health, Maine Department of Mental Health and Mental Retardation.

Everett, B., and Nelson, A. (1992) We're not cases. And you're not managers. An account of a client/professional partnership developed in response to a "borderline" diagnosis. *Psychosocial Rehabilitation Journal,* 15(4):49–60.

Friday, J. (1986) *Case managers for the chronically mentally ill: Assessing and improving their performance.* Atlanta, Georgia: Southern Regional Educational Board.

Furlong-Norman, K. (ed.) (1991) From the editor. *Community Support Network News,* 7(3):2.

Goering, P.N., Huddart, C., Wasylenki, D., and Ballantyne, R. (1989) The use of rehabilitation case management to develop necessary supports: community rehabilitation services. In Farkas, M.D., Anthony, W.A. (eds.), (1989) *Psychiatric Rehabilitation Programs: Putting Theory into Practice,* pp. 197–206. Baltimore and London: Johns Hopkins University Press.

Goering, P.N., and Stylianos, S. (1988) Exploring the helping relationship between the schizophrenic client and the rehabilitation therapist. *American Journal of Orthopsychiatry,* 58:271–280.

Goering, P., Wasylenki, D., Farkas, M., Lancee, W., and Ballantyne, R. (1988) What difference does case management make? *Hospital and Community Psychiatry,* 39:272–276.

Goering, P., Wasylenki, D., Lancee, W., and Freeman, S.J.J. (1984) From hospital to community: six-month and two-year outcomes for 505 patients. *The Journal of Nervous and Mental Disease,* 172(11):667–673.

Goering, P., Wasylenki, D., and MacNaughton, E. (1992) Planning mental health services: current Canadian initiatives. *Canadian Journal of Psychiatry,* 37:259–263.

Goering, P., Wasylenki, D., St. Onge, M., Paduchak, D., and Lancee, W. (1992) Gender and the evaluation of a hostel outreach program. *Hospital and Community Psychiatry,* 43(2): 160–165.

Harris, M. (1988) New directions for clinical case management. In Harris, M. Bachrach, L.L. (eds.), *Clinical Case Management, New Directions for Mental Health Services.* San Francisco: Jossey-Bass.

Harris, M., and Bergman, H.C. (1987) Case management with the chronically mentally ill: a clinical perspective. *American Journal of Orthopsychiatry,* 57:296–302.

Herz, M.I. (1984) Recognizing and preventing relapse in patients with schizophrenia. *Hospital and Community Psychiatry,* 35:344–349.

Intagliata, J. (1982) Improving the quality of community care for the chronically mentally disabled: the role of case management. *Schizophrenia Bulletin,* 8(4):655–674.

Intagliata, J., Willer, B., and Ergi, G. (1986) Role of the family in case management of the mentally ill. *Schizophrenia Bulletin,* 12:699–708.

Johnson, P., and Rubin, A. (1983) Case management in mental health: a social work domain? *Social Work,* 28:49–55.

Kanter, J. (1989) Clinical case management: definition, principles and components. *Hospital and Community Psychiatry,* 40:361–368.

Kanter, J. (1987) Mental health case management: a professional domain? *Social Work,* September/October: 461–462.

Krauss, J.B. (1989) New conceptions of care, community, and chronic mental illness. *Archives of Psychiatric Nursing,* 3(5):281–287.

Lamb, H.R. (1982) *Treating the Long-Term Mentally Ill.* San Francisco: Jossey-Bass.

Lamb, H.R. (1980) Therapist-case managers: more than brokers of services. *Hospital and Community Psychiatry,* 31:762–764.

Levine, I.S., and Fleming, M. (1985) *Human Resource Development: Issues in Case Management.* Rockville, Maryland: Center for State Human Resource Development, Community Support and Rehabilitation Branch, National Institute of Mental Health.

Levine, M. (1979) Case management: lessons from earlier efforts. *Evaluation and Program Planning,* 2:235–243.

Modrcin, M., Rapp, C.A., and Chamberlain, R. (1985) Case management with the psychiatrically disabled: curriculum and training program. Lawrence, Kansas: University of Kansas, School of Social Welfare.

Mound, B., Gyulay, R., Khan, P., and Goering, P. (1991) The expanded role of nurse case managers. *Journal of Psychosocial Nursing,* 29(6):18–22.

Reinke, B., and Greenley, J.R. (1986) Organizational analysis of three community support program models. *Hospital and Community Psychiatry,* 37(6):624–629.

Robinson, G.K., Bergman, G.T., and Scallet, L.J. (1989) Choices in case management: a review of current knowledge and practice for Mental Health Programs. Rockville, MD: National Institute of Mental Health.

Rog, D.J., Andranovich, G.D., and Rosenblum, S. (1987) Intensive case management for persons who are homeless and mentally ill: a review of community support program and Human Resource Development program efforts. Washington, D.C.: COSMOS Corporation.

Schwaber, E. (1981) Narcissism, self-psychology and the listening perspective. *Annual of Psychoanalysis,* 9:115–131.

Schwartz, S.R., Goldman, H.H., and Churgin, S. (1982) Case management for the chronically mentally ill: models and dimensions. *Hospital and Community Psychiatry,* 33(12):1006–1009.

Sherman, P.S., and Porter, R. (1991) Mental health consumers as case management aides. *Hospital and Community Psychiatry,* 42(5):494–498.

Solomon, P. (1992) The efficacy of case management services for severely mentally disabled clients. *Community Mental Health Journal,* 28(3):163–180.

Stein, L., and Test, M.A. (1980) Alternative to mental hospital treatment. I. conceptual model: Treatment program, and clinical evaluation. *Archives of General Psychiatry,* 37:392–397.

Thornicroft, G. (1991) The concept of case management for long-term mental illness. *International Review of Psychiatry,* 3:125–132.

Turner, J.C., and TenHoor, W.J. (1978) The NIMH community support program: pilot approach to a needed social reform. *Schizophrenia Bulletin,* 4:319–348.

Wasylenki, D. (1992) Psychotherapy of schizophrenia revisited. *Hospital and Community Psychiatry,* 43(2):123–127.

Wasylenki, D., Goering, P., Lancee, W., Fischer, L., and Freeman, S.J.J. (1985) Psychiatric aftercare in a metropolitan setting. *Canadian Journal of Psychiatry,* 30(5):329–336.

Wasylenki, D., Goering, P., and MacNaughton, E. (1992) Planning mental health services: background and key issues. *Canadian Journal of Psychiatry,* 37(3):199–205.

Weil, M., Karls, J., et al. (1985) *Case Management in Human Service Practice.* San Francisco, California: Jossey-Bass.

24

Prevention

WILLIAM R. BREAKEY

The proposition that it is better to prevent illness than to allow it to occur with its associated suffering, loss of function, and need for treatment, is one of the basic premises of public health that requires no justification. The great historic reductions in morbidity from infectious diseases such as tuberculosis, poliomyelitis, or rubella, or nutritional disorders such as scurvy, rickets, or iodine-deficiency goiter, result from well-organized programs for prevention rather than from improved treatment. The prevention of heart disease, cancer, and AIDS are among the most important challenges for public health in the 1990s, the focus of great public concern and major scientific effort.

The same challenge confronts psychiatry: there is no other realistic way to tackle the enormous burden of psychiatric disorder worldwide (Sartorius and Henderson, 1992). The Epidemiologic Catchment Area study found that approximately 20 percent of Americans suffer from a psychiatric disorder at any given time. There is no reason to believe that prevalences are lower in any other country. America is relatively richly supplied with mental health professionals and services; attempting to meet the need for treatment in countries with less highly developed treatment systems poses major challenges. Effective methods for prevention provide the only hope. The high prevalence of specific psychiatric disorders is not the only cause for concern. Pardes and colleagues (1989) point out that ten of the leading causes of death are associated with risk-taking or unhealthy behaviors such as alcohol and drug abuse, smoking, violence, overeating, lack of exercise, or maladaptive response to stress. Preventing these disorders requires a change in motivation and behavior—which reemphasizes the interaction of physical and mental health concerns and the need for taking a broad view of disease prevention and health promotion.

Community psychiatrists, adopting a public health orientation, have always believed that prevention is an important objective, and in the 1950s and 1960s, with somewhat naive optimism as to what could be accomplished, prevention was seen as one of the primary goals for community psychiatry programs. In spite of this intent, the federal CMHC program only provided scant resources for prevention, and the activities that were mounted were poorly evaluated and probably of limited effectiveness (Cooper, 1990). In most community psychiatry programs for adults today, state priorities for serving the most severely mentally ill people have come to outweigh most other priorities, and prevention is generally less strongly emphasized in planning and program development. In programs for children and adolescents, prevention programs clearly have a central role. Child psychiatrists have a keen awareness of the developmental consequences of adverse circumstances or emotional disorders in early life (Chapter 26; Kasdin, 1993; Lorion and Ross, 1992; Offord, 1987). Nonetheless, a preventive orientation must be maintained; existing knowledge of prevention should be used effectively and new knowledge developed. The need for research and development in prevention has been stressed repeatedly (Neighbors, 1990; NIMH, 1993; Institute of Medicine, 1994). The National Institute of Mental Health, through its Office of Prevention, has developed a series of Preventive Intervention Research Centers (Koretz, 1991). Research in the field is active and is expanding in many ways conceptually ahead of current practice (Institute of Medicine, 1994).

Concepts and Definitions

Preventive interventions can be defined as measures designed to prevent or delay the onset of a disease or symptoms, provided for people who are currently free of that disease or those symptoms. A widely used classification of preventive measures was developed by the 1957 Commission on Chronic Illness, as follows:

- *Primary* prevention is the prevention of occurrence of a disorder that had not previously existed in an individual up to that point.
- *Secondary* prevention is the reduction of the extent of morbidity in a population by detecting disease early in its course and preventing its further development.
- *Tertiary* prevention is the implementation of procedures or interventions that prevent chronicity or disability.

More recently, in an extensive review of research in the prevention of psychiatric disorders, the Institute of Medicine (IOM) has advocated that the term *prevention* be used only for the prevention of occurrence of new cases of a disorder (primary prevention), proposing that interventions formerly designated secondary or tertiary prevention should be more properly considered as aspects of good treatment. The IOM (1994) adopts a different classification, first proposed by Gordon (1983), that focuses on the targeting and delivery of preventive interventions:

- *Universal* interventions, directed at whole populations;
- *Selective* interventions, directed at groups with known risk factors;
- *Indicated* interventions, for people who have clinical evidence that they, individually, are at special risk.

Both of these schemas have strengths in conceptualizing the scope and potential for prevention in psychiatry, and both will be employed in this chapter.

Principles of preventive medicine have been established for decades, with their most clearly effective applications in infectious and nutritional diseases. These same principles have been applied successfully in those psychiatric disorders that have clear organic etiologies. Other psychiatric conditions for which the disease model seems to have great utility, notably schizophrenia and the major affective disorders, are still of unclear etiology, and rational primary preventive interventions are not yet available. As knowledge advances in the genetics and pathobiology of the major mental illnesses, and the role of other risk factors is elucidated, however, preventive measures will become possible. In other disorders more usefully viewed from a dimensional or behavioral perspective, or in disorders in which a life-story perspective provides the best explanatory model (McHugh and Slavney, 1983), it makes greater sense to think of causative processes rather than causative agents. These processes—dynamic elements in the person's cognitive, affective, and behavioral development—may occur over periods of years in an individual's life-span, so that preventive interventions need to be differently conceptualized.

Risk Factors and Protective Factors

Underlying all discussion of prevention is the concept of risk. Individuals are subject to a number of risk factors: biological, environmental, psychological, and social. Risk factors may include one's own genetic constitution, one's past and present physical environment, the psychological and social environment in which one grew up and currently lives, and specific physical or psychological insults one may have suffered *in utero* or at any subsequent point. Current illness may have its origins in events that occurred many years ago. Childhood environmental influences may be risk factors for psychiatric disorder in later life.

The discovery of risk factors is one of the principal tasks of epidemiology. Data showing that African Americans are at increased risk for essential hypertension have led to blood pressure screening programs in African-American communities. Studies of elderly people show that those who are taking psychotropic medications are at increased risk of falling and thus sustaining fractures. Preventive measures ("fall precautions") are for this reason focused on this group to reduce the risk of injuries in hospital. Intravenous drug use is a risk factor for HIV infection, so that interventions to prevent AIDS, such as needle-exchange programs, are specially targeted at drug users in order to diminish the risk of infection.

Although knowledge of risk implies some understanding of cause, it is not necessary to understand etiology or disease mechanism before implementing preventive measures, if careful empirical observation leads to the discovery of risk factors. The classical example of this was the prevention of cholera by John Snow during an epidemic in London in 1849. His careful observations indicated that persons drawing water from the Broad Street pump were at greatest risk of becoming ill. He removed the pump handle to hasten the end of the epidemic without understanding the bacterial origin of the disease (Snow, 1965).

As a contemporary example of how risk factors can be elucidated and applied, Kellam and colleagues have confirmed that childhood behavior patterns predict problems such as antisocial behavior in adolescence and adult life. Their continuing research is exploring how implementing preventive programs in childhood can have positive effects in reducing the incidence of problem behaviors in later life. The intervention is designed to reduce certain behavior patterns (e.g., aggressiveness, shyness, and poor school performance) in small children. This is the *proximal* preventive aim. The ultimate objective, the *distal* preventive aim, is the reduction of pathology in later life. Understanding risk permits the development of models for preventive interventions and, conversely, systematic testing of these interventions can provide confirmation of etiologial theories (Kellam and Rebok, 1992).

Other factors within the person or in the physical or emotional environment may act as protective factors. It is known, for example, that children growing up in economically impoverished and socially deprived environments are at greater risk than children from economically and socially advantaged communities of developing antisocial patterns of behavior in adult life (Kolvin et al., 1988). The deprived childhood environment thus constitutes a risk factor. However, individuals vary in their life courses—not all become antisocial. Individual protective factors evidently operate to ensure that most children develop normally, even in adverse environments. Rutter (1985) refers to the ability to withstand stress as *resilience* and traces its development to many factors in the environment of the growing person, from early childhood onward, including the previous experiences of the person, the support provided by family and others, the particular meaning of stressors to the individual, and opportunities to develop self-esteem and a sense of mastery.

The Institute of Medicine report (1994) provides an overview of current information on risk factors for a number of psychiatric disorders. For Alzheimer's disease, they review the considerable evidence that has accumulated for a genetic etiology in some families, noting that other cases occur without a family history. It appears that other factors are of importance, at least in these non-familial cases. Other research has demonstrated somewhat weaker associations with three "malleable" risk factors: lower level of education, smoking, and history of head trauma, but the report acknowledges that these offer little scope for preventive interventions.

In relation to schizophrenia, a number of risk factors have also been identified. Genetic factors have been clearly implicated in a series of research studies over several decades; the risk of developing schizophrenia is elevated in first-degree relatives of schizophrenics relative to the general population, and the concordance rate in monozygotic twins is four times that of dizygotic twins. However, this genetic factor does not explain all the risk—other factors are of importance. Over many years, controversy has surrounded the undisputed finding that low socioeconomic status is a risk factor (Cohen, 1993). The controversy concerns whether poverty is a cause or a consequence of schizophrenia; the epidemiological data would support either explanation. Dohrenwend and his colleagues designed an ingenious method to tease apart the effects of inheritance from those of environment and concluded that the low economic status is a consequence rather than a cause of schizophrenia (Dohrenwend et al., 1992). Another series of investigations has shown that insults to the fetus in the second trimester of pregnancy are associated with the development of schizophrenia later in life. Other than encouraging good nutrition and health habits for women in pregnancy, universally accepted measures for many reasons, there are as yet no risk factor data on schizophrenia that provide a basis for designing more specific preventive interventions.

Studies of risk factors in alcoholism provide greater opportunity for prevention. Family history of alcohol use disorders is a clear risk factor, and it is possible that certain forms of alcohol dependence, but not all forms, have genetic predisposition. Certain biological markers have been identified, but the risk factors with greatest usefulness for prevention are in the psychosocial sphere. The Institute of Medicine report summarizes current knowledge in terms of six risk factors that have potential utility for prevention: history of alcoholism in a close relative; one of several biological markers; antisocial behavior or aggressiveness and shyness in childhood; low adaptability and poor stress tolerance; exposure to norms that foster alcohol abuse; and easy access to alcohol.

For depressive disorders, for which both genetic and environmental factors have demonstrated importance in etiology, five risk factors have been identified: mood disorder in a parent or close relative; a severe stressor; low self-esteem; being female; and living in poverty. Good intelligence, easy temperament, a strong sense of self, and good interpersonal relationships have been found to be protective factors.

It is apparent that many of the risk factors for mental disorders are very nonspecific. Limited education, for example, is a risk factor for Alzheimer's disease, but also for antisocial behavior. Poverty is a risk factor for depression, schizophrenia, and intravenous drug use.

Primary, Secondary and Tertiary Prevention

The traditional schema for categorizing preventive interventions, based on recommendations of the Commission on Chronic Illness (1957), embodies a concept of the course of illness which includes onset (incidence), course (prevalence), and chronicity (disability).

Primary Prevention

Primary prevention leads to a reduction in incidence. The eradication of smallpox, confirmed in 1979, was a major triumph of primary prevention on a global scale. Fluoridation of drinking water to prevent dental caries or eliminating tobacco smoking to reduce the incidence of lung disease are other examples.

The most successful primary prevention programs for psychiatric disorders have been for diseases with exogenous organic etiologies. In the realm of nutrition, the prevention and treatment of hypothyroidism, including adding iodine to table salt in areas with low levels of natural iodine, has virtually eliminated cretinism, a major cause of mental retardation in earlier generations. Adequate nutrition to eliminate pellagra has eradicated pellagra psychosis. The treatment of syphilis with penicillin before it reaches the tertiary stage has led to the virtual disappearance of general paresis of the insane, which was a major contributor of chronic patients in mental hospitals 50 years ago. In the current era, the devastation caused by the HIV pandemic is widely recognized, and the prevention of AIDS is one of the most formidable public health challenges. Preventing AIDS will prevent the resulting psychiatric complications of secondary affective disorder and dementia (Chapter 29).

One reason that physicians in general and psychiatrists specifically have been less interested in prevention than might be expected is that when effective primary preventive measures are feasible, they often fall outside the realm of clinical practice, and even outside the realm of health care. For example, preventing water-borne diseases is in the hands of water engineers who design distribution and purification systems. Similarly, measures to prevent mental retardation in many cases fall outside the scope of mental health agencies—for example in lead paint abatement and the prevention of head injuries. Primary prevention of the adverse psychological effects of poverty, racism, family violence, and poor education lies in areas of social policy beyond the power of psychiatrists to change. When preventive interventions fall in the realm of health care, they again are often outside the purview of psychiatrists (Sartorius and Henderson, 1992). Improved access to prenatal care, genetic counseling, early identification by pediatricians of inborn metabolic disorders, and the prevention of delirium and dementia in the elderly (Rabins, 1992) are all examples, reinforcing the importance of psychiatrists' maintaining active dialogue with specialists in other medical fields.

Secondary Prevention

Secondary prevention, the reduction of prevalence by reducing the duration of illness, generally takes the form of implementing a screening program to detect illness at an early stage, followed by appropriate and energetic treatment. One example is tuberculin testing to detect the presence of tuberculosis before clinical diagnosis is possible, so that treatment can be initiated when it is most effective and before the disease can be transmitted. By this means, the number of active or advanced cases in the community is reduced. Serological screening for prostate cancer so that treatment can be instituted before the cancer has metastasized is another example. Blood pressure screening permits the institution of antihypertensive treatment at an early stage in the progression of essential hypertension (proximal goal) and prevents later complications such as heart failure and stroke (distal goal).

This paradigm requires an effective screening method or tool, an effective intervention, and a means of using the screening data to target the intervention to individuals at risk. In the realm of mental disorders, there has been progress in all of these areas, but there are only a few situations in psychiatry in which the complete process is systematically implemented. The best examples are in the prevention of developmental disability. For decades it has been standard practice to test newborns' urine to detect phenylketonuria. If this metabolic defect is detected at an early stage, introduction of a phebylalanaine-free diet prevents the development of the disorder and its associated mental disabilities. This intervention has essentially eliminated phenylketonuria in the developed world (Medical Research Council, 1993) Another example is the *in utero* detection of chromosomal disorders, such as trisomy-21 which is associated with Down Syndrome. This procedure provides parents with information needed to decide whether to terminate a pregnancy that would result in a cognitively disabled child.

Depression Screening Days and Anxiety Screening Days provide an example of the widespread use of screening methods for secondary prevention of psychiatric disorder in adult life. At these events, paper-and-pencil screening tests for depression or anxiety are offered in shopping malls, hospitals, and other public places. People who screen positive are then guided and encouraged in seeking appropriate psychiatric evaluation and treatment.

Screening tests for psychopathology for use in general clinical settings such as primary care clinics or internists' office practice have been developed and used widely in research but are still under-used in clinical practice. The General Health Questionnaire (GHQ) provides an excellent example. This is a self-administered paper-and-pencil questionnaire that requires about 5 minutes to complete. It was designed to detect cases of probable psychiatric disorder in British general practice settings, so that general practitioners could pursue further inquiry to establish a psychiatric diagnosis and institute proper treatment or referral (Goldberg, 1972). The GHQ does not provide a diagnosis, but it does provide a general measure of distress and dysphoria, with high levels of sensitivity and specificity. It has been widely used as a screener in epidemiological research, but it has not been clearly established that its use by general practitioners is effective in initiating early treatment and preventing more serious pathology. An American preventive trial using this instrument was disappointing because the GHQ results provided to internists had very little influence on their treatment of individual patients, even where the results were strongly suggestive of "caseness" (Shapiro et al., 1987). The PRIME-MD (Primary Care Evaluation of Mental Disorders) is a more recently developed American screening tool (Spitzer et al., 1994). This instrument provides a simple screen for the five most commonly occurring disorders in primary care settings: depression, anxiety, somatoform disorders, substance use disorders, and eating disorders. It consists of a brief self-administered patient questionnaire and clinician evaluation guide. The clinician uses the latter instrument to inquire in more detail about conditions for which the patient gave positive responses in the patient questionnaire.

Other secondary prevention methods include screening patients routinely for alcohol use disorders using the CAGE or other screener (Mayfield et al., 1974); educating school teachers to identify children who show signs of emotional disorder who can then be referred to appropriate mental health services; and telephone counseling services, or "hot lines," through which people in crisis can seek help and possibly prevent a more serious outcome, such as a suicide.

Tertiary Prevention

Tertiary prevention is concerned with the prevention of chronicity, complications, or disability. Examples in the realm of physical disorders include physical therapies to improve function in a limb following a fracture and careful wound care and foot care for diabetics to prevent infections.

Techniques for relapse prevention in schizophrenia provide a good example of tertiary prevention in psychiatry. A program of research spanning two decades demonstrated that the likelihood of relapse for a person with schizophrenia is greater in families that have higher levels of "expressed emotion" (EE), characterized by high levels of criticism and negative comments in the home. This research led to the development of an intervention based on education and discussion groups for the families of schizophrenic patients which was successful in reducing the number of relapses (Leff, 1994).

Tertiary prevention is also directed at the functional impairments associated with chronic psychiatric disorders. These impairments result from the effects of several factors. The intrinsic psychopathology associated with illnesses such as schizophrenia is of primary importance, but the unwanted effects of pharmacological treatments, such as akathisia, hypersomnolence, extrapyramidal motor symptoms, or memory impairment further contribute to the disability. In addition, social and psychological influences are of major importance (Wing and Brown, 1970; Gruenberg, 1974). These include the stultifying environment of long-term hospital wards, but also unstimulating or infantilizing community residential alternatives, social isolation, stigmatizing public attitudes, and the effects of poverty. Tertiary preventive measures are directed at reducing the risk of these complications. Whether the person is mentally ill, developmentally disabled, or chronically addicted, the social breakdown syndrome has similar manifestations, and similar psychosocial rehabilitation measures are indicated. Rehabilitation programs (Chapter 21) provide carefully titrated stimulation for chronically disabled people, focusing on the maintenance and restoration of function, empowerment, and the promotion of self-esteem, all with the aim of reducing handicap, disability, and stigma. Psychiatrists play a major role through the careful use of psychotropic medications, employing minimum doses to achieve a therapeutic effect with minimal adverse effects such as cognitive slowing or dyskinesia.

Other clinical interventions help reduce stigma and combat the tendency for social withdrawal. Group techniques that enable patients to cope with symptoms such as hallucinations in their everyday lives and that cultivate self-esteem may help patients overcome the sense of shame associated with mental illness. Shame and embarrassment lead to greater social isolation, which in turn can lead to increased idiosyncracy, greater stigma, and further diminution of self-esteem.

Functional Categorization of Preventive Interventions

Gordon's operational categorization draws attention to the practical consideration of targeting preventive measures. *Universal* measures are directed to whole populations. The many examples in public health include water fluoridation, prenatal care, childhood immunization, gun control, radiation monitoring, or anti-smoking propaganda. *Selective* measures are applied to populations at special risk and include immunizations for persons traveling to areas of the world with high prevalence of certain infectious diseases, needle exchange programs for intravenous drug users, and protective clothing for people working in certain industries. *Indicated* measures are directed at individuals who have clinical evidence that they are at special risk, such as prophylactic antibiotics for immunosuppressed individuals or cholesterol-lowering agents for people with hypercholesterolemia who are at risk of heart disease.

All three types of preventive intervention may be of value in relation to certain diseases. Huntington's disease, which has both neurological and psychiatric manifestations, provides an example. Prevention is possible because DNA analysis can detect carriers of the dominant gene at an early age, before the illness emerges and before the person has had any children. *Universal* public education measures encourage potential carriers to present themselves for screening. *Selective* screening of persons in affected families permit a determination of their carrier status. Counseling for carriers who must make decisions about child-bearing is an *indicated* preventive intervention (Folstein, 1989; Harper, 1991).

Universal Measures

There is as yet limited opportunity for employing universal interventions for the prevention of psychiatric disorders that are comparable in their specificity to the chlorination of water to prevent enteric infections or the immunization of children to prevent poliomyelitis. There are, however, examples in the areas of substance abuse and developmental disability. Warning labels on alcoholic beverage containers and educational programs against substance abuse in schools and elsewhere are universal measures to prevent drug and alcohol use disorders and their sequelae. Certain programs to reduce exposure to exogenous poisons, such as reducing lead in gasoline and removing lead paint from dwellings, are universal measures for the prevention of developmental disabilities.

Other universal preventive measures that are proposed in relation to mental health are considerably more general in their scope, do not focus on the prevention of specific disorders, and are more properly considered as *mental health promotion* efforts, with the aim of enabling people to cope better with the stresses of everyday life. The possibilities are myriad, including teaching of parenting skills; providing opportunities for children to exercise choices, confront potential dangers, and develop mastery; fostering supportive family environments; and providing positive educational experiences. Insofar as these activities increase a person's ability to cope with life's problems more effectively or to develop personality strengths, they can be considered aspects of mental health promotion and universal measures for the prevention of emotional or behavioral difficulties. Stress reduction in the workplace and measures to combat racism, to promote the equality of women, and to combat child abuse all have obvious face validity as universal preventive measures.

In the 1960s and 1970s, community psychiatrists emphasized mental health consultation as an approach to altering stressful environments, and this universal approach has been widely used in schools and other organizations. The role of the consultant in this model is to work with the consultee in such a way that the organization can be changed for the better, with creation of an environment that is expected to be more conducive to positive mental health. A less stressful environment, it was supposed, would produce less psychopathology. The principal proponent of this approach was Gerald Caplan in the 1960s and 1970s, who developed a theory, based on psychoanalytic principles, relating to the unconscious dynamics in organizations that can prevent change and create stress (Caplan, 1964).

Selective Measures

Selective measures are employed with the intention of identifying persons who are at special risk and directing preventive measures specifically at those individuals. For example, education regarding the danger of drinking alcohol during pregnancy and the risk of fetal alcohol syndrome is particularly aimed at women in the child-bearing age group who drink alcohol, and most specifically at women in the early stages of pregnancy (Smith and Coles, 1991). In the area of child mental health, specific groups have been identified who are at special risk of emotional disturbance or conduct disorders, and interventions have been planned to give them extra support and services. Examples include Mexican-American infants, African-American preschoolers in poverty, and teenage mothers. Evaluation has demonstrated the effectiveness of these interventions (Price et al., 1988).

Other selective prevention programs assist people in specific stressful situations to cope more effectively, so that transient and normal reactions are not prolonged into more serious and lasting disorders. In many cases ''survivors groups'' are the means for achieving this. Survivors of natural or man-made disasters, sexual assaults, or other victimization benefit from such interventions. Bereavement is a particularly stressful transition experienced by most people at some time, with a demonstrated risk of depression (Parkes, 1965; Institute of Medicine, 1984). Widow-to-widow groups are widely employed to assist persons to cope with grief and have demonstrated effectiveness in preventing depression in this stressful situation (Vachon et al., 1980). Other groups provide support for parents who have lost a child.

Indicated Measures

There are a number of situations in community psychiatry where preventive interventions can be applied in the presence of specific clinical indications. One of the most straightforward is the prevention of complications of chronic alcohol intoxication or withdrawal. Thiamine in given to patients with chronic alcohol intoxication to prevent further neurological damage which might result in Wernicke's encephalopathy or Korsakoff Syndrome, and in the setting of withdrawal from alcohol, benzodiazepines or similar sedating drugs are prescribed to prevent delirium tremens.

One of the major complications of community-based care for people with severe and persistent mental illnesses is substance abuse and dependence. Indicated preventive measures in community psychiatry programs therefore include measures to motivate and assist people with mental illnesses to avoid these added problems. Such measures include focused educational programs to ensure that they are aware of the dangers, and the provision of other recreational opportunities, specifically for the individuals at risk (Chapter 28).

A further example of opportunity for indicated prevention is in the prevention of homelessness in people who are chronically mentally ill. A history of childhood disruption, substance dependence, and social isolation are all risk factors for homelessness (Breakey and Fischer, 1995). Knowledge of these risk factors enables service providers for severely mentally ill individuals to implement special preventive measures to help avoid homelessness in those at risk (Chapter 28).

Conclusion: Implications for Community Psychiatry

What are the implications for community psychiatrists and for community mental health programs? It must be acknowledged that with the unremitting pressures for fiscal restraint, and directives from state funding agencies to set priorities for treatment of the severely mentally ill, few modern community psychiatry programs in recent years have explicitly established programs for prevention. Prevention at this level is an undertaking for the whole community through its various political, economic, educational, and social agencies. It is also true that well-evaluated methods for prevention that can be applied in a community psychiatry setting are still limited. Nonetheless, many of the activities of community psychiatrists and community mental health programs have preventive impact, which may at times not be acknowledged (Table 24–1). Community psychiatrists contribute to prevention through their own clinical activities as they improve their service systems for earlier and more effective treatment of illnesses, thereby reducing prevalence and preventing complications. They also are active in prevention through interactions with other health care sectors as they work with primary-care agencies, well baby clinics, or nursing homes. The public education activities of community psychiatrists have clear preventive implications. Many community psychiatrists are involved in a variety of community organizations as board members, consultants, trainers, or advisors. These can include schools, youth centers, women's counseling programs, advocacy organizations for homeless people, senior centers, and many others. Commonsense, if not science as yet, gives these activities validity as having a preventive role in building up healthy communities, reducing stress in people's lives, or increasing resiliency.

Table 24–1   The preventive activities of the community psychiatrist

Activity	Preventive Impact
As a Clinician:	
Skilled and careful use of psychotropic drugs	Reduce risk of side-effects
Active rehabilitation for disabled patients	Prevent social deterioration
Ensuring that women have proper prenatal care;	Reduce risk of fetal abnormalities and cognitive disabilities
Ensuring that patients' children have proper nutrition and pediatric care	Reduce risk of childhood illness and developmental delays
Ensuring that patients' children live in a stable and supportive emotional climate and are receiving proper parenting and education	Reduce risk of antisocial behaviors and educational disadvantage
Identify patients at risk of homelessness and provide additional supports	Prevent homelessness
Through Contacts with Other Physicians:	
Facilitating referrals to improve access to psychiatric treatment	Reduce risks associated with untreated mental illness
Providing screening tools	Facilitate recognition of treatable disorders
Destigmatizing mental illness and psychiatry	Reduce barriers to help-seeking
As an Educator:	
Public relations efforts to encourage early diagnosis and treatment	Reduce risks associated with untreated mental illness
Educational programs directed at parents, teachers, and community residents that improve child care	Reduce risk of developmental problems
In Collaboration with Other Community Organizations:	
Anti-drug campaigns	Primary prevention of substance abuse
Anti-violence campaigns	Reduce risk of head injury and associated psychopathology
Anti-stigma programs	Reduce barriers to seeking care
Depression/anxiety screening days	Promote early diagnosis and treatment

Summary

It is important that a community psychiatrist have a preventive perspective. The principles of prevention outlined here are incorporated in many community psychiatry activities. The technology of prevention in mental health is still in its infancy, and preventive intervention research to provide more powerful tools for prevention should be given high priority (Institute of Medicine, 1994). This should not deter community psychiatrists from pursuing those approaches to prevention that have commonsense validity and apparent effectiveness.

References

Breakey, W.R., and Fischer, P.J. (1995) Mental illness and the continuum of residential stability. *Social Psychiatry and Psychiatric Epidemiology,* 30:147–151.

IV

Services for Special Populations

25

The Dually Diagnosed

ROBERT E. DRAKE
FRED C. OSHER
STEPHEN J. BARTELS

This chapter reviews the literature on co-occurring severe mental illness and substance use disorder, often termed *dual diagnosis.* The review is restricted to patients with severe mental disorders, such as schizophrenia or bipolar disorder. It covers several aspects of substance abuse among patients with severe mental disorder: prevalence and etiology, clinical correlates, course and outcome, assessment, and treatment. Within each of these categories, practical clinical implications are emphasized.

Prevalence and Etiology

Severe mental disorders are frequently complicated by comorbid disorders: medical illnesses, mental retardation, or substance abuse. Co-occurring substance use disorder is the most frequent and clinically significant (Minkoff and Drake, 1991). The Epidemiologic Catchment Area (ECA) study confirmed the extent of comorbidity of substance use disorders with severe mental illnesses in the community. Nearly half of the individuals with a lifetime diagnosis of schizophrenia or schizophreniform disorder in the ECA study also met criteria for some form of substance abuse or dependence (Regier et al., 1990). The ECA study also confirmed that individuals with multiple disorders are more likely to be in treatment than those with single disorders, so rates of comorbidity are higher in some clinical settings.

The rates of diagnosed comorbidity in mental health settings continue to rise as clinicians become more aware of the high prevalence of substance abuse and dependence and more skilled at identifying multiple disorders (Lehman et al., 1989). In addition, at least two factors may have contributed to a real increase in the prevalence of substance abuse among psychiatric patients. First, an entire generation of young adults with severe mental illness in the United States has become ill and grown up during the era of deinstitutionalization. While residing predominantly in the community rather than in hospitals, they have had few vocational, recreational, and social opportunities but have experienced regular exposure and ready access to alcohol and other drugs (Lamb, 1982; Pepper et al., 1981). Second, during the same years that the deinstitutionalization policy has been implemented, availability of and experimentation with illegal drugs has increased dramatically in the United States. In the early 1960s only 2 percent or less of the population had experimented with illegal drugs, but by 1985 almost half of all young adults had tried various psychoactive substances other than alcohol (National Institute on Drug Abuse, 1989). Although these rates have declined since 1985, many mentally disabled young people have abused drugs for several years prior to the development of their psychiatric disorders (Barbee et al., 1989; Breakey et al., 1974; Caton et al., 1989). Furthermore, they have often used new types of drugs (such as LSD in the 1960s, PCP in the 1970s, and potent forms of cocaine in the 1980s) that distort symptoms, obscure diagnosis, adversely affect the course and treatment of major mental illness, and may precipitate or induce psychiatric disorders (Breakey et al., 1974; Dixon et al., 1990).

Although people with severe mental illnesses probably experiment with alcohol and other drugs for the same reasons as others in society, several additional factors have been hypothesized to contribute to their high rate of substance use disorders: downward social drift into poor urban living settings; attempts to alleviate (or self-medicate) the symptoms of mental illness, the side effects of psychotropic medications, or the dysphoria associated with mental illness; and attempts to establish an identity other than that of mental patient (Minkoff and Drake, 1991). Speculations regarding the etiology of substance use disorders for this population have often identified factors that are associated with early experimentation (such as social pressure), short-term effects (such as relief from anxiety), self-reports regarding reasons for use (such as relief from medication effects), and clinical correlates (such as antisocial behavior). For example, clinicians often speak loosely of self-medication even when history clearly indicates that the substance abuse preceded the psychiatric disorder by many years.

Attempts to discern causality from these approaches are difficult and should be treated with caution. More research is needed but is likely to find that substance use disorders in severely mentally ill persons, as in others, are determined by a complex set of biopsychosocial factors. In the meantime, attempts to understand causality should be separated from studies of the factors that sustain problematic use. For example, physiological reinforcement mechanisms, associative learning phenomena, poor cognitive, social, and vocational functioning, and the lack of significant social and material resources appear to be related to sustained abuse and dependence, regardless of the reasons for initial use.

Correlates of Substance Abuse in People with Severe Mental Illnesses

Cross-sectional studies indicate that substance use disorder among people with severe mental illness is associated with several manifestations of poor adjustment. These include increases in psychiatric symptoms, psychosocial instability, medical problems, homelessness, and institutionalization. Substance abuse has been linked with exacerbations of psychiatric symptoms or more severe chronic symptoms in many studies (Carey et al., 1991; Dixon et al., 1990; Drake and Wallach, 1989). Alcohol abuse may also be correlated with depression in schizophrenia (Bartels et al., 1992). In addition to psychiatric symptoms, substance abuse is also associated with disruptive behaviors such as hostility, aggression, and criminal behavior (Drake and Wallach, 1989; McCarrick et al., 1985; Safer, 1987; Yesavage and Zarcone, 1983).

Dually diagnosed patients have greater difficulty than those with single disorders managing the practical aspects of their lives, such as money and housing, and are particularly prone to unstable housing arrangements and homelessness (Belcher, 1989; Drake and Wallach, 1989; Drake et al., 1991; Lamb and Lamb, 1990). They also are prone to more HIV risk behavior and are thus more likely to become infected (Cournos et al., 1991). Finally, dually diagnosed patients tend to be noncompliant with treatment (Drake and Wallach, 1989; Kashner et al., 1991) and to receive emergency services and institutional care in hospitals and jails rather than housing and day treatment supports (Bartels et al., 1993).

Because most studies are cross-sectional, cause and effect are difficult to sort out. While assigning causal significance to substance abuse is tempting, many other factors could explain the relationships between substance abuse and poor adjustment. For example, the same patients who abuse alcohol are prone to abuse other, potentially more toxic drugs, to be noncompliant with medications, and to be living in stressful circumstances without a strong support network (Drake et al., 1989). They may also have been different premorbidly from patients with the same disorders who do not abuse drugs (Breakey et al., 1974). Laboratory experiments are somewhat helpful in clarifying effects, but the circumstances, quality, and quantity of use in laboratory situations may be quite different from typical patterns of use in the community (Dixon et al., 1990).

A similarly complex set of factors leads to difficulty for this group of patients in establishing good relationships with service providers. Undoubtedly, acute and chronic intoxication exacerbate the effects of severe mental illness in compromising the patient's capacity to trust and to develop a therapeutic relationship. In addition, dually diagnosed patients are seen as difficult to treat and are often poorly served by or extruded from mental health, substance abuse, and housing programs. A variety of other factors related to funding, training, philosophy, and administration make it difficult for dually diagnosed patients to fit into the existing mental health or substance abuse treatment systems (Ridgely et al., 1987). For example, the training of clinicians, the structure of mental health programs, and the incentives of public funding may all conspire against mental health providers in their attempts to address substance abuse.

Course and Outcome

Longitudinal data are accumulating rapidly regarding the course and outcome of comorbid severe mental illness and substance use disorder (Drake et al., in press). Short-term studies (one year or less) indicate that dually diagnosed persons are prone to negative outcomes. They are more difficult to engage in services, even with a team approach and assertive outreach (Arana et al., 1991), but newer dual-diagnosis programs have been successful in engaging them (Mercer-McFadden and Drake, 1995). Their substance abuse is relatively unchanged over one year of treatment (Bond et al., 1991; Lehman et al., 1993). They are prone to leave residential treatment early or to relapse to substance abuse soon after discharge to the community (Bartels and Thomas, 1991). Finally, a variety of short-term outcome studies show that they are prone to homelessness, psychiatric hospitalization, and incarceration (Bartels et al., 1993; Belcher, 1989; Drake et al., 1991b; Safer, 1987).

Long-term outcomes (greater than one year) are less well studied. One investigation of schizophrenia found that former substance abusers were no more symptomatic than non-drinkers (Zisook et al., 1992). A similar study showed that former substance-abusing patients had a low rate of hospitalization but did use housing supports and day treatment services at a high rate compared to patients who had never abused (Bartels et al., 1993). Neither of these studies followed patients prospectively, so patients with more negative outcomes could have been lost from the samples.

A recent 7-year follow-up study of severely mentally ill patients in Boston found that the overall rate of substance use disorder in the sample did not change significantly over the 7 years (Bartels et al., 1995). The 7-year follow-up assessed their patterns of alcohol use over a 6-month period. Although approximately one-third of the original dually diagnosed subgroup were not abusing alcohol or other drugs at follow-up, nearly as many patients who had not been abusing substances at baseline were assessed as having active substance use disorders at that time. These findings may reflect high rates of concurrent recovery and development of new cases of substance use disorder over the 7 years. A more likely explanation, however, is that because substance use disorder is chronic, with exacerbations and remissions, a 6-month window identifies many who are not currently abusing but also are not in stable recovery. Six months has been proposed as a minimal interval to discern stable remission (Vaillant, 1983), but it may not be sufficient for this population. For example, many patients who appear to be moderate drinkers during a 6-month assessment interval show clear evidence of abuse outside of that interval (Drake and Wallach, 1993).

Several recent studies of dual-diagnosis programs, which integrate substance abuse and mental health treatments within the same setting, indicate more positive outcomes (Drake et al., in press). These studies show a steady rate of reduction in substance use, with a cumulative group of patients attaining stable abstinence during each year of consistent treatment (Drake et al., 1993c; Durrell et al., 1993; McHugo et al., 1995; Mueser et al., in press).

Assessment

Thorough assessment includes three overlapping but conceptually separable issues: detection, diagnosis, and treatment planning (Drake and Mercer-McFadden, 1995).

Detection refers to the identification of abuse or dependence, and of harmful or dangerous use that does not yet qualify for a diagnosis (Babor et al., 1989). Diagnostic issues include not only the identification of DSM-III-R substance use disorders, but also the difficulties of assigning other psychiatric diagnoses in the presence of substance use disorder. Treatment planning emphasizes a thorough analysis of the biopsychosocial factors that sustain substance use disorder. Assessment and treatment planning prepare the patient for participating in an appropriate intervention.

Detection

Failure to detect substance abuse in psychiatric settings can result in misdiagnosis and overtreatment of psychiatric syndromes with medications. Appropriate interventions such as detoxification, substance abuse education, and substance abuse counseling are neglected and inappropriate treatment plans developed. Nevertheless, numerous studies show that substance use disorder is typically underdiagnosed in acute care psychiatric settings (Ananth et al., 1989; Drake et al., 1990; Galletly et al., 1993; Stone et al., 1993). Among the factors that account for this high rate of non-detection are mental health clinicians' inattention to substance abuse; patients' denial, minimization, or inability to perceive the relationships between substance use and problems in living; and the lack of reliable and valid methods of detection in this population (Drake et al., 1993a).

Several critical steps will improve the detection of substance abuse and dependence and of potentially harmful use in psychiatric settings. Most important, mental health clinicians need to have a high index of suspicion regarding substance use. Suspicion should be modified by base rates of substance use disorder in the population and by clinical correlates. For example, the rate of substance use disorder in schizophrenia is greater than 50 percent when other risk factors such as youth, male gender, medication noncompliance, a history of disruptiveness, and unstable housing are present (Drake et al., 1993a). Rates of abstinence are also high in this population, and there is little evidence that psychiatric patients are able to sustain moderate use without incurring problems (Drake and Wallach, 1993). Clinicians should therefore pay attention to all patients who use alcohol or other drugs. Even small amounts of psychoactive substances may be harmful in people who already have brain disorders (Drake et al., 1989; Lieberman et al., 1990).

Clinicians should be trained to detect substance abuse and dependence in standardized ways. Even brief measures, such as the CAGE, MAST, and DAST, may detect the majority of mentally ill persons who abuse alcohol and other drugs (Drake et al., 1990). Other detection methods include breathalyzers, urine screens, physical exams, and information from collaterals (Drake et al., 1993a). Laboratory methods, such as urine drug tests, may be particularly important when illicit drugs, such as crack cocaine, are involved (Galletly et al., 1993; Stone et al., 1993).

Clinicians should be aware that the adverse effects of alcohol and other drugs are often denied, minimized, or misperceived by psychiatric patients, most of whom have had unusual cognitive and affective experiences without using drugs (Drake et al.,

1990; Test et al., 1989). The types of consequences they experience may also be different from the general population, since patients with severe mental disabilities often do not drive cars, have marriages, and work. Instead, warning signals such as poor response to treatment, problems with family, or unstable housing should warrant continuing reevaluation (Drake et al., 1993a). Longitudinal observation by trained clinicians, such as case managers who observe their patients and interact with their support network in the community, is most likely to detect adverse effects related to alcohol or other drugs (Drake et al., 1990).

Diagnosis

Diagnosis of dual disorders is complicated and controversial (Lehman et al., 1989). Alcohol and drug use disorders can often be diagnosed with greater certainty than other co-existing psychiatric syndromes (Kofoed, 1991). Persistent substance use that results in social, vocational, psychological, or physical problems should be considered abuse or dependence according to DSM-III-R criteria. For psychiatric patients, relatively small amounts of substances may result in psychological problems or decompensation, or may evolve into a clear use disorder, because of their vulnerability to the effects of psychoactive substances (Dixon et al., 1990; Drake et al., 1989). Therefore, all patients who use alcohol and other drugs should be followed longitudinally to identify potential negative effects that are not readily apparent to the patient. If questions about adverse effects exist, a trial of abstinence may clarify the situation.

Diagnosing other psychiatric disorders in the face of substance abuse is more complicated (Kofoed, 1991). Psychoactive substances can induce or mimic almost any psychiatric syndrome, and patients who present with concurrent syndromes often have little history of being substance-free for extended periods of time. Recent evidence suggests that a high proportion of the psychiatric syndromes presenting in the context of substance abuse may be transitory and will disappear over time with abstinence (Lehman et al., 1994). While scientific evidence indicates that making a diagnosis should be deferred, other factors such as the need to treat, communicate, and charge for services push clinicians toward making a diagnosis rapidly. Perhaps a reasonable compromise for the present is to consider all psychiatric diagnoses made in the context of substance abuse provisional; the diagnoses and their associated treatments should be reconsidered at regular intervals, especially during periods of abstinence from psychoactive substances.

Treatment Planning

Assessment goes beyond detection and diagnosis to a process that involves the patient in reviewing all the data and in specifying a strategy for further exploration or change. Treatment planning includes a thorough biopsychosocial review: historical information, family history, current frequency and patterns of use, physiological factors, cognitive-behavioral expectancies related to the use of different substances, environmental cues, social networks, other social and behavioral patterns that sustain abuse, interrelationships between substance use, medications, and psychiatric illness, and previous attempts to control or treat substance use (Donovan, 1988). Treatment planning involves a continuous, dynamic, and longitudinal process, in which the clinician and patient collaborate over time (Kofoed, 1991). For example, as new information is learned through trials of controlled intake or abstinence, the plan is updated.

The biopsychosocial model of addiction renders inadequate those reductionistic views of addiction (e.g., present vs. absent) that lead to simplistic approaches to treatment (e.g., one approach for all). Empirical research supports the view that multiple variables are involved and need to be addressed in treatment (Donovan et al., 1986). A thorough assessment that includes treatment planning should specify: (a) the behavioral, psychological, physiological, and environmental conditions that are associated with the problem's occurrence and maintenance, (b) an appropriate set of interventions, based on systems involved and stage of treatment (see below), and (c) criteria for evaluating outcome (Donovan, 1988).

A well-done evaluation and planning meeting increases the patient's motivation for the interventions (Miller and Rollnick, 1991). Thus, for example, an educational group and a change of living situation may be adequate treatment for a young schizophrenic man who becomes angry and belligerent when he drinks but has no family history of alcoholism, no evidence of the alcohol dependence syndrome, and only began to drink when he moved into an apartment setting in which most of the residents are heavy drinkers. On the other hand, a middle-aged schizophrenic man who has been drinking heavily in isolation for many years and now has severe dependence and cognitive impairments due to alcohol will need a more intensive intervention.

Treatment

Over the past 10 years, several innovative models for the treatment of dual disorders have emerged (Carey, in press; Drake et al., 1993b; Fariello and Scheidt, 1989; Minkoff, 1989; Minkoff and Drake, 1991; Ridgely et al., 1987) and several attempts to identify critical interventions and emerging treatment principles have appeared (Carey, 1989; Drake et al., 1993b; Nikkel and Coiner, 1991; Osher and Kofoed, 1989). Successful programs now exist in the mental health treatment system, in the substance abuse treatment system, as collaborations across the two systems, and in new hybrid settings. Despite their differences, programs that address the severely mentally disabled population share several commonalities.

Integrated Treatment

This approach combines mental health and substance abuse treatments in the same setting in a concurrent and coordinated fashion (Minkoff and Drake, 1991). For historical reasons, the mental health and substance abuse treatment systems in the United States are quite separate, and traditional approaches to dual disorders have straddled uncomfortably across the two systems of care. Extruding patients from each system because of the other disorder or attempting to treat only one disorder or the two disorders in sequence remain common but generally ineffective approaches (Ridgely et al., 1990).

Another common approach involves concurrent, parallel treatments in the two systems. Although there are no data from controlled studies, many clinicians and researchers have observed that parallel treatment is difficult for several reasons (Galanter et al., 1988; Kline et al., 1991; Ridgely et al., 1990; Wallen and Weiner, 1989). It places on the patient the burden of integrating two systems with disparate philosophies, treatments, and clinicians. It allows each system to continue to provide a standard form of treatment and to resist modifications that are specific for subgroups. And it maximizes the potential for miscommunications and noncompliance. Too often the patient becomes lost between the two systems.

To address these problems, integrated treatment programs that focus on dually diagnosed patients have developed in many settings (Minkoff and Drake, 1991; Ridgely et al., 1987; Teague et al., 1990). Integrated programs do more than combine two forms of treatment. Clinicians typically modify previous beliefs and behaviors to become flexible dual-diagnosis specialists who are expert in several areas: motivating patients for active treatment, using techniques of close monitoring (including involuntary interventions), leading dual-diagnosis groups, linking with self-help groups, and providing longitudinal stage-wise treatment (see below) (Drake et al., 1993b).

The superior effectiveness of integrated programs has been well demonstrated in a variety of open clinical trials (Drake et al., 1995). For example, Kofoed and coworkers (1986) treated dually diagnosed patients in a group setting and found that the one-third who remained in treatment for one year reduced their days in the hospital. Drake and colleagues (1993c) found that over half of schizophrenic patients with alcoholism achieved stable remission from alcoholism during 4 years in an integrated treatment program that included assertive case management and substance abuse treatment. Durrell and colleagues (1993) followed 43 patients with dual disorders for 18 months or longer and found that two-thirds reduced their substance use.

In most community mental health settings, substance abuse treatment can be integrated as a component of comprehensive treatment at relatively low cost (Fox et al., 1992). Substance abuse treatment can be provided on an individual basis by clinical case managers and therapists and in groups by case managers or other mental health staff. The expense of instituting such a system involves mostly training the current workforce; whereas, the expense of creating comprehensive services in conjunction with a substance abuse treatment program is usually prohibitive.

Longitudinal Stage-Wise Treatment

The development of addictions generally takes several years, and the process of recovery also takes place over years (Vaillant, 1983). Clinicians should therefore be prepared to address dual disorders continuously over years rather than intermittently for weeks or months. Although the short-term outcomes for people with dual disorders are relatively poor, their long-term outcomes in a program that offers specific dual-diagnosis treatment may be quite favorable (Drake et al., in press).

Substance use disorder, like major mental illness, can be conceptualized as a chronic, relapsing illness that is treatable in stages. Osher and Kofoed (1989) conceptualized four stages: *engagement, persuasion, active treatment,* and *relapse prevention.* These stages refer to overlapping processes: developing a trusting relationship, or working alliance, with the patient (engagement); helping the patient to perceive and acknowledge the adverse consequences of substance use in his or her life and to develop motivation for recovery (persuasion); helping the patient to achieve stable recovery, whether that is controlled use or abstinence (active treatment); and helping the patient to maintain a stable recovery (relapse prevention).

During each stage of treatment, a range of treatment options is available, and specific plans should reflect patients' preferences (Drake and Noordsy, 1994). Treatment is assertive during the engagement stage, with a strong emphasis on outreach, practical assistance, and building a relationship (Drake et al., 1991a). During persuasion, dual-diagnosis groups, multiple family groups, or individual interactions can be used to help the patient to understand the relationship between problems of living and the use of psychoactive substances, and to develop and enhance motivation for change (Noordsy and Fox, 1991). Once the patient is committed to an active strategy of change, clinicians help to devise an individualized strategy that addresses all of the systems that sustain abuse or dependence. Active treatment may include cognitive-behavioral interventions, social network interventions, dual-diagnosis groups, and sometimes involves self-help groups. Relapse prevention is also highly individualized, taking advantage of whatever format serves best to remind the patient of vulnerability and risk factors.

A stage model of treatment is used for heuristic purposes rather than because treatment proceeds in a linear or invariant pathway. Patients typically cycle back and forth between engagement and persuasion early in treatment and may also relapse from active treatment or relapse prevention stages. Over time, however, they typically make progress through the stages (McHugo et al., 1995).

More important, the stage model usefully guides clinicians in planning and deciding what interventions are appropriate at a particular point in time. Consider, for example, the issue of abstinence-orientation, a philosophy that often causes friction between clinicians. Insisting on abstinence when the patient is in the engagement stage of treatment will frequently drive the patient from treatment, whereas successful engagement can often take place without interrupting the substance abuse or during intervals, such as hospitalizations, when the abuse is interrupted by natural consequences. During the persuasion stage, the existence of a working alliance may allow the clinician to discuss abstinence, but insisting on abstinence with a patient who is not yet acknowledging a substance abuse problem may again be counterproductive. During the active treatment stage, most patients accept the goal of abstinence; placing them in treatment programs and housing programs that insist on abstinence is usually helpful (Drake et al., 1991a; Noordsy and Fox, 1991). Similarly, abstinence orientation is entirely consistent with the comprehensive treatment plan when a patient is in the relapse prevention stage.

Summary and Conclusions

Substance use disorders (abuse and dependence) are extremely common (approximately 50 percent) among people with severe mental illnesses in community mental health settings. The rate is probably even higher among high-risk groups, such as young men with a history of violence or homelessness, and among patients in acute care settings. Psychiatric patients with dual disorders constitute an extremely heterogeneous population, which makes assessment a complex task. Nevertheless, detection, diagnosis, and treatment planning can be improved considerably by attending to standard procedures.

Substance use disorder among severely mentally ill patients is correlated with poor adjustment in several domains and with negative short-term outcomes. Nevertheless, specific treatments that integrate mental health and substance abuse treatments for patients with dual disorders are effective. Substance abuse treatment should be provided in stages, over the long term, by dual-diagnosis experts.

References

Ananth, J., Vanderwater, S., Kamas, M., Brodsky, A., Gamal, R., and Miller, M. (1989) Missed diagnosis of substance abuse in psychiatric patients. *Hospital and Community Psychiatry,* 40:297–299.

Arana, J.D., Hastings, B., and Herron, B. (1991) Continuous care teams in intensive outpatient treatment of chronic mentally ill patients. *Hospital and Community Psychiatry,* 42:503–507.

Babor, T.F., De Lafuente, J.R., Saunders, J., and Grant, M. (1989) *AUDIT: The alcohol use disorders identification test, guidelines for use in primary care.* Geneva: World Health Organization.

Barbee, J.G., Clark, P.D., Crapanzano, M.S., Heintz, G.C., and Kehoe, C.E. (1989) Alcohol and substance abuse among schizophrenic patients presenting to an emergency service. *Journal of Nervous and Mental Disease,* 177:400–407.

Bartels, S.J., Drake, R.E., and McHugo, G.J. (1992) Alcohol use, depression, and suicide in schizophrenia. *American Journal of Psychiatry,* 149:394–395.

Bartels, S.J., Drake, R.E., and Wallach, M.A. (1995) Long-term course of substance use disorders among patients with severe mental illness. *Psychiatric Services,* 46:248–251.

Bartels, S.J., Teague, G.B., Drake, R.E., Clark, R.E., Bush, P., and Noordsy, D.L. (1993) Service utilization and costs associated with substance abuse among rural schizophrenic patients. *Journal of Nervous and Mental Disease,* 181:227–232.

Bartels, S.J., and Thomas, W.N. (1991) Lessons from a pilot residential treatment program for people with dual diagnoses of severe mental illness and substance use disorder. *Psychosocial Rehabilitation Journal,* 15:19–30.

Belcher, J.R. (1989) On becoming homeless: a study of chronically mentally ill persons. *Journal of Community Psychology,* 17:173–185.

Bond, G.R., McDonel, E.C., Miller, L.D., and Pensec, M. (1991) Assertive community treatment and reference groups: an evaluation of their effectiveness for young adults with serious mental illness and substance abuse problems. *Psychosocial Rehabilitation Journal,* 15:31–43.

Breakey, W.R., Goodell, H., Lorenz, P.C., McHugh, P.R. (1974) Hallucinogenic drugs as precipitants of schizophrenia. *Psychological Medicine,* 4:255–261.

Carey, K.B. (1989) Emerging treatment guidelines for mentally ill chemical abusers. *Hospital and Community Psychiatry,* 40:341–342, 349.

Carey, K.B. (in press) Substance use reduction in the context of outpatient psychiatric treatment: A collaborative, motivational, harm reduction approach. *Community Mental Health Journal.*

Carey, M.P., Carey, K.B., and Meisler, A.W. (1991) Psychiatric symptoms in mentally ill chemical abusers. *Journal of Nervous and Mental Disease,* 179:136–138.

Caton, C.L.M., Grannick, A., Bender, S., and Simon, R. (1989) Young chronic patients and substance abuse. *Hospital and Community Psychiatry,* 40:1037–1040.

Cournos, F., Empfield, M., Horwath, E., McKinnon, K., Meyer, I., Schrage, H., Carrie, C., and Agasin, B. (1991) HIV seroprevalence among patients admitted to two psychiatric hospitals. *American Journal of Psychiatry,* 148:1225–1229.

Dixon, L., Haas G, Weiden, P., Sweeney, J., and Frances, A. (1990) Acute effects of drug abuse in schizophrenic patients: clinical observations and patients' self-reports. *Schizophrenia Bulletin,* 16:69–79.

Donovan, D.M. (1988) Assessment of addictive behaviors: implications of an emerging biopsychosocial model. In Donovan, D.M., Marlatt, G.A. (eds.), *Assessment of Addictive Behaviors,* pp. 3–48. New York: Guilford Press.

Donovan, D.M., Kivlahan, D.R., and Walker, R.D. (1986) Alcoholic subtypes based on multiple assessment domains: validation against treatment outcome. In Galanter, M. (ed.), *Recent Developments in Alcoholism,* 4:207–222. New York: Plenum Press.

Drake, R.E., Alterman, A.I., and Rosenberg, S.R. (1993a) Detection of substance use disorders in severely mentally ill patients. *Community Mental Health Journal,* 29:175–192.

Drake, R.E., Antosca, L., Noordsy, D.L., Bartels, S.B., and Osher, F.C. (1991a) New Hampshire's specialized services for people dually diagnosed with severe mental illness and substance use disorder. In Minkoff, K., Drake, R.E. (eds.), *Dual Diagnosis of Major Mental Illness and Substance Disorder,* pp. 57–67. San Francisco: Jossey-Bass.

Drake, R.E., Bartels, S.J., Teague, G.B., Noordsy, D.L., and Clark, R.E. (1993b) Treatment of substance abuse in severely mentally ill patients. *Journal of Nervous and Mental Disease,* 181:606–611.

Drake, R.E., McHugo, G.J., and Noordsy, D.L. (1993c) Treatment of alcoholism among schizophrenic outpatients: four-year outcomes. *American Journal of Psychiatry,* 150:328–329.

Drake, R.E., and Mercer-McFadden, C. (1995) Assessment of substance use among persons with chronic mental illness. In Lehman, A., Dixon, L. (eds.), *Double Jeopardy: Chronic Mental Illness and Substance Abuse,* pp. 47–62. New York: Harwood Academic Publishers.

Drake, R.E., Mueser, K.T., Clark, R.E., and Wallach, M.A. (in press) The natural history of substance disorder in persons with severe mental illness. *American Journal of Orthopsychiatry.*

Drake, R.E., and Noordsy, D.L. (1994) Case management for people with coexisting severe mental disorder and substance use disorder. *Psychiatric Annals,* 24:427–431.

Drake, R.E., Osher, F.C., Noordsy, D.L., Hurlbut, S.C., Teague, G.B., and Beaudett, M.S. (1990) Diagnosis of alcohol use disorder in schizophrenia. *Schizophrenia Bulletin,* 16: 57–67.

Drake, R.E., Osher, F.C., and Wallach, M.A. (1989) Alcohol use and abuse in schizophrenia: a prospective community study. *Journal of Nervous and Mental Disease,* 177:408–414.

Drake, R.E., and Wallach, M.A. (1989) Substance abuse among the chronic mentally ill. *Hospital and Community Psychiatry,* 40:1041–1046.

Drake, R.E., and Wallach, M.A. (1993) Moderate drinking among people with severe mental illness. *Hospital and Community Psychiatry,* 44:780–782.

Drake, R.E., Wallach, M.A., Teague, G.B., Freeman, D.H., Paskus, T.S., and Clark, T.A. (1991) Housing instability and homelessness among rural schizophrenic patients. *American Journal of Psychiatry,* 148:330–336.

Durrell, J., Lechtenberg, B., Corse, S., and Frances, R.J. (1993) Intensive case management of persons with chronic mental illness who abuse substances. *Hospital and Community Psychiatry,* 44:415–416, 428.

Fariello, D., and Scheidt, S. (1989) Clinical case management of the dually diagnosed patient. *Hospital and Community Psychiatry,* 40:1065–1067.

Fox, T., Fox, L., and Drake, R.E. (1992) Developing a statewide service system for people with co-occurring severe mental illness and substance use disorder. *Innovations and Research,* 1(4):9–13.

Galanter, M., Castenada, R., and Ferman, J. (1988) Substance abuse among general psychiatric patients: Place of presentation, diagnosis, and treatment. *American Journal of Drug and Alcohol Abuse,* 142:211–235.

Galletly, C.A., Field, C.D., and Prior, M. (1993) Urine drug screening of patients admitted to a state psychiatric hospital. *Hospital and Community Psychiatry,* 44:587–589.

Kashner, T.M., Rader, L.E., Rodell, D.E., Beck, C.M., Rodell, L.R., and Muller, K. (1991) Family characteristics, substance abuse, and hospitalization patterns of patients with schizophrenia. *Hospital and Community Psychiatry,* 42:195–197.

Kline, J., Bebout, R., Harris, M., and Drake, R.E. (1991) A comprehensive treatment program for dually diagnosed homeless people in Washington, D.C. In Minkoff, K., Drake, R.E. (eds.), *Dual Diagnosis of Major Mental Illness and Substance Disorder,* pp. 95–106. San Francisco: Jossey-Bass.

Kofoed, L. (1991) Assessment of comorbid psychiatric illness and substance disorders. In Minkoff, K., Drake, R.E. (eds.), *Dual Diagnosis of Major Mental Illness and Substance Disorder,* pp. 43–55. San Francisco: Jossey-Bass.

Kofoed, L.L., Kania, J., Walsh, T., and Atkinson, R.M. (1986) Outpatient treatment of patients with substance abuse and coexisting psychiatric disorders. *American Journal of Psychiatry,* 143:867–872.

Lamb, H.R. (1982) Young adult chronic patients: the new drifters. *Hospital and Community Psychiatry,* 33:465–468.

Lamb, H.R., and Lamb, D.M. (1990) Factors contributing to homelessness among the chronically and severely mentally ill. *Hospital and Community Psychiatry,* 41:301–305.

Lehman, A.F., Herron, J.D., Schwartz, R.P., and Myers, C.P. (1993) Rehabilitation for young adults with severe mental illness and substance use disorders: a clinical trial. *Journal of Nervous and Mental Disease,* 181:86–90.

Lehman, A.F., Myers, C.P., and Corty, E. (1989) Assessment and classification of patients with psychiatric and substance abuse syndromes. *Hospital and Community Psychiatry,* 40: 1019–1025.

Lehman, A.F., Myers, C.P., Corty, E., and Thompson, J. W. (1994) Prevalence and patterns of "dual diagnosis" among psychiatric inpatients. *Comprehensive Psychiatry,* 35:1–5.

Lieberman, J.A., Kinon, B. J., and Loebel, A.D. (1990) Dopaminergic mechanisms in idiopathic and drug-induced psychoses. *Schizophrenia Bulletin,* 16:97–110.

McCarrick, A.K., Manderscheid, R.W., and Bertolucci, D.E. (1985) Correlates of acting out behaviors among young adult chronic patients. *Hospital and Community Psychiatry,* 44: 259–261.

McHugo, G.J., Drake, R.E., Burton, H.L., and Ackerson, T.M. (in press) A scale for assessing the stage of substance abuse treatment in persons with severe mental illness. *Journal of Nervous and Mental Disease.*

Mercer-McFadden, C., and Drake, R.E. (submitted) *A review of 13 NIMH demonstration projects for young adults with severe mental illness and substance abuse problems.* Rockville, MD: Community Support Program, Center for Mental Health Services, U.S. Department of Health and Human Services.

Miller, W.R., and Rollnick, S. (1991) *Motivational Interviewing: Preparing People to Change Addictive Behavior.* New York: Guilford Press.

Minkoff, K. (1989) An integrated treatment model for dual diagnosis of psychosis and addiction. *Hospital and Community Psychiatry,* 40:1031–1036.

Minkoff, K., and Drake, R.E. (eds.) (1991) *Dual Diagnosis of Major Mental Illness and Substance Disorder.* San Francisco: Jossey-Bass.

Mueser, K.T., Drake, R.E., and Miles, K.M. (in press) The course and treatment of substance use disorder in patients with severe mental illness. *National Institute of Drug Abuse (NIDA) Research Monographs.* Rockville, MD: U.S. Department of Health and Human Services.

National Institute of Drug Abuse (1989) *National household survey on drug abuse, population estimates 1988.* DHHS Publication Numer (ADM) 89–1636. Washington, D.C.: U.S. Govt. Print. Office.

Nikkel, R., and Coiner, R. (1991) Critical interventions and tasks in delivering dual diagnosis services. *Psychosocial Rehabilitation Journal,* 15:57–66.

Noordsy, D.L., and Fox, L. (1991) Group intervention techniques for people with dual disorders. *Psychosocial Rehabilitation Journal,* 15:67–78.

Osher, F.C., and Kofoed, L.L. (1989) Treatment of patients with psychiatric and psychoactive substance abuse disorders. *Hospital and Community Psychiatry,* 40:1025–1030.

Pepper, B., Kirshner, M.C., and Ryglewicz, H. (1981) The young adult chronic patient: overview of a population. *Hospital and Community Psychiatry,* 32:463–469.

Regier, D.A., Farmer, M.E., Rae, D.S., Locke, B.Z., Keith, S.J., Judd, L.J., and Goodwin, F.K. (1990) Comorbidity of mental disorders with alcohol and other drug abuse: results from the Epidemiologic Catchment Area (ECA) study. *Journal of the American Medical Association,* 264:2511–2518.

Ridgely, M.S., Goldman, H.H., and Willenbring, M. (1990) Barriers to the care of persons with dual diagnoses: organizational and financing issues. *Schizophrenia Bulletin,* 16:123–132.

Ridgely, M.S., Osher, F.C., and Talbott, J.A. (1987) *Chronic mentally ill young adults with substance abuse problems: treatment and training issues.* Baltimore, MD: University of Maryland Mental Health Policy Studies Center.

Safer, D.J. (1987) Substance abuse by young adult chronic patients. *Hospital and Community Psychiatry,* 38:511–514.

Stone, A.M., Greenstein, R.A., Gamble, G., and McLellan, A.T. (1993) Cocaine use in chronic schizophrenic outpatients receiving depot neuroleptic medication. *Hospital and Community Psychiatry,* 44:176–177.

Teague, G.B., Schwab, B., and Drake, R.E. (1990) *Evaluating programs for young adults with severe mental illness and substance use disorder.* Arlington, VA: National Association of State Mental Health Program Directors.

Test, M.A., Wallish, L., Allness, D.J., and Burke, S.S. (1989) Substance use in young adults with schizophrenic disorders. *Schizophrenia Bulletin,* 15:465–476.

Vaillant, G.E. (1983) *The Natural History of Alcoholism.* Cambridge, MA: Harvard University Press.

Wallen, M.C., and Weiner, H.D. (1989) Impediments to effective treatment of the dually diagnosed patient. *Journal of Psychoactive Drugs,* 21:161–168.

Yesavage, J.A., and Zarcone, V. (1983) History of drug abuse and dangerous behavior in inpatient schizophrenics. *Journal of Clinical Psychiatry,* 44:259–261.

Zisook, S., Heaton, R., Moranville, J., Kuck, J., Jernigan, T., and Braff, D. (1992) Past substance abuse and clinical course of schizophrenia. *American Journal of Psychiatry,* 149:552–553.

26

Community Service Systems for Children and Adolescents

MICHAEL BOGROV
RAYMOND L. CROWEL

Children's mental health services are somewhat like the weather. There is much talk, but until recently very little action. . . . The most recent estimates suggest that two thirds of the seriously mentally ill children and adolescents do not even get services, and countless others get inappropriate services.

(Knitzer, 1984)

Although in many ways the state of children's community mental health services has changed little since Knitzer's observation, there have been dramatic changes in certain aspects. These changes include an emphasis on the least restrictive setting, the introduction of care management, and the increased influence of the many stakeholders in the system. Mental health services have had to respond to state reform initiatives, such as family preservation, and other system reforms, as well as changes in funding and legal mandates. Prevention and early intervention approaches, as well as an expanded continuum of services, have resulted in improved services to children with serious emotional disturbances, but have presented challenging problems for clinicians. This chapter provides an overview of the issues, goals, and progress made in the field.

Children's community mental health in general, and community child psychiatry in particular, advocates a community-based, systems focused, population-oriented, multidisciplinary approach to the mental health needs of children. Community child psychiatry is not specifically differentiated as a subspecialty within child and adolescent psychiatry because much of the field acknowledges the importance of these aspects of care. The difference, however, is in the degree of emphasis, the manner of application, and the level of integration of the various components.

Children's mental health service needs differ markedly from those of adults. To begin with, the target populations are very different: adult services focus primarily on the chronically mentally ill, whereas children's services are broader-based. In addition,

other agencies have strong interest in children's mental health services because of
shared goals, and they are becoming more involved in the design of systems and
determination of the intended impact. Perhaps the biggest difference is that, whereas
the goal for adults is generally to promote independent living, the goal with children
is for them to remain with or return to their families, and to the support systems in
which they are involved.

Community child psychiatry advocates not simply community-based treatment, but
a recognition of the importance of this multilevel system as both a resource and a risk
factor in a child's life. In contrast to interventions that remove a child from his or her
natural support system, there is an emphasis on maintaining the child at home and
using the available natural support systems. Hospitalization and residential treatment
are important clinical options, but in a community orientation they are interventions
of last resort. In less restrictive interventions, such as outpatient therapy or day programs, every attempt is made to utilize the community in the treatment model, make
the interventions relevant to the child's natural environment, and advocate for each
child's community to be as responsive to the child's needs as possible. (Stroul, 1988)

Community child psychiatry recognizes that each component of the child's system
influences outcomes. The goal is not simply to diminish those influences, but to utilize
them in prevention and treatment. Using a systems approach, it is not enough for only
one small component of the system to be addressed. The goal of community child
psychiatry is to build and forge linkages within the overall system, making it more
responsive to all children, and particularly to those children with serious emotional
disturbances.

Children's community mental health is multidisciplinary at each level of intervention. In regard to the individual child, there is a recognition that children with serious
emotional disturbances often have educational, recreational, language, social, or physical problems also. From a population-based perspective, there is a need to utilize all
available providers in order to meet the projected service demands. From a system
point of view, the goal is an understanding and coordination of each agency's goals
and operating procedures in order to develop an integrated service system for children.

History

In 1896, the first clinic for children was founded by William Lightner at the University of Pennsylvania, with a focus on helping children with school problems. By the
start of the twentieth century the mission had expanded to include discovering the
causes of juvenile delinquency and developing successful interventions. Under the influence of William Healey, the first child-focused multidisciplinary team consisting of
a physician, a psychologist, and a social worker was employed by the Illinois Juvenile Psychopathic Institute in 1909. A further boost in the development of the child
guidance movement occurred when the National Committee for Mental Hygiene's
1915 survey of school children revealed the extent of mental health problems in chil-

dren and the meager services and resources available to meet those needs. Even so, it was not until 1922 that the first child guidance clinics were funded by the Committee's own demonstration grants and programs. The child guidance movement and the use of multidisciplinary teams were given a stronger base with the founding of the American Orthopsychiatry Association in 1924.

There has long been a historical interest in developing a national model for helping children with serious emotional disturbances. In 1930, the White House Conference on Children called for national and state agencies to provide for the development of a comprehensive plan on behalf of handicapped children (Joint Commission on the Mental Health of Children, 1969). Under NIMH, established in 1949, the child guidance model continued its development and evolution until the advent of community mental health centers in late 1960s. Contemporary mental health centers, though markedly expanded in scope and approaches, still contain many of the ideas and approaches of the child guidance movement, most notably the use of multidisciplinary teams (Achenbach, 1974).

Legislative mandates on other child-serving agencies have also influenced the development of mental health services. One such mandate was the 1974 Education for All Handicapped Children Act, referred to most commonly as PL 94-142. In this sweeping legislation, children who were categorized as ''severely emotionally disturbed'' were guaranteed access to all services necessary to obtain an education. This law galvanized an advocacy force seeking to ensure that children with special needs would receive adequate and commensurate services in the least restrictive setting. It also brought child and adolescent psychiatrists into the educational mainstream.

In addition to the legislative process and the child guidance movement, another significant influence on the field has been the reliance on public funding for services, and associated demands for accountability. This has contributed to an increased emphasis on time-limited diagnostic and treatment services, in contrast to long-term dynamic therapy. As a consequence, and in conjunction with scientific and philosophical changes in the field, innovative and less restrictive approaches were developed, and the spectrum of treatment models expanded considerably. In 1969, the Joint Commission on Mental Health of Children specifically referred to a *continuum of care,* which was reinforced in 1978 by the President's Commission on Mental Health (Behar, 1984).

Perhaps the most significant influence on the development of community mental health services for children in the United States was the Child and Adolescent Service System Program (CASSP). CASSP was established by the National Institute of Mental Health to help develop the infrastructure for providing child mental health services. The philosophy of CASSP was that interventions should be child and family centered, community based, and culturally competent. As a result of this program's growth, there is now a well-articulated *system of care* approach which applies these fundamental tenets, and which is the basis of much of the current work in the field of community child psychiatry (Stroul et. al., 1994).

A Public Health Approach

Epidemiology

Offord and Fleming (1991) note three administrative implications of epidemiological findings in child psychiatry. First, given that 12 percent of the child population suffers from one or more psychiatric disorders, and 3 percent can be considered seriously emotionally disturbed (Knitzer, 1982), a broad array of personnel other than simply mental health clinicians will have to be utilized in the intervention system. Second, given the vast need and the limitation of resources, specialized services should be specifically targeted to those children most in need and most likely to benefit. Third, the high prevalence rates indicate that prevention programs are essential to addressing the problem of childhood mental illness.

A major goal for epidemiology is to identify factors that increase or decrease risk of morbidity. Risk factors, which can be genetic, biological, environmental, familial, or ecological, have been defined as "those factors that increase a child's likelihood developing an emotional or behavioral disorder when compared with a child from the general population (Garmezy, 1983). Protective factors are defined as "those factors that modify, ameliorate, or alter a person's response to some environmental hazard that predisposes to a maladaptive outcome" (Rutter and Quinton 1984). These can be characteristics of the child, the child's family, or the community in which the child lives.

Prevention Programs

In community child psychiatry there is a strong emphasis on prevention programs. This emphasis is essential both for practical and for philosophical reasons. Practically, it is unlikely that there will ever be enough clinicians to treat children after they have developed a disorder, so that it is much more realistic to use resources for primary prevention to reduce the incidence of emotional problems. There are also questions of whether it is more difficult to treat some disorders after they are established. Philosophically, it is not clear that the current means of allocating resources actually target the appropriate children (Behar, 1990), or that earlier interventions may be more likely to do so.

Community psychiatrists must therefore have an awareness of risk and protective factors in order to develop preventive programs that have a community-wide impact (Lorion and Ross, 1992). For example, there is ample evidence that children of parents with psychiatric illness are at greater risk of psychiatric disorder themselves (Rutter and Quinton 1984). Screening for parents who have evidence of a genetically transmitted psychiatric disorder is an example of an appropriate preventive intervention. As another example, community psychiatry programs have developed crisis response teams to support communities or schools at greatest risk for exposure to violence and have utilized wraparound services to alleviate some of the worst impacts of poverty

(Behar, 1992), based on the knowledge that exposure to violence and poverty are significant risk factors for emotional and conduct disorders. Reducing out-of-home placements is an example of an intervention derived from an understanding that removing a child from the home has been identified as a contributor to risk for psychiatric disorder (Rutter, 1979).

Programs that are based on an understanding of protective factors have also been developed. Social competence is a protective factor; in the school-age period, affective education and training in social problem solving are competency-enhancing interventions. Family protective factors include a supportive relationship with at least one consistent, caring parent and adequate resources to stimulate the child's healthy growth and development; preventive interventions can include programs for children of divorce or parent training (Rae-Grant et al., 1989). Community factors, as demonstrated by Werner and Smith (1982), include the support provided by extended family and other supportive adults. In response, self-help and support groups have been utilized for mothers of preschool children and children of divorce, and similar efforts have decreased the social isolation of parents at risk for abusing their children.

Prevention programs have been categorized by their methodological approach, such as providing positive competencies, increasing self-help and supportive systems, and addressing systems changes (Stroul and Friedman, 1986), as presented above, and by their target populations, such as specific age groups, high-risk groups, and communities (Offord, 1987). Head Start is an example of a program that has targeted a specific age group, disadvantaged preschool children, that is at risk for a specific psychiatric risk factor, mental retardation (Offord, 1987). High-risk programs have targeted hospitalized children, children with chronic medical illness, siblings of delinquent children, and children of substance-abusing parents (OSAP, 1991). Community-wide programs have included modifying the manner in which children make the transition from one school to another, specific strategies in particular settings, or reducing opportunities for at-risk behaviors, such as the use of drugs or alcohol (OSAP, 1991).

Systems of Care

The concept of a *system of care* acknowledges that each service agency (i.e., mental health, child welfare, juvenile justice) may have a continuum of services, but together, along with the families they serve, these agencies form a system. The system not only includes program and service components, but also integrating mechanisms, arrangements, structures, or processes, to ensure that the services are provided in a coordinated, cohesive manner. There are many reasons for this approach: Children can get lost ''between the cracks'' of multiple agencies; funding for necessary services may be tied to a specific program so that children may not qualify because of their sponsoring agency; or all of the necessary services may be provided, but there may be duplication, lack of focus, or conflict between the different agencies.

A system of care is not merely a set of services or programs. The concept provides

Table 26–1   Ten guiding principles of a system of care (Stroul and Friedman, 1986)

1. Emotionally disturbed children should have access to a *comprehensive array* of services that address the child's physical, emotional, social, and educational needs.
2. Emotionally disturbed children should receive *individualized* services in accordance with the unique needs and potentials of each child, and guided by an individualized service plan.
3. Emotionally disturbed children should receive services within the least restrictive, *most normative environment* that is clinically appropriate.
4. The *families* and surrogate families of emotionally disturbed children should be full participants in all aspects of the planning and delivery of services.
5. Emotionally disturbed children should receive services that are *integrated*, with linkages between child-caring agencies and programs, and mechanisms for planning, developing, and coordinating services.
6. Emotionally disturbed children should be provided with case management or similar mechanisms to ensure that multiple services are delivered in a *coordinated* and therapeutic manner, and that they can move through the system of services in accordance with their changing needs.
7. *Early identification and intervention* for children with emotional problems should be promoted by the system of care in order to enhance the likelihood of positive outcomes.
8. Emotionally disturbed children should be ensured *smooth transitions to the adult service system* as they reach maturity.
9. The rights of emotionally disturbed children should be protected, and *effective advocacy* efforts for emotionally disturbed children and youth should be promoted.
10. Emotionally disturbed children should receive services *without regard to race, religion, national origin, sex, physical disability, or other characteristics*, and services should be sensitive and responsive to cultural differences and special needs.

a philosophical approach to working with the most challenging children across multiple agencies. Stroul and Friedman (1986) have outlined ten "guiding principles" of a system of care (Table 26–1), several of which merit further elaboration. The provision of individualized services requires that children not be plugged into existing standardized treatment programs, but that a very specific set of interventions should be designed for one child at a time (Burchard et al., 1993). Resources dedicated to the care of children must remain flexible so that they can be utilized in an individualized manner. Collaborating staff must adopt a "whatever is necessary" approach to addressing problems and needs that fall outside of traditional roles.

Emphasizing the least restrictive, most normative environment is in marked contrast to the idea of extricating a child from his natural surroundings in order to provide treatment. Rather than bringing the child to a residential program, for example, it is as if the residential program were brought to the child and his family. There is an acknowledgement in practice that the most important and potentially beneficial influence on the child is his family and home.

The use of a strengths-based, ecological orientation is an important principle of care. "While traditional assessments tend to emphasize pathology and service needs, assessments for individualized care emphasize the child's and family's assets as well as deficits" (Stroul and Friedman, 1986). In other words, rather than simply trying to find out what is wrong, there is an equally concerted effort to find out what is right with the child and family. There is an implicitly decreased emphasis on blame or correction, and an increased emphasis on empowerment. The ecological orientation requires that resources be sought within the child's own domain, rather than provided from within a program's purview, and that these be the building blocks for a successful intervention.

Closely related to strengths-based ecological approaches are principles of cultural sensitivity and responsiveness. There needs to be an in-depth understanding and respect for the ways in which cultures differ in their expression of symptomatology, their attitudes and values regarding normalcy and help-seeking, and their preferred methods of intervention. These considerations must be addressed with considerable caution in order to avoid stereotyping, while ensuring that the individuals' desires and needs are truly understood and appropriately addressed.

Finally, another dramatic attitudinal shift required with the system of care orientation is that care be "unconditional." The commitment to the child is absolute, and service teams do whatever is necessary in the interest of the child. This is in marked contrast to the traditional abstinence or administrative discharges based primarily on a family's or child's noncompliance.

A system of care should include case management, self-help and support groups, advocacy, transportation, legal services, and volunteer programs. Again, considering these components as essential to care requires a paradigm shift. It must be recognized that what helps to keep children in the system and to provide communication among the various services is as critical as the specific interventions themselves (Homonoff and Maltz, 1991).

The Role of Families in the System of Care

Community psychiatry must be sensitive to variations in the structure and definition of family. All too often, families have been either ignored or viewed as the origins of much child pathology. In a successful system of care, however, the family is regarded not only as vital to successful treatment outcomes, but as a legitimate and necessary member of the treatment team.

Families have their own areas of expertise and skills, and they can bear much of the responsibility for executing the treatment plan. Collins and Collins (1990) has identified five important factors in enhancing the parent-professional relationship: acceptance of parents as full-fledged members of treatment teams; professional willingness to share all relevant information; two-way, jargon-free communication; focus of treatment planning on strengths and assets of child and family as well as needs; and joint decision making between parents and professionals.

The definition of family may include not only two-parent, biological, nuclear families, but may also be extended to include fictive kin or neighbors (Franklin, 1989). The family may be blended, single-parent, or "non-traditional" in many ways. All of these forms of families are included in a comprehensive approach.

Interagency Coordination

Children with serious emotional disturbances are likely to be receiving intensive services from multiple agencies; the more agencies with which a child is involved, and the greater the intensity of services provided, the higher the likelihood that the child will have a serious emotional disturbance. Thus the need for interagency coordination is crucial. Without sufficient coordination, given the historic fragmentation of children's service agencies, severely emotionally disturbed children are likely to be poorly served because of the considerable gaps in the services they receive (Stroul and Friedman, 1986). For this reason, community child psychiatry programs must foster strong working relationships with other child care agencies. These include, at a minimum, schools, primary health care providers, child welfare agencies, juvenile justice systems, adult community psychiatry programs, and substance abuse services. The ultimate goal is not simply collaboration, but for all of these agencies to constitute one seamless system of care (Lourie, 1994).

There are several basic elements to good interagency working relationships. Community child psychiatry programs should help ensure that each of these elements exists with each agency. All agencies should be familiar with the basic issues faced by other agencies. Thus, child welfare workers should have a concept of general mental health principles, and mental health clinicians should have a working knowledge of abuse, neglect, foster care, juvenile justice, education, and other issues that are the primary focus of concern for the other agencies. In addition to a basic familiarity with other agencies, each agency should have a well-developed screening and referral program, preferably designed in collaboration with other service agencies and with attention to barriers that an outside agency might encounter. There should be the capacity for case consultation between agencies, and for interagency support in planning crisis response in areas where one agency may have expertise. There needs to be coordination of interventions and a mechanism for ongoing feedback regarding all of the services. Additionally, there should be interagency flexibility to address problems that fall outside the normal service roles of agencies in the system.

The Mental Health Continuum of Care

As a part of the broader system of care, the mental health services continuum provides for assessment and treatment interventions in the setting most appropriate for individual children and families. Settings can range from the outpatient clinic to the home to the day program to the inpatient unit. For severely mentally disturbed children, specific criteria should be established for placement on the continuum.

Assessment is probably the most important component of a mental health service continuum. It often sets the tone for the entire service system in that it describes the child for all involved and aligns the system with a certain trajectory. Assessment must be comprehensive, incorporating data from all available sources. Offord and Fleming (1991) reported that rates of childhood disorder depend greatly on the informant; each component of the service system has a unique perspective on the child. In giving due weight to input from all the data sources, a message is given to all that their perspectives are valued and that they are part of the intervention team. It also serves a crucial educational function by reflecting to others how their observations can be understood.

Outpatient services. Outpatient services have traditionally been the primary intervention for child psychiatry, but home-based services are increasingly popular and among the fastest-growing sectors in the continuum of care. One significant factor in this growth is the cost of out-of-home residential placements and an attempt to find alternatives. Home-based programs are predicated on a high intensity of service, with maximum accessibility and optimal involvement with parents and children. They target children at risk for out-of-home placement and are crisis-oriented. In light of the demand, in-home services are typically time-limited, with small caseloads (Hinkley and Ellis, 1985). To some extent, in-home services, such as the well-known Homebuilders model, provide the traditional mental health interventions in a different setting (Knitzer, 1982) but also rely heavily on social casework, referral, and advocacy services. There is evidence that interventions such as these are effective in reducing residential placement and are also cost-effective.

Day programs. In a similar attempt to be cost-effective, to maintain children in the least restrictive environment, and to draw on the strengths and resources of the families, day programs are utilized increasingly. Day programs provide a high-intensity service in a therapeutic setting on a daily basis while maintaining the child at home within the family. Partial hospitalization programs for children range from long-term programs in collaboration with school systems, to full day, intermediate term interventions, to part day or after-school programs. Such programs usually combine a special education approach, individual, group, and family therapies, recreational activities, and skill-building interventions. Depending on what other elements there are in the system of care, long-term day programs can provide an alternative to residential placement; short-term day programs can serve as either a step-down or step-up unit as an alternative to hospitalization. The part-day programs are particularly useful for maintaining children in the least restrictive setting while providing therapeutic services and support on a daily basis, and they are particularly helpful for working parents.

Emergency services. Emergency services have historically in many cases been the first point of contact for children with severe emotional disturbances, but they have not always been well incorporated into the mental health system. There are many ways, however, that they can serve an integrated function. They can provide a range of services from prevention to stabilization. Services can include crisis prevention, 24-hour phone lines, outpatient services, mobile units, and back-up to in-home services, including provision of a therapist to go into the home.

Schools

It is essential that community child psychiatry programs develop close working relationships with schools. Schools not only have a significant impact on children with serious emotional disturbance, they are often the initial site of detection and referral. Seriously emotionally disturbed children are at higher risk for disciplinary interventions, retention, and exhibition of high-risk behaviors such as truancy, school refusal, and violence (Rutter et al., 1979). Many interventions require coordination between the mental health program and the school and efficient interactions between the teachers and mental health professionals. For outpatients, there needs to be coordination with the school around medication administration, behavioral expectations and interventions, and the logistics of appointments. The last may be as simple as ensuring that the child does not miss the same class each time, or more complex, such as arranging for transportation to the clinic.

In order to facilitate effective collaboration, not only should teachers know how to access mental health services, they must have an understanding of how to screen for emotional problems. They should understand that poor academic performance or disruptive behavior may be a first indicator of psychiatric problems. In fact, most teachers readily identify openly disruptive behaviors; additional education is needed to assist them in identifying more internalizing behaviors, such as depression and anxiety. Incorporating a mental health component into the school's response to absenteeism or aggression, for example, may help detect potentially amenable emotional disturbance.

"Inclusion" of disturbed children in regular classrooms requires attention to the school environment, which can be a critical and powerful protective factor in the clinical outcomes of both severely mentally disturbed and at-risk children (Rutter, 1979). It is important to address such issues with school staff, but this is a particularly sensitive issue to raise and requires the utmost tact and attention to the consultative process. Raising the level of awareness of developmental issues, and in particular keeping the exchange of information practical and collegial, are essential for success.

Social Services

Community child psychiatry also has significant overlap of areas of concern with departments of social services. The more obvious issues are those of physical abuse and neglect, sexual abuse, foster care, and family preservation, but social service agencies are the focal point for many child-based policies. They are often the principal agencies through which society expresses its attitude toward children. The numbers of children who are victims of abuse are staggering. Almost 6 children per thousand are victims of physical abuse, while the figure for sexual abuse is 2.5 per thousand. It is estimated that one million children each year in the United States are victims of neglect. Each year 173,000 children are injured or impaired, and there are between 2,000 and 5,000 deaths as a result of abuse.

There are several approaches to prevention in the area of child abuse. These include parent education programs, broad-based media campaigns or crisis hotlines, and targeting of high-risk families. In addition to primary prevention programs, mental health and social service agencies can work together to raise the community level of awareness of abuse, its causes, and the required response upon its detection. Children who are victims of abuse benefit if all of the agencies involved in the response coordinate the investigative procedure. This includes not only child protective services and mental health services, but the courts and primary-care and pediatric services. It has been demonstrated that children benefit from a comprehensive approach that minimizes the number of investigative interviews (Baker, 1989).

Earlier strategies for the treatment of child abuse have focused on psychotherapy, though more recent approaches emphasize engaging the families of these children (Brunk et al., 1987). The need for this new approach is reflected in the high rates of psychopathology among the parents of abused children, including depression and substance abuse. Histories frequently reveal that the parents themselves have been abused. Child psychiatry programs can be most effective if they work with agencies that are already mandated to intervene with parents. In this way there is a greater likelihood of success and continuity of care with a group that is otherwise difficult to engage.

Foster Care and Family Preservation

Coordination between mental health clinicians and foster care and family preservation programs is important because the rates of psychiatric disorder among foster care children are far higher than in the general population. Even if the children placed in foster care were at no greater risk than their peers prior to the events that resulted in a placement, the typical sequence of events and the separation from family are quite stressful. Children have often been the victims of significant physical, emotional, or sexual abuse, neglect, or a traumatic life event that leaves the biological family unable to care for the child. It has been demonstrated that children placed outside the home will be at higher risk of emotional problems if they do not have a stable placement (Rutter and Quinton 1984); ensuring that foster parents are aware of the stresses involved in caring for a child in need, and that they are are provided with an adequate support system, is in the best interest of the child. In addition, foster parents must be prepared to become partners with the many agents intervening on behalf of the child, not only the foster care program staff, but mental health providers, special educators, pediatricians, and the child's biological parents.

The interface between foster care and mental health programs includes the adequate screening of children, training of foster parents, informed child-centered planning for case disposition, and coordination of interventions with foster care workers. Many interventions are now provided that were once considered innovative, but have been shown to be essential, such as respite planning and in-home services. The Homebuilders model (Kinney et al., 1977) is one example of an approach targeted toward maintaining the child in the family of origin. The in-home services are typically multifaceted, including skill training, helping families obtain resources, and counseling. Services are based on need rather than categorical placement, and workers have small caseloads so as to allow for the intensity of service. Most use a time-limited intervention with follow-up and evaluation.

Child community psychiatry programs and social service agencies can also be partners in addressing the issues of homelessness. Identifying children at risk for an especially adverse response to homelessness, or helping to identify hidden strengths or resources such as a stable family member, are appropriate mental health contributions. Simply identifying the link between the child's presentation and homelessness can be a significant intervention.

Juvenile Justice

Criminal activity is one of the most pressing problems faced by child and adolescent psychiatry. The extent of the problem is clear. Thirty percent of all persons arrested nationally in 1990 were under the age of 21; the crime index of arrests for serious crimes shows that 43 percent were committed by persons under the age of 21 and 28 percent by persons under the age of 18; 1.75 million juveniles were arrested in 1990; in 1985, 83,000 children, on average, were held daily in detention and correctional facilities; the cost of vandalism in schools alone is $200 million each year (Zigler et al., 1992). Homicide has become a national epidemic. Overall, it is the second leading cause of injury-related deaths among all children and adolescents in the United States (Hammond and Yung 1993). Among African Americans aged 15–34, homicide was the leading cause of death in 1992 (National Center for Health Statistics, 1992). The extent of the problem is great, but many mental health professionals are ambivalent about working with offenders (American Psychiatric Association, 1993).

Not least among the many difficulties inherent in the area is the multiplicity of symptoms and neuropsychiatric issues associated with aggressive and assaultive behavior. The problem of differential diagnosis is important to both juvenile authorities and mental health providers. Many psychiatric disorders, such as depression or psychosis, can result in antisocial activities and aggression (Lewis, 1991).

Within the juvenile justice system there are several opportunities to introduce therapeutic strategies into an essentially punitive structure. Coordination with the juvenile courts is important to utilize effectively the mechanisms of court referrals and court-ordered treatment. Juvenile service workers provide crucial links in screening and referral. Probationary strategies need to be combined with treatment in appropriate cases and should be incorporated into an overall treatment plan. In a number of places a more ecological approach has been developed and found to be effective (Bordin et al., in press). In its "Willie M." program, the state of North Carolina, in response to a class action suit, allocated $27 million to provide community-based programs for previously institutionalized children. In the majority of these cases, "the threat of violence decreased dramatically," and 80 percent of children were rated as receiving "some . . . [or] significant benefit." (Keith, 1988).

Primary Health Care

Primary health care is a critical component of any system of care, and primary-care providers can serve as resources for mental health providers in several ways. Primary-care providers are crucial in that they provide a familiar and non-stigmatized point of contact for families who have known them over time. Often they can provide important additional history, such as early developmental progress, which may be relevant to particular emotional disturbances. In addition, primary-care providers have access to siblings who may be significantly at risk. In managed care systems, the primary-care practitioner is often the gatekeeper for psychiatric services, and frequent updates may be required to maintain the child in treatment. In some settings, the pediatrician provides lab work or monitors medications. At a minimum, the primary-care provider can assist by reinforcing compliance with treatment plans and by monitoring progress.

Coordination between primary-care providers and mental health services must be mutually supportive. A community child mental health program can offer, for example, information, education, and support for managing the child in the pediatrician's office, or the program can assist in family and other interagency issues (Rafferty, 1991).

Legal Issues

Many legal issues arise in the care of children with severe emotional disturbances. Legal issues often take on an interagency focus as many of the questions cross agency lines. This reinforces the need for cross-agency training so that the resolution of legal questions does not become a barrier to care.

The most important legal questions usually have to do with consent to treatment and confidentiality. Particularly for children who are in the custody of another agency, the question of who can authorize treatment requires clear guidelines, and the answer may be dependent on the level of intervention intended. For example, authorization for the use of medication is more crucial than for behavioral therapy. Providing for an emergency placement, including hospitalization or residential treatment, requires a still higher level of consent. Each state has specific guidelines for a minor's consent or assent to treatment. Just as with a guardian's consent, the child's rights are dependent on the intervention proposed. The questions are particularly important when they concern a minor's emancipation. Similarly, issues of confidentiality are considerable when working across a system of care. The extent to which agencies can and should have clinical information, and under what circumstances, are usually complicated and tension-producing questions for those involved.

Legal questions can be raised concerning issues outside the mental health system. Many parents will turn to the clinician for assistance in understanding the special education referral process. An understanding of the law may be one of the most powerful interventions a mental health provider can offer. Other examples include reporting of abuse or neglect, accessing residential placement, or advocating for the least restrictive placement for institutionalized children. The community child psychiatrist must also be familiar with the state's provisions for children who are in need of guardianship or extra supervision.

Cultural Competence

There is ample evidence that different cultural groups vary in their risk for certain disorders or risk factors. It has become equally clear that ethnicity should be a factor in designing treatment programs. The integration of these issues into the development of mental health services is referred to as *cultural competence*. Cross and colleagues (1989) define cultural competence in this way:

> The word *culture* is used because it implies the integrated pattern of human behavior that includes thoughts, communications, actions, customs, beliefs, values and institutions of a racial, ethnic, religious, or social group. The word *competence* is used because it implies having the capacity to function in a particular way: the capacity to function within the context of culturally integrated patterns of human behavior as defined by the group.

A culturally competent system values diversity, has the capacity for cultural self-assessment, is conscious of the dynamics inherent when cultures interact, has institutionalized cultural knowledge, and has developed adaptations to service delivery reflecting an understanding of cultural diversity. This ideal is generally not attainable without an overt and concerted effort on the part of mental health administrations (Hanley, 1995).

Within a culturally competent system, therapists are especially sensitive to the risk of misinterpretation based on differences in the use of language, religious differences, or values in parenting styles. Inherent in culturally competent systems is the professional's awareness of his or her own culture and potential biases toward other ethnic groups. At management and policy levels, the culturally competent system addresses issues of diversity in hiring and promotion of staff, and ensures that services are acceptable to these being served (Chapter 11).

The Psychiatrist in the System of Care

From a community mental health perspective, and particularly within a system of care, the community child psychiatrist must adapt to a changing role. While previously authority was vested by virtue of a title, a psychiatrist's influence is increasingly derived from the relationships built within the multidisciplinary team of professionals representing several agencies.

The roles of the psychiatrist are still many. Some remain an absolute province, such as prescription of medications. The most crucial role derives from the psychiatrist's training in diagnosis and synthesis of information. The process of ascertaining the phenomenology of a complex problem and organizing the information, recommending interventions, and assessing prognosis remains an invaluable mechanism for understanding a child's difficulties. It provides perspective for a team and an excellent means for determining efficacy. Through this type of effort, the psychiatrist can become an integral and essential team member, using knowledge of medications and neurobiological, genetic, and psychodynamic models to add an additional perspective, rather than diminishing other equally vital views of the child.

Psychiatrists' roles have been limited in the past, and will continue to be limited, by virtue of availability. Availability may be limited for many reasons such as time constraints, limited number of child psychiatrists, and financial disincentives. Solving this problem requires that child community psychiatrists understand, join forces with, and make use of all the components of the system. This means accepting an even greater leadership role in developing and managing a system of care that provides comprehensive services to children. Training for child psychiatrists should include a clear understanding of how to work effectively within a system of care, an in-depth understanding of and respect for the roles of other agencies and families in the system, and an increase in direct community-based experience.

References

Achenbach, T. (1974) *Developmental Psychopathology.* New York: Ronald Press.

American Psychiatric Association (1993) *Violence and Youth: psychology's response. Volume I: Summary Report of the APA Commission on Violence and Youth.* Washington, DC: American Psychiatric Association.

Baker, P. (1989) *Clinical Interviews with Children and Adolescents.* New York: W.W. Norton Co.

Behar, L. (1984) An integrated system of services for seriously disturbed children. Presented at the ADAMHA/OJJDP State of the Art Research Conference on Juvenile Offenders with serious Alcohol, Drug Abuse and Mental Health Problems. Rockville, MD: ADAMHA.

Behar, L. (1990) Financing mental health services for children and adolescents. *Bulletin of the Menninger Clinic,* 54:127–139.

Behar, L. (1992) *Fort Bragg child and adolescent mental health demonstration project.* Raleigh, North Carolina, Division of Mental Health, Developmental Disabilities, and Substance Abuse Services, Child and Family Services Branch.

Borduin, C.M., Mann, B.J., Cone, L.T., and Henggeler, S.W. Multisystemic treatment of serious juvenile offenders. (1995) *Journal of Consulting and Clinical Psychology,* 63:569–578.

Brunk, M., Henggeler, S.W., and Whelan, J.P. (1987) Comparison of multisystemic therapy and parent training in the brief treatment of child abuse and neglect. *Journal of Consulting and Clinical Psychology,* 55:171–178.

Burchard, J.D., Burchard, S.N., Sewell, R., and VanDenBerg, J. (1993) *One Kid at a Time. Evaluative Case Studies and Description of the Alaska Youth Initiative Demonstration Project.* Burlington, VT: Department of Psychology, University of Vermont.

Collins, B., and Collins T. (1990) Parent-professional relationships in the treatment of seriously emotionally disturbed children and adolescents. *Social Work,* 35:522–527.

Cross, T.L., Bazron, B.J., Dennis, K.W., and Isaacs, M.R. (1989) *Towards A Culturally Com-*

petent System of Care: A Monograph on Effective Services for Minority Children Who Are Severely Emotionally Disturbed. Washington DC: CASSP Technical Assistance Center.

Franklin, N.B. (1989) *Black Families in Therapy.* New York: Guilford Press.

Garmezy, N. (1983) Stressors of childhood. In Garmezy, N., Rutter, M. (eds.), *Stress, Coping and Development in Children.* Minneapolis: McGraw-Hill.

Hammond, W., and Yung, B. (1993) Psychology's role in the public health response to assaultive violence among young African-American men. *American Psychologist,* 48:142–154.

Hanley, J. (1995) On cultural competence in southern states. Personal Communication.

Hinckley, E.C., and Ellis, W.F. (1985) An effective alternative to residential placement: home-based services. *Journal of Clinical Child Psychology,* 14:209–213.

Homonoff E.E., and Maltz P.F. (1991) Developing and maintaining a coordinated system of community-based service to children. *Community Mental Health Journal,* 27:347–358.

Joint Commission on the Mental Health of Children (1969) *Crisis in Child Mental Health: Challenge for the 1970s.* New York: Harper and Row.

Keith, C.R. (1988) Community treatment of violent youth: seven years of experience with a class action suit. *Journal of the American Academy of Child Adolescent Psychiatry,* 27: 600–604.

Kinney, J.M., Madsen, B., Fleming, T., and Haapala, D.A. (1977) Homebuilders: keeping families together. *Journal of Consulting and Clinical Psychology,* 45:667–673.

Knitzer, J. (1982) Unclaimed children: the failure of public responsibility to children and adolescents in need of mental health services. Washington DC: Children's Defense Fund.

Knitzer, J. (1984) Developing systems of care for disturbed children. Rochester, N.Y., Institute for Child and Youth Policy Studies.

Lewis, D.O. (1991) Conduct Disorder. In Lewis, M. (ed.), *Child and Adolescent Psychiatry: A Comprehensive Textbook.* Baltimore: Williams & Wilkins.

Lorion, R.P., and Ross, J.G. (eds.) (1992) OSAP special issue: Programs for change: Substance Abuse Prevention Demonstration Models. *Journal of Community Psychology.* Brandon, VT.

Lourie, I. (1994) *Principles of Local System Development.* Chicago: Kaleidoscope.

National Center for Health Statistics (1992) Annual Report. Rockville, MD.

Office for Substance Abuse Prevention, U.S. Department of Health and Human Services. (1991) *The future by design: a community framework for prevention of alcohol and other drug problems through a systems approach.* DHHS Publication No. (ADM) 91-1760. Rockville, MD.

Offord, D.R. (1987) Prevention of behavioral and emotional disorders in children. *Journal of Child Psychology and Psychiatry,* 28:9–19.

Offord, D.R., and Fleming, J.E. (1991) Epidemiology. In Lewis, M. (ed.), *Child and Adolescent Psychiatry: A Comprehensive Textbook.* Baltimore: Williams & Wilkins.

Rae-Grant, N., Thomas, B.H., Offord, D.R., and Boyle, M.H. (1989) Risk, protective factors, and prevalence of behavioral and emotional disorders in children and adolescents. *Journal of the American Academy of Child Adolescent Psychiatry,* 28:262–268.

Rafferty, F.T. (1991) Effects of health delivery systems on child and adolescent mental health care. In Lewis, M. (ed.), *Child and Adolescent Psychiatry: A Comprehensive Textbook.* Baltimore: Williams & Wilkins.

Rutter, M., Maughan, B., Mortimori, P., and Auston, J. (1979) *Fifteen Thousand Hours: Secondary Schools and Their Effects on Children.* London: Open Books.

Rutter, M. (1979) Protective factors in children's responses to stress and disadvantage. In Kent, M.W., Rolf, S.E.J.E. (eds.), *Primary Prevention of Psychopathology: Social Competence in Children, Vol. 3.* Hanover: University of New England.

Rutter, M., and Quinton, D. (1984) Parental psychiatric disorder: effects on children. *Psychological Medicine,* 14:853–880.

Stroul, B.A., and Friedman, R.M. (1986) *A System of Care for Severely Emotionally Disturbed Children and Youth.* Washington DC: CASSP Technical Assistance Center.

Stroul, B. (1988) *Series on Community-Based Services for Children and Adolescents Who Are Severely Emotionally Disturbed.* Washington, DC: CASSP Technical Assistance Center.

Stroul, B.A., Lourie, I.S., Goldman, S.K., and Katz-Leavy (1994) *Profiles of Local Systems of Care.* Washington, DC: CASSP Technical Assistance Center.

Werner, E.E., and Smith, R.S. (1982) *Vulnerable But Invincible: A Longitudinal Study of Resilient Children and Youth.* New York: McGraw Hill.

Zigler, E., Taussig, C., and Black, K. (1992) Early childhood intervention: a promising preventative for juvenile delinquency. *American Psychologist,* 47:997–1006.

27

Community Services for Older Persons

SUSAN W. LEHMANN
PETER V. RABINS

With the exception of dementia and its psychiatric complications, older persons suffer from the same types of mental disorders as younger persons. Many treatment issues are independent of age, and many standards of mental health practice can be implemented regardless of age; however, psychiatric disorders in the elderly often co-exist with medical, social, and functional impairments that are uncommon in younger patients. This chapter will address the design and implementation of psychiatric services for the elderly that incorporate these special needs and will review several aspects of serious and persistent mental illnesses in older persons that are uniquely relevant in their treatment.

Epidemiology and Access to Care

Community studies have generally found that the prevalence rates of schizophrenia, bipolar disorder, and major depression are lower among the elderly than among middle-aged individuals. In the Epidemiologic Catchment Area (ECA) study of the National Institute of Mental Health, the one-month prevalence rate for schizophrenia was 0.1 percent for persons over age 65, but 0.6 to 0.8 percent for persons between 18 and 64 years. Similarly, among persons 65 years and older, prevalence rates of major depression were found to be one-third of the rate found for the 45- to 64-year-old age group. These results have been challenged on many fronts: greater reluctance of the elderly to acknowledge psychiatric symptoms, difficulty identifying psychiatric disorder in persons with medical illness, high concentrations of depression among older persons in settings such as nursing homes that are not usually included in epidemiologic samples, and different symptom patterns in the elderly. The original report of the ECA study itself acknowledged the possibility that some form of cognitive impairment, such as pseudodementia from severe depression, may have falsely lowered the prevalence rates of serious mood disorder in the older group (Regier et al., 1988). To date, however, no data have been generated to refute these lower prevalences. However, other smaller community-based studies have noted a high frequency of clinically significant depressive *symptoms* among elderly persons (approximately 15 percent). This has led some to speculate that the formal diagnostic categories of major depression and dysthymia do not include the majority of older persons suffering from disabling depressive symptoms (Blazer et al., 1987; Blazer, 1994). The prevalence of cognitive disorder clearly rises with age, so that both delirium and dementia are most common in individuals 75 years of age and older (Regier et al., 1988).

Epidemiologic studies confirm that the elderly mentally ill are less likely to receive needed services than younger individuals. Over 12 percent of the population in the United States is over age 65, but less than 5 percent of people over age 65 receive outpatient mental health services (Lebowitz et al., 1987; Light et al., 1986). Of subjects in New Haven and Baltimore in the ECA study, only 4–15 percent of persons age 65 or older with a psychiatric disorder had made ambulatory mental health visits in the past 6 months. In contrast, 20 percent of persons age 45–64, and 17–24 percent of persons age 25–44 with psychiatric disorders had made mental health visits in the preceding 6 months (Shapiro, et al., 1984). At the same time the elderly population in America is growing rapidly. It is estimated that by 2030 one in five Americans will be age 65 and older. Furthermore, more older people are living into their eighties and nineties. By the year 2000, it is estimated that 35 million Americans will be over age 65, and almost half of them will be 75 years or older (Kasper, 1988). Thus, even if the prevalence of serious mental illness is somewhat lower among older persons, the elderly remain a markedly underserved group.

The dramatic reduction in the number of long-term beds in state psychiatric hospitals in the past 20 years has significantly affected needs for housing. Many severely and persistently mentally ill persons who at one time lived for years and even decades in psychiatric hospitals are now living in nursing homes, in private board and care homes, in adult foster care situations, and in public housing for the elderly. In recent years a number of studies have shown that psychiatric symptoms are widespread and underdiagnosed among elderly residents in these settings. H. Richard Lamb (1979) called board and care homes "the new asylums in the community." Rovner and colleagues (1986) found that over 90 percent of residents in a community nursing home had a mental disorder diagnosable by DSM-III criteria. In a study of elderly residents of urban public housing, the one-month prevalence of DSM-III psychiatric disorders was 31.4 percent (Roca et al., 1990). In the past, psychiatrists have worked in hospitals, private offices, and outpatient clinics, but few have seen patients in nursing homes, much less in private homes. Clearly, there is a need for psychiatrists to become involved in delivering mental health care to elderly patients at nontraditional sites.

We believe that plans for community-based psychiatric service for the elderly should focus on at least five important goals: (1) to alleviate significant psychiatric symptoms and their related morbidity; (2) to promote individual independence in a safe environment; (3) to decrease social isolation and promote increased social contacts; (4) to provide support services to caregivers; and (5) to improve quality of life for elders. In order to achieve these goals, community psychiatric services for the elderly must include the following important components: (1) identification of cases (referral network); (2) diagnosis and treatment; (3) education of those who refer and care for the elderly; (4) support for caregivers; and (5) an array of community support services.

An important issue in improving access to care is to improve coordination of care among the programs serving older patients. Light and colleagues (1986) found that community mental health centers with specialized programs for the elderly had significantly higher utilization rates by older patients than did centers without such programs. Utilization rates by older patients were highest at community mental health centers that also had developed coordinated links with other community agencies serving the psychosocial needs of the elderly. These community agencies, such as adult protective services, visiting nurse associations, and home health services, are often under the auspices of local area agencies on aging. This should make coordination easier to achieve, although inter-agency tensions sometimes prevent this.

Overcoming Barriers to Care

Breaking down barriers of stigma is not easy; efforts to educate and improve communication with non-psychiatric physicians about mental illness is vital. A number of investigators have found that older people are more likely to present mental health complaints to their general medical physician than to seek out psychiatric care (Waxman et al., 1984; German et al., 1985). In addition, it has been estimated that the prevalence of major depressive disorders is 10 percent among medical outpatients with chronic diseases (Borson et al., 1986). Family physicians and internists need to be educated about the symptoms of depression which may manifest as gastrointestinal distress, headaches, fatigue, insomnia, anxiety, or other somatic symptoms. Many physicians may be reluctant to refer their elderly patients to psychiatrists because of mental health biases and misconceptions (e.g., "Psychiatrists don't really help people") and undue pessimism (e.g., "It's normal to be depressed when you have as many problems as she has"). Yet failure to treat depressive disorder in older patients with co-existent medical illness is associated with patient failure to improve in physical functioning (Harris et al., 1988). Thus, a crucial aspect of community psychiatric services for the elderly is establishing referral networks and links with internists, family physicians, and others who may be treating older patients.

In addition, older persons themselves are often reluctant to seek mental health care because of concerns about the stigma of mental illness. Today's cohort of elderly individuals was born in the first several decades of this century. They grew up before Social Security, Medicare, and Medicaid existed, when individuals had to rely almost solely on the goodwill of family, church, and charity during times of hardship. They also lived through the Great Depression of the early 1930s and two world wars. Many were raised with beliefs that one should "pick one's self up by the boot straps," and that to ask for help with mental problems would be indicative of personal and moral failure. They also came into adulthood at a time when the family physician was often seen as a member of the family who could be turned to for any medical problem. As a result it is not surprising that older people with psychiatric or emotional problems are more likely to present first to internists and family physicians and may refuse to seek help for psychiatric symptoms.

The Psychiatrist's Role in Community Psychiatric Service

A comprehensive psychiatric evaluation and proper diagnosis is essential to developing an appropriate plan for treatment. The psychiatrist's medical background makes him or her uniquely trained to interface between the medical, neurological, pharmacologic, and psychosocial issues that often co-exist with or complicate psychiatric symptoms. In addition to treating elderly patients in traditional private offices, clinic settings, and community mental health centers, psychiatrists also function as liaison consultants to general physicians on medical and surgical hospital services, and increasingly as consultants to nursing homes, life care communities, or other resident communities for the elderly. However, with increasing scarcity of resources (both clinical and financial), the psychiatrist may not always be the one providing the direct treatment of the patient. Often the psychiatrist may be supervising other mental health professionals such as psychiatric nurse clinicians and social workers, who also provide supportive therapy and family therapy.

The psychiatrist must work closely with all other physicians involved in the care of the patient. It is not uncommon for older patients to count among their regular physicians cardiologists, ophthalmologists, orthopedists, rheumatologists, oncologists, GI specialists, and neurologists, in addition to internists or family physicians. Close communication among all health professionals treating a given patient is essential for avoiding polypharmacy and for minimizing the chances of adverse psychiatric and biologic effects of medication. For instance, elderly patients on digoxin or coumadin who are subsequently started on fluoxetine for depression will need to have digoxin or coumadin levels monitored more closely to prevent possible toxicity. Similarly, the elderly patient on lithium carbonate whose primary-care physician recommends a nonsteroidal anti-inflammatory drug for arthritis will need more frequent checking of lithium levels and possible lowering of the dose to prevent lithium toxicity.

It is also important to establish good rapport with all family members and significant others involved in the day-to-day life of the psychiatrically ill older individual. Family members and home care assistants are important sources of historical information as well as being sources for information on response to treatment. They may provide information about previous interests and activities which might become part of the treatment goals. Moreover, they may assist in providing transportation to appointments and encourage or supervise adherence to recommended treatment plans.

In addition to providing diagnosis and treatment of psychiatric symptoms, the psychiatrist is often called on by family and others to provide guidance on issues related to guardianship, competency, and nursing home placement for an elderly individual. Expertise in these area is not common in those who do not treat the elderly.

Psychiatric Outreach to the Elderly

Transportation is a barrier to receiving psychiatric care for many mentally ill elderly people. Limited finances, cognitive impairment, physical disability, or inability to drive or use public transportation make it difficult for many older people to get access to traditional psychiatric care. In-home services and on-site programs (nursing homes, senior centers) described below can be used to address this issue in part. Telephone contact is sometimes crucial to ongoing care. Psychiatric home visits and outreach programs are increasingly being used to meet the mental health needs of various older populations.

In one innovative program in Baltimore County, small teams made up of a psychiatrist, psychiatric nurses, and psychiatric social workers make home visits to homebound elderly people with psychiatric disorders for evaluation and to promote ongoing treatment. In this program, most of the patients have a late-life-onset psychiatric disorder (usually major depression or anxiety disorder). Cases are often referred for evaluation from other agencies for the elderly such as Visiting Nurse Associations or local senior center staff, but cases may also be generated by family members (De Renzo et al., 1991). In addition, there have been a number of reports of psychiatric outreach programs to elderly residents in urban public housing. In one such program in Baltimore City, a team of two nurses and two psychiatrists provide psychiatric evaluation and treatment to residents who are referred by building management staff. This program, known as PATCH (for psychogeriatric assessment, treatment, and teaching in public housing) was developed in 1987 (Roca et al., 1990). Another outreach program has been described in Central City in San Francisco in which a multidisciplinary team of psychiatrists, nurse clinicians, social workers, and aides provide outpatient mental health services to elderly people living in federally subsidized housing (Heim, 1985).

Community Support Services for the Elderly

While always a mobile society, Americans have become much more likely to move since the second world war. This has undoubtedly affected the family life of many older individuals. While the majority of elderly persons still live within one hour's drive of a child (Kovar, 1986), many older individuals have children and other family members who live significant distances away. This is likely the first cohort of the elderly for whom this is true and is a change from their experiences during their youth when close geographic ties among family members were the rule. Thus, loss of family social supports and loneliness are common psychosocial factors that compound the stresses of retirement, widowhood, and physical disability.

Many community services are available to combat the isolation that can result from loss of family support. Senior centers are gaining in popularity as places where seniors can form new friendships, exercise, learn new leisure hobbies, hear interesting lectures, and take organized bus trips. They tend to be located in or near residential neighborhoods and therefore tend to attract seniors with similar socioeconomic backgrounds. Most senior centers are open 5 days per week and offer lunch. Many churches also have clubs or senior groups with similar programs. For older patients whose physical abilities are more limited by medical problems and/or cognitive impairment, medical day care programs should be considered. These programs have on-site nurses who can monitor medications and vital signs in addition to providing structured activities and socialization. Many medical day care programs also provide transportation and are usually open during normal working hours, a boon to working families caring for an elderly relative. However, fees for medical day care can vary considerably and often are not covered by medical insurance.

Increasingly, for older people who cannot get out, in-home services are becoming available to help maintain them safely in their homes. These include Meals-on-Wheels, a service that delivers a hot mid-day meal and occasionally a cold supper to housebound persons aged 60 and older. Meals-on-Wheels is funded under the Older Americans Act (OAA) of 1965. In addition, many private agencies as well as some public agencies are now providing in-home services such as *visiting nurses* who may monitor medication compliance and vital signs and/or provide short-term specialized nursing care; *personal care aides* to assist in bathing, dressing, and light housekeeping services; *companions* who provide safe supervision and socialization; and *friendly visitors,* lay volunteers who register with local senior centers and the local Office on Aging and who will visit older persons at home once a week for general conversation or to help with simple errands. These services can be crucial supplements to the outpatient psychiatric treatment of older patients with early dementia or major depression who are temporarily (or permanently) unable to care for themselves independently and safely at home.

Mental health professionals treating older patients in the community need to be aware of the range of community services that their patients may need, including respite programs and support services for care-givers. The difficulties of providing regular personal and physical care to persons with chronic physical or psychiatric illness is a concern that is receiving more attention today. Care-givers themselves experience very high rates of depression, anger, and loss, as well as fatigue, isolation, loss of financial supports, and financial strain (Rabins et al., 1982). It is often most fruitful to address these issues with family or professional care-givers while also treating the patient's psychiatric or behavior disorder. In addition, care-givers benefit from local support groups such as Alzheimer's disease and Parkinson's disease support groups. Medical day care programs, as noted earlier, may provide needed day-time respite and support for care-givers of persons with dementia. Many nursing homes now also provide short-term (i.e., days to weeks) respite care, which can enable a caregiver to take a much-needed break. Service providers also need to be aware of local services that can be contacted if there are concerns about elder abuse, financial exploitation of an older person by friends or family, or incapacity of an older person to care for himself. These services are usually provided by public departments of social services.

Finally, mental health professionals who treat elderly persons in the community must be able to call on emergency and/or intensive psychiatric care options. Inpatient psychiatric hospitalization is a necessity for patients who are suicidal or whose judgment is so impaired by psychotic symptoms or cognitive decline that outpatient treatment is not safe for them or others. Inpatient psychiatric treatment is usually the best and safest avenue for treatment of patients with severe depression, the frail elderly, and patients with multiple medical problems. However, another option for intensive psychiatric treatment is partial hospitalization. As overall lengths of stay in psychiatric inpatients units are decreasing, many psychiatric hospitals are establishing partial hospitalization programs in which patients are treated intensively during weekdays but return to their own homes for the evenings and during weekends. This model of care is usually less expensive than traditional inpatient treatment but can be as effective as inpatient treatment for many patients. However, partial hospitalization is only appropriate for patients who are not a danger to themselves or others, who have a stable home situation, and who have a reliable means of transportation to and from the hospital each day (Chapter 18).

Clinical Considerations

Special Disorders

Schizophrenia.   Schizophrenia is a life-long illness for most individuals, although the follow-up studies of Harding and coworkers (1987) suggest that long-term outcome is not as universally bad as was once feared. Nonetheless, this work and follow-up studies in other countries demonstrate that most individuals with schizophrenia severe enough to be hospitalized during their youth are left with residual social, psychological, and cognitive impairments (Cohen, 1990). Hallucinations and delusions persist in some patients and require active neuroleptic therapy, although often at doses lower than are required by younger patients. Persistent ''negative'' symptoms of apathy, disinterest, negativism, and social isolation are prevalent and require active psychosocial programs.

Schizophrenia can also begin in later life (Rabins et al., 1984). Late-onset schizophrenia is often characterized by florid delusions and hallucinations, particularly of the paranoid type. This disorder is significantly more common in women than men (with ratios of 2:1 to 8:1 being reported). Late-onset schizophrenia occurs in individuals with relatively intact personality and affects individuals who have often been seen as somewhat eccentric. It is often associated with sensory impairments such as limited hearing and vision.

For the elderly, the goal of treatment is long-term maintenance of function rather than short-term rehabilitation and job training. Many elderly individuals with schizophrenia are likely to live alone, often in public housing apartments. At times paranoid delusions may attract the attention of the building manager, who may initiate a request for psychiatric evaluation. In such cases outreach psychiatric visits may be necessary, not only to treat disabling symptoms, but also to prevent eviction. Congregate living settings such as foster homes and group homes can provide adequate care for many individuals with residual symptoms, but others require more restrictive environments; they appear to do best in long-term care settings such as state hospital units or nursing homes. Although improved service programs for this group of individuals are clearly needed, this area has rarely been studied.

Major depression.   Major depression is often the most common problem seen in the elderly in community mental health settings (Blazer et al., 1987). The co-occurrence of medical illness sometimes makes diagnosis more complex and complicates therapy because it requires that the clinician distinguish between somatic symptoms derived from physical illness or medications and hypochondriacal symptoms or delusions (Siris and Rifkin, 1981). The bizarre nature of many somatic depressive delusions and the lack of evidence of any abnormality after careful physical assessment should reassure the clinician that treatment for depression is appropriate. A number of studies have suggested that the frequency of relapse increases with increasing age; chronic relapsing depression is thus one aspect of geriatric care (Hinrichsen, 1992).

A common issue in treating elderly depressed patients is the high prevalence of side effects from anti-depressant drugs. Older persons are particularly sensitive to anticholinergic side effects (such as constipation, urinary retention, and memory impairment) and to developing orthostatic hypotension. Of these possible adverse effects, orthostatic hypotension is of greatest concern because it can lead to falls. Most clinicians advise against the use of drugs such as amitriptyline and imipramine, which have relatively high anticholinergic activity and relatively high propensity to cause orthostatic hypotension. We recommend sertraline, nortriptyline, desipramine, or fluoxetine as first-line treatment of major depression in older persons. In addition, because of its relative safety and because depression can be life-threatening in the elderly, ECT plays an important part in the therapy of some individuals.

Mania.   Mania is relatively uncommon in the elderly. There appear to be few significant differences between early- and late-life mania, and the therapy is similar (Dhingra and Rabins, 1991). Most clinicians recommend using lower doses of lithium with the goal of obtaining lower maintenance lithium blood levels in the elderly. We suggest blood levels between 0.5 and 0.8 for most older individuals.

Anxiety disorders.   Both generalized anxiety disorders and panic disorders can be seen in older individuals. The ECA study found that anxiety disorders are the most common psychiatric problems in the community across all age groups. The data also suggest they are both underdiagnosed and undertreated (Regier et al., 1988). Principles of treatment of anxiety disorders are essentially the same for older persons as for younger ones. However, benzodiazepines must be prescribed more cautiously, as will be discussed below.

Substance abuse.   Few elderly people are currently in treatment for alcohol or illicit drugs abuse, but the number is clearly increasing. While the addicting disorders are lifelong for most individuals, evidence suggests that many persons die of causes both directly and indirectly related to their addiction disorder before entering old age. Many chronically addicted patients also develop marked medical sequelae such as cirrhosis or severe gastrointestinal bleeding, which limit their ability to abuse drugs or alcohol later in life. In general, the elderly ingest less alcohol and are less likely to be heavy drinkers and more likely to be abstainers than the young. Social problems among elderly alcoholics differ from those seen among the young in that alcohol is more likely to provoke health and marital problems and is less likely to cause legal and job-related difficulties. Also, the effects of alcohol are more easily misattributed to dementia or other medical illness in the elderly (Schuckit, 1982). These factors probably lead to underdiagnosis (West et al., 1984). Late-onset alcoholism is more common in women than in men and is associated with change in psychosocial circumstances in many individuals (Wattis, 1983).

Clinical experience suggests that benzodiazepines have high addiction potential in the elderly at relatively low doses. Because of the high frequency of coexisting medical illness, withdrawal protocols should be very slow and may require inpatient treatment.

Dementia.   Dementia affects approximately 5 percent of individuals over 65 but increases dramatically in prevalence in very late life; it affects approximately 20 percent of 80-year-olds and 30 percent of 90-year-olds. At least 50 percent of patients with dementia who present to the medical health care system have behavioral, emotional, or psychiatric symptoms such as hallucinations and delusions (Rabins et al., 1982). Caring for a demented family member can be very stressful and demanding. In addition, many of the difficulties that care-givers experience result from their own emotional distress as well as directly from the behavioral and cognitive changes that occur in the demented patient. It is important for mental health professionals to teach family and professional care-givers about management strategies as well as about having their own emotional needs met (Mace and Rabins, 1981). Psychoactive medications may be needed to manage the hallucinations, delusions, agitation, and depression experienced by patients.

Medical day care can be an essential component in the treatment of the demented person and can help delay the need for nursing home placement. The patient benefits from a stimulating, structured program while the care-giver benefits from needed respite from daytime care. The treatment of dementia should include family support groups, which are an important source of help for care-givers. Groups specifically established to help with Alzheimer's disease, Parkinson's disease, and Huntington's disease have chapters nationwide.

Delirium.   Delirium is most prevalent in the elderly. The diagnostic hallmark of delirium is an altered level of consciousness or attention. This means that individuals with delirium are not only cognitively impaired but appear drowsy, inaccessible, or inattentive. Delirium is certainly most common in hospital settings. Studies have demonstrated that 30 to 50 percent of patients aged 70 or older admitted to general medical wards showed evidence of delirium at some point (Lipowski, 1987). However, delirium can develop in an outpatient setting due to psychotropic medication, non-psychotropic medication, and/or underlying metabolic abnormalities. These symptoms may first come to the attention of the mental health clinician. Delirium requires careful medical assessment since it is often caused by treatable and reversible diseases or conditions.

Mental retardation.   Few systems have been developed to care for the elderly mentally retarded with mental illness. Community surveys suggest that more than 5 percent of the population has been functioning adequately throughout adult life with borderline or mild mental retardation (Bassett and Folstein, 1991). Stressors associated with aging—such as changing medical, cognitive, social, and financial conditions—may unmask symptoms and dysfunction in this group for the first time in their life. Psychiatric illness can co-occur with mental retardation as well (Menolascino and Potter, 1989).

The illness or death of elderly parents who have been life-long care-givers may lead to the first presentation of a person with life-long cognitive limitations in their sixth or seventh decades. Elderly parents who care for aging children with mental retardation have needs that are similar to the care-giver of other chronically ill individuals (Seltzer and Krauss, 1989).

Symptom Issues in the Elderly

Suicide.   Suicide rates are higher among the elderly than in any other age group, with elderly white males comprising the single highest risk group (Conwell et al., 1991). Studies continue to suggest that most individuals who commit suicide—perhaps 90 percent—have a major mental illness including substance abuse (Conwell et al., 1991). In addition, with increasing age more suicide victims are widowed rather than single, separated, or divorced. Chronic physical illness and loss are important risk factors and are the most common precipitants to suicide in the elderly. Thus, clinicians must have a high index of suspicion and inquire about suicidal thoughts in any older individual being evaluated for a psychiatric problem. Because suicide attempts in the elderly are commonly successful, the elicitation of suicidal thoughts should lead to a consideration of inpatient hospitalization, although this is not always necessary. Careful documentation that explains why a decision was made is important.

Persistent grief.   The elderly suffer many losses through death of family, friends, and acquaintances. It is uncommon for individuals to present to mental health services primarily for therapy of grief, but some individuals do have persistent or paralyzing symptoms. The mainstays of therapy are supportive and exploratory psychotherapy along with short-term, symptom-oriented pharmacologic treatment. Many bereaved persons also suffer from concomitant sleep disorders. We recommend short-term benzodiazepine use for this symptom, although in individuals with persistent grief and depressive symptomatology an anti-depressant may treat both the sleep disorder and mood symptoms.

Self-neglect.   An uncommon psychiatric condition which occurs mostly among the elderly and which is seen by psychiatric services that treat the elderly has been called "the Diogenes Syndrome" or the "Senile Breakdown Syndrome" (Macmillan and Shaw, 1966). Individuals with these behaviors hoard large amounts of useless or minimally useful material, neglect their health, and remain indoors and socially isolated. They frequently deny symptoms of primary psychiatric disorder, are often cognitively normal, and refuse any psychosocial help or intervention. Because this is a behavior rather than a diagnosis, this "syndrome" can be seen in individuals who suffer schizophrenia, dementia, personality disorder, or alcoholism, but no specific diagnosis can be made in many cases. Clearly treatment of an underlying psychiatric disorder should be given to such persons. Public health authorities are often involved because the hoarding behavior has become a health hazard. Forced clean-up by judicial or public health authorities is often the only effective intervention.

Ethical issues.   There are few ethical issues unique to the elderly mentally ill. Nevertheless, questions of capacity to choose one's own living situation when judgment is impaired by a psychiatric illness, questions about how active a clinician should be in involving family members, and questions about when to force a medical assessment in a person with psychiatric illness who is refusing needed medical care are examples of common dilemmas. Good clinical practice mandates balancing the patient's autonomy against several factors: the capacity to decide, distortion of judgment caused by a psychiatric condition, and danger to the individual, to others in the immediate environment, and to society at large (Applebaum and Roth, 1981).

Psychodynamic issues.   In working with older persons and their families, certain psychotherapeutic issues often emerge. These often include life-long relationship issues between parents and children, and among siblings who have now aged. In addition, there may be new stresses between the generations induced by physical dependency, increasing financial dependency, or decreasing ability of parents to provide emotional, psychological, or financial support to their children. Marital issues are common as well, as spouses adjust to the changes brought on by retirement and unanticipated disability.

Implications for the Future

Will future cohorts of the elderly differ significantly from current cohorts? There is little data on which to base a prediction but several issues are of note. Certainly the need for psychiatric services for older individuals will increase in the future as today's "baby boom" generation ages. In addition, with continued advances in health care, more and more people can be expected to live to old age. Thus it is likely that there will be more senior citizens with aged parents of their own. However, if current societal trends continue, high divorce rates, geographic mobility, and disintegration of strong nuclear families may all continue, leading to further isolation and less family support for older individuals in the future.

While illicit drug and alcohol use have always been significant societal problems, they have clearly increased in prevalence among young and middle-aged individuals in the past 20 years. It is likely that this cohort behavior will be carried into late life, and that drug and alcohol service for the elderly will need to be increased.

If there is somewhat less stigma about psychiatric treatment among younger and middle-aged individuals, perhaps this will carry over into the next elderly cohort's opinions about psychiatric treatment and make it easier for services to meet needs. Moreover, today's middle-aged individuals have already distinguished themselves by their political activism. As this politically astute cohort ages, one can hope there will be more pressure from consumers for the development of services that meet the needs of older individuals.

Housing has become a central focus of comprehensive mental health service planning in recent years and will remain important in years to come. Some housing sites such as nursing homes and retirement communities are unique to the elderly and will require special consideration. Flexibility in delivery of services and expansion of psychiatric service availability in nontraditional locations will remain the hallmark of psychiatric services for the elderly.

A current trend that is likely to continue is the emphasis on outpatient rather than inpatient treatment for psychiatric problems. Expansion of outpatient services has shortened hospital stays for medical, surgical, and psychiatric patients. As a result, patients are being discharged to community-based care with greater degrees of psychiatric and medical morbidity. These trends are unlikely to reverse themselves since inpatient care delivery is unlikely to become less costly. As the percentage of elderly persons in the population continues to grow, there will be an increasing need for community psychiatrists to be knowledgeable about the special needs of this population.

References

Applebaum, P.S., and Roth, L.H. (1981) Clinical issues in the assessment of competency. *American Journal of Psychiatry,* 128:1462–1467.

Bassett, S.S., and Folstein, M.F. (1991) Cognitive impairment and functional disability in the absence of psychiatric diagnosis. *Psychological Medicine,* 21:77–84.

Blazer, D., Hughes, D.C., and George, L.K. (1987) The epidemiology of depression in an elderly community population. *The Gerontologist,* 27:281–287.

Blazer, D.G. (1994) Is depression more frequent in late life? *American Journal of Geriatric Psychiatry,* 2:193–199.

Borson, S., Barnes, R.A., Kukull, W.A., Okimoto, J.T., Veith, R.C., Inui, T.S., Carter, W., and Raskind, M.A. (1986) Symptomatic depression in elderly medical outpatients. I. Prevalence, demography, and health service utilization. *Journal of the American Geriatric Society,* 34:341–347.

Cohen, C.I. (1990) Outcome of schizophrenia into later life: an overview. *Gerontologist,* 30: 790–797.

Conwell, Y., Olsen, K., Caine, E.D., and Flannery, E.D. (1991) Suicide in later life: psychological autopsy findings. *International Psychogeriatric,* 3:59–66.

De Renzo, E.G., Byer, V.L., Grady, H.S., Matricardi, E.J., Lehmann, S.W., and Gradet, B.L. (1991) Comprehensive community-based mental health outreach services for suburban seniors. *The Gerontologist,* 31:836–840.

Dhingra, U., and Rabins, P.V. (1991) Mania in the elderly: A 5–7 year follow-up. *Journal of the American Geriatrics Society,* 39:581–583.

German P.S., Shapiro, S., and Skinner, E.A. (1985) Mental health of the elderly: use of health and mental health services. *Journal American Geriatrics Society,* 33:246–253.

Harding, C.M., Brooks, G.W., Ashikaga, T., Strauss, J.S., and Breier, A. (1987) The Vermont longitudinal study of persons with severe mental illness. *American Journal of Psychiatry,* 144:727–735.

Harris, R., Mion, L.C., Patterson, M.B., and Frengley, J.D. (1988) Severe illness in older patients: the association between depressive disorders and functional dependency during the recovery phase. *Journal American Geriatrics Society,* 36:890–896.

Heim, P. (1985) Psychiatric outreach to the mentally disabled elderly living independently. *Psychiatric Annals,* 15:673–677.

Hinrichsen, G.A. (1992) Recovery and relapse from major depressive disorder in the elderly. *American Journal of Psychiatry,* 149:1575–1579.

Kasper, J. (1988) *Aging Alone: Profiles and Projections.* A Report of The Commonwealth Fund Commission on Elderly People Living Alone. New York, U.S. Offset Corporation.

Kovar, M.G. (1986) Aging in the eighties, age 65 years and over and living alone, contacts with family, friends, and neighbors. *Advance Data from Vital and Health Statistics,* 116: 1–6.

Lamb, H.R. (1979) The new asylums in the community. *Archives General Psychiatry,* 36:129–134.

Lebowitz, B.D., Light, E., and Bailey, F. (1987) Mental health center services for the elderly: The impact of coordination with area agencies on aging. *The Gerontologist,* 27:699–702.

Light, E., Lebowitz, B.D., Bailey, F. (1986) CMHC's and elderly services: An analysis of direct and indirect services and service delivery sites. *Community Mental Health Journal,* 22: 294–302.

Lipowski, Z.J. (1987) Delirium (acute confusional states). *Journal American Medical Association,* 258:1789–1792.

Mace, N., and Rabins, P.V. (1981) *The 36-Hour Day: A Family Guide to Caring for Persons with Alzheimer's Disease, Related Dementing Illnesses and Memory Loss in Late Life.* Baltimore: Johns Hopkins Press.

Macmillan, D., and Shaw, P. (1966) Senile breakdown in standards of personal and environmental cleanliness. *British Medical Journal,* 2:1032–1037.

Menolascino, F.J., and Potter, J.F. (1989) Mental illness in the elderly mentally retarded. *Journal of Applied Gerontology,* 8:192–202.

Rabins, P.V., Mace, N.L., and Lucas, M.J. (1982) The impact of dementia on the family. *Journal American Medical Association,* 248:333–335.

Rabins, P.V., Pauker, S., and Thomas, J. (1984) Can schizophrenia begin after age 44? *Comprehensive Psychiatry,* 25:290–293.

Regier, D.A., Boyd, J.H., Burke, J.D. Jr., Rae, D.S., Myers, J.K., Kramer, M., Robins, L.N., George, L.K., Karno, M., and Locke, B.Z. (1988) One-month prevalence of mental disorders in the United States. *Archives General Psychiatry,* 45:977–986.

Roca, R.P., Storer, D.J., Robbins, B.M., et al. (1990) Psychogeriatric assessment and treatment in urban public housing. *Hospital & Community Psychiatry,* 41:916–920.

Rovner, B.W., Kafonek, S., Filipp, L., Lucas, M.J., and Folstein, M.F. (1986) Prevalence of mental illness in a community nursing home. *American Journal of Psychiatry,* 143:1446–1449.

Schuckit, M.A. (1982) A clinical review of alcohol, alcoholism, and the elderly patient. *Journal Clinical Psychiatry,* 43:396–399.

Seltzer, M.M., and Krauss, M.W. (1989) Aging parents with adult mentally retarded children: risk factors and sources of support. *American Journal Mental Retardation,* 94:303–311.

Shapiro, S., Skinner, E.A., Kessler, L.G., Von Korff, M., German, P.S., Tischler, G.L., Leaf, P.J., Benham, L., Cottler, L., and Regier, D.A. (1984) Utilization of health and mental health services. *Archives General Psychiatry,* 41:971–978.

Siris, S.G., and Rifkin, A. (1981) The problem of psychopharmacotherapy in the medically ill. *Psychiatric Clinics of North America,* 4:379–390.

Wattis, J.P. (1983) Alcohol and old people. *British Journal of Psychiatry,* 143:306–307.

Waxman, H.M., Carner, E.A., and Kelin, M. (1984) Underutilization of mental health professionals by community elderly. *The Gerontologist,* 24:23–30.

West, J.L., Maxwell, D.S., Noble, E.P., and Solomon, D.H. (1984) Alcoholism. *Annals of Internal Medicine,* 100:405–416.

28

Homelessness and Mental Health Services

PAMELA J. FISCHER
PAUL COLSON
EZRA SUSSER

And homeless near a thousand homes I stood,
And near a thousand tables pined and wanted food.
(*William Wordsworth*)

The increase in numbers of homeless people in recent years is unprecedented, as is their rapid dispersal from pockets of the largest American cities, such as New York's Bowery, to every community, however small (cf. London, 1907). Likened to "counting the grains of sand on the beach, as the tide moves in or out" (Snyder, 1984), accurate estimation of the size of the homeless population is fraught with problems unlikely to be resolved, so that a measure of the magnitude of the homelessness problem is best obtained not so much from the numbers of individuals who are homeless, but from the broad range of people who become homeless, the impact that homelessness has on those who are directly affected and on their entire communities, and the scale of the services needed to address their problems (Breakey and Fischer, 1990).

The homeless population changes with the social and economic climate of the country. Until recently, alcoholic men clustered on skid rows comprised the bulk of the homeless population, but homelessness today defies easy categorization. Its heterogeneity may best be described in terms of subgroupings linked by impoverishment. Overarching sociodemographic characteristics include youthfulness, overrepresentation of racial and ethnic minorities, particularly blacks and Hispanics, and an increasing proportion of women and children. In common with the former skid row populations, homeless people of today report eroded social relations, poor health, and frequent passage through the criminal justice system relative to the general population.

Several subgroups of particular interest with respect to their needs for service can be discerned within the homeless population. One such subgroup consists of the chronic alcoholics who, a generation ago, would have drifted to skid rows. Another subgroup consists of drug abusers, typically younger than the chronic, deteriorated alcoholics. People with mental illnesses have come to personify homelessness in the public eye since Reich and Siegel (1978) noted the transformation of New York's Bowery—perhaps the most infamous American skid row—into a "psychiatric dumping ground," linking the burgeoning "new" American homeless population with changes in mental health service policies (Lamb, 1984). It has been suggested that families with young children may be the fastest growing subgroup of the contemporary homeless population. "Runaways," children who have left their families, and "throwaways," who have been abandoned by their families, represent a subgroup of major concern; this group is heavily involved in drug and alcohol abuse, prostitution and other antisocial activities and at high risk for hepatitis and HIV infection (Hermann, 1988; Solarz, 1988)

It can be useful to lump homeless people into subgroups defined by their demographic characteristics (e.g., homeless families) or by their disorders (e.g., homeless mentally ill) for specific purposes such as defining service needs. In this discussion, we also consider characteristics that crosscut subgroups, affecting individuals' prospects for both entering and overcoming homelessness. Mental illness and substance abuse have been used to define specific groups, but also contribute to homelessness in all groups along with poverty, the experience of violence, and lack of adequate social support. In the following, we will discuss these issues and relate them to community treatment schemes.

The difficulties experienced in attempting to serve the homeless population adequately may have as much to do with the nature of assistance offered as with the characteristics of the recipients. As traditional forms of mental health treatment have often proven inadequate, new models have emerged for reaching these very disadvantaged and often difficult-to-serve patients. The second section of this chapter describes these evolving service strategies, identifying common themes and describing model programs. The final section focuses on strategies for preventing homelessness among the mentally ill, with special attention to the role of housing and HIV prevention.

Estimates of Prevalence

Although homeless populations exhibit high rates of broadly defined mental disorders, the precise magnitude of alcohol, drug, and mental disorders remains controversial because of methodological problems in this field of research. A comprehensive review of the literature since 1980 documented rates of mental health problems ranging from 2 to 90 percent, rates of alcohol problems from 4 to 86 percent, and rates of drug abuse from 1 to 70 percent (Fischer, 1991). Building on this review, Lehman and Cordray (1993) combined prevalence estimates using meta-analytic techniques to produce a narrower range of estimates, 47 to 50 percent having any mental health problem (28 to 71 percent Axis I disorders with 13 to 26 percent reported as severe and persistent), and 30 to 73 percent having any substance use disorder (26 to 67 percent alcohol, 11 to 48 percent drug use disorders). This variability can be further reduced, however, by focusing on the more rigorous studies and on specific disorders (Susser et al., 1993).

Many homeless people have more than one disorder. As many as a third of homeless adults are reported to have concurrent alcohol and drug problems, up to 25 percent have alcohol and mental disorders, around 3 percent have both mental and drug disorders, and perhaps 7 percent suffer alcohol, drug, and mental problems concurrently. The pattern of comorbidity suggests that men are more likely than women to be alcoholics without a concomitant mental illness, whereas women are more likely than men to have a mental disorder without substance abuse. Dually diagnosed homeless individuals may be the most disabled by virtue of their disorders and disadvantages because of barriers to categorical treatment (Caton et al., 1994).

It is understandable that homeless people experience high rates of emotional distress and demoralization. Studies that have used nonspecific measures of depression and distress have found rates of positive scores on such measures well in excess of rates in general populations. In studies contrasting homeless samples to domiciled comparison populations, the homeless individuals exhibit symptoms of emotional distress 2 to 8 times more frequently than the general population (Koegel et al., 1988; Breakey et al., 1989; Gelberg and Linn, 1989).

Specific Disorders

Major mental illnesses.   Prevalence rates of specific psychiatric disorders vary in different subgroups, and from place to place, but a broad consensus has emerged from a series of research studies over the past decade (Koegel et al., 1988; Breakey et al., 1989; Susser et al., 1989; Smith et al., 1992, 1993). Data from the Baltimore Homeless Study are typical: Approximately 35 percent of men and 48 percent of women were found to have a major mental illness. Schizophrenia was diagnosed in 9 percent of men and 16 percent of women, and major affective disorders in 17 percent of men and 25 percent of women.

Diagnosis alone is not sufficient to define a group of persons with special treatment needs who meet a definition of ''severely mentally ill.'' However, few studies of the homeless mentally ill have attempted to assign severity ratings. Davies and her colleagues (1987) found that three-fifths of those with psychiatric disorders in a Pittsburgh single room occupancy hotel (SRO) were judged to be moderately to extremely ill. About two-thirds of clients of the Health Care for the Homeless program with psychiatric or emotional disorders were judged to have moderate to severe disabling impairments (Wright and Weber, 1987). One-third of homeless mentally ill adults in Baltimore were deemed severely dysfunctional according to DSM-III Axis V ratings by examining psychiatrists: 56 percent of schizophrenics, 40 percent of persons with bipolar disorders, 12 percent of persons with major depression (unipolar), and 25 percent of persons with other major mental illnesses. Combining a major mental illness diagnosis with either a rating of severe dysfunction or a history of extensive hospitalization, 13 percent of homeless men and 24 percent of homeless women were designated as severely mentally ill. Based on diagnosis and symptom severity, 28 percent of homeless adults in Los Angeles were considered chronically mentally ill, and half of those were also chronic substance abusers (Koegel et al., 1988).

Alcohol use disorders.   The association of alcoholism and homelessness has long been recognized. Although the skid row public inebriate is no longer stereotypical, alcoholism remains the most pervasive health problem of homeless people (Institute of Medicine Committee on Health Care for Homeless People, 1988; Fischer, 1989). Studies using nonhomeless comparison groups demonstrate the magnitude of the problem. The prevalence of alcoholism among homeless men in Baltimore was 5 times higher, and among homeless women, 15 times higher, than in domiciled men and women sampled in the Baltimore ECA study. In Los Angeles, lifetime prevalence rates of alcohol abuse and dependence were 2.5 times greater among homeless individuals than men in the Los Angeles ECA household sample (Koegel and Burnam, 1987, 1988). Bassuk and Rosenberg (1988) determined that the female heads of homeless families were more than twice as likely to be alcohol abusers (12 percent) as a comparison group of housed indigent women in Boston (5 percent). Compared to housed families enrolled in income maintenance programs in New York, homeless families seeking emergency assistance were 2 to 4 times more likely to report problems with substance abuse in themselves or their families (Knickman and Weitzman, 1989).

There is evidence that homeless alcoholics experience the more severe forms of alcoholism. In the database from the national VA Homeless Chronically Mentally Ill Veterans Program, substance abuse problems were the single most common health problem found among veterans, with many having "oriented their lives around substance abuse for many years" (Rosenheck et al., 1988). The alcohol dependence syndrome accounted for 82 percent of the total DSM-III alcohol use disorders in homeless men and 52 percent in homeless women in Baltimore. Compared to domiciled alcoholics, homeless alcoholics have been found to exhibit more severe patterns of drinking as measured by duration, regularity, frequency, amount, and symptoms of dependence.

Other drug use disorders.   Patterns of abuse of drugs other than alcohol by homeless people have been studied much less intensively than mental illness or alcoholism, and drug use has commonly been lumped with alcohol as "substance abuse." In addition, polydrug use makes classifying users into discrete categories difficult, and the inability to differentiate between casual drug use and dependence makes interpretation of rates of drug problems in homeless populations difficult.

Reliable estimates suggest that 25 to 50 percent of homeless people use illicit drugs and that their rates of use exceed those reported for the general population (Fischer, 1989, 1991; Lehman and Cordray, 1993). For example, psychiatrists in Baltimore diagnosed drug use disorders in 22 percent of homeless men and 17 percent of homeless women (Breakey et al., 1989). Whether this degree of substance abuse reflects the stress of the homeless lifestyle or whether it represents one of the causes of homelessness, there is no doubt that, as in the case of alcohol, drug use impedes recovery from homelessness.

The impact of drug use can be gauged through changing patterns of drug use and health consequences to drug users. More than half of drug users in a Boston shelter in the mid-1980s reported marijuana use and a third used amphetamines; fewer than a tenth reported use of cocaine (8 percent), opiates (4 percent) or barbiturates (1 percent); a third of drug users reported daily use (Schutt and Garrett, 1986). However, when the shelter users were reexamined the following year, the rate of marijuana use was found to have increased by 23 percent, while use of cocaine (19 percent) and opiates (10 percent) more than doubled (Schutt, 1988). Indeed, Susser and colleagues (1989) report that as early as 1985, cocaine had become the drug of choice in New York City shelters, noting that ''27 percent had used it more than 50 times; 25 percent had used it during the past month.'' Substantial numbers of homeless drug users report habitual intravenous use of drugs such as heroin (Breakey et al., 1989; Rosenheck et al., 1988).

The link between IV drug use and AIDS is likely to increase seropositivity among the homeless (Goldfinger et al., 1994; Zolopa et al., 1994). In a study of psychiatric patients in a men's shelter, 19 percent were found to be infected with HIV; chart information suggests that half may have become infected through injection drug use (IDU) (Susser et al., 1993). A subsequent study of IDU in this population suggests that the subjects' homeless condition may be related to practices such as needle sharing and use of shooting galleries, which carry high risk for HIV transmission. Similarly, homeless youth are also at high risk for HIV infection and other sexually transmitted diseases due to drug use and prostitution (Robertson, 1988, Rotheram-Borus et al., 1991).

Other disorders.   Personality disorders, anxiety disorders, phobias, and a variety of depressive syndromes are also very frequent in homeless people. Personality or characterological problems are particularly salient to homelessness because they interfere badly with an affected individual's ability to function successfully. Studies that have examined samples of men and women in shelters for single homeless people report prevalence rates of personality disorder varying from 21 percent (Bassuk et al., 1984) to 42 percent (Breakey et al., 1989). When homeless mothers in Massachussetts family shelters were examined, 71 percent were diagnosed with personality disorders (Bassuk et al., 1986). In the Los Angeles Skid Row Study, Koegel and his colleagues (1988) found antisocial personality disorders in nearly a third of the sample—a rate substantially greater than that observed in the ECA household population. The most frequently diagnosed DSM-III personality disorders in the Baltimore Homeless Study were of the paranoid, schizoid, and antisocial types, affecting 28 percent of men and 22 percent of women. This group was found to be less likely to have completed high school, more likely never to have married, and less likely to have friends than other homeless adults. The findings were consistent with the interference with formation of supportive and lasting personal relationships associated with these disorders.

Correlates of Mental Disorders

Demographic correlates. Where sex comparisons are drawn, prevalence estimates in homeless populations reflect gender-associated relationships reported in the general population. The Baltimore Homeless Study found that although the prevalence of schizophrenia and bipolar disorders in women was double that in men, the rates for major depression (unipolar) and other major mental illnesses were the same. Alcoholism is to be found in all age groups and in both sexes, but studies consistently report substantially higher prevalence rates for alcoholism in men than in women (Fischer, 1991; Smith et al., 1993), and homeless alcoholics tend to be older than other homeless people. Although rates of drug abuse in older homeless people are substantial, suggesting that prolonged drug abuse may increase risk of homelessness, drug abusers cluster in the younger age groups of the homeless. Robertson and her colleagues (1989) found that homeless adolescents were 5 times more likely to have DSM-III diagnoses of drug abuse or dependence than a comparison sample of high-risk nonhomeless adolescents.

Poverty. Higher prevalence rates of mental illnesses in lower socioeconomic groups in the community have been documented for many years (Hollingshead and Redlich, 1958; Cohen, 1993), which raises the question of whether the homeless are different in this respect from other poor, but domiciled, groups. A comparison of data from the Baltimore Homeless Study with data from the Baltimore ECA sample shows that although the prevalence of schizophrenia, for example, was 3 times greater in poor (1.8 percent) than in non-poor domiciled subjects (0.6 percent), this rate is still very much less than that in the Baltimore homeless (10.5 percent). The magnitude of the difference would suggest that the homeless population, in this respect, is qualitatively different.

Public income support programs appear to be having relatively little impact. Mulkern and her colleagues (1985) reported that respondents with high probability of mental disorder were more likely to be receiving some form of public support, but only 6 percent received SSI benefits. These findings were confirmed in Baltimore: In spite of apparently better access to public funds, three-fifths of those with major mental illnesses reported monthly incomes of less than $150, and four-fifths reported monthly incomes less than $300. In three counties in California, mentally ill homeless respondents were more likely to be in receipt of some form of public support than other homeless persons, but the rates of benefits were extremely low. Only 12 percent of the seriously mentally disordered received SSI or SSDI; only 22 percent received Medi-Cal or Medicare (Vernez et al., 1988).

Social support.   Social support is an area that has not been clearly delineated by research findings. Through the mid-1980s, the homeless were often viewed as isolates and loners; this picture was reinforced by research studies suggesting that large numbers had no friends or relatives (see Bassuk et al., 1984; Rossi et al., 1986; Roth et al., 1985). However, through use of a more inclusive definition of social support, Sosin and his colleagues (1988) found less striking differences between homeless and domiciled respondents. There is evidence of greater disaffiliation among disordered subgroups, particularly mentally ill homeless persons (Vernez et al., 1988) and those with alcohol problems (Koegel et al., 1988; Mundy et al., 1990). It remains unclear, however, whether these problems in the social networks are cause or effect of the homeless experience. The case for a causal role is advanced by evidence that early problems in the social network may increase later vulnerability to homelessness. For example, almost half of former psychiatric patients in a New York City shelter sample had been placed away from their families as children (Susser et al., 1987). Nearly two-fifths of a Minneapolis sample of homeless adults had a history of placement as a child (Piliavin et al., 1988).

Violence.   Exposure to violence and victimization early in life, defined broadly to include adverse childhood conditions as well as specific abusive experiences, establishes patterns of behavior that contribute to adult vulnerability to a host of adverse experiences, including homelessness (Fischer, 1992). Childhood antecedents, especially abuse and out-of-home placements, have been identified as risk factors for homelessness (Caton et al., 1994; Piliavin et al., 1988; Susser et al., 1987, 1991; Weitzman et al., 1990, 1992; Wood et al., 1990; Zozus and Zax, 1991). There is evidence that dysfunctional childhoods, including disruptions of families of origin, parental histories of problem behaviors, and physical and sexual abuse, produce patterns of learned helplessness, disaffiliation, and cycles of abuse where homelessness is one outcome.

    The extent of violent behavior among the mentally ill has long been debated. Recent studies suggest that violence is largely restricted to a subset of the population, particularly those who abuse substances, are experiencing psychotic symptoms, or are noncompliant with medication (Link et al., 1992; Torrey, 1994). Such antisocial behaviors tend to reinforce public prejudices about the mentally ill and add to the stigmatization of this group. Victimization, defined more conventionally as experiencing criminal acts against the person and property, is also a frequent occurrence among homeless people. Furthermore, victimization is associated with dysfunction: Higher rates are reported by homeless individuals who have mental illness and substance abuse problems as well as those with childhood abuse histories. Unfortunately, reported childhood violence, along with current experiences with violence, are pervasive enough to warrant diagnosis of post-traumatic stress disorder in substantial proportions of homeless populations (North and Smith, 1992).

Implications for Services

Planning mental health services for this population presents many challenges (Lamb et al., 1994; Brickner et al., 1990; Institute of Medicine Committee on Health Care for Homeless People, 1988) and must take into consideration the wide variety of disorders and patient characteristics. The groups that need services range from middle-aged men with chronic drinking problems, to young women who are suffering from after-effects of victimization, to children with behavioral disturbances. No single service strategy could suffice to address these diverse needs. Nonetheless, some common themes have emerged. Clinicians who work with homeless people have reshaped services in similar ways for different disorders and different subgroups.

Characteristics of Homeless People that Affect Service Provision

The most obvious characteristics shared by homeless people which affect their service needs are their transience and the hardship of their living circumstances. In addition, however, they often manifest distrust of formal service systems, a lack of effective social supports, and extreme poverty.

Distrust. Service programs for homeless people must be prepared to encounter distrust of formal services by many of the potential recipients and must adjust their expectations and approaches accordingly. They should not expect that all who need services will seek them, nor should they expect that proffered help will in all cases be gratefully accepted. Those whose needs seem greatest may be the most reluctant to seek help. The distrust of many homeless people of helpers and helping agencies likely has several roots. It may be related to prior experiences with mental health services that were perceived as unhelpful (Schutt and Garrett, 1992; Cohen et al., 1984; Goldfinger and Chafetz, 1984; Ball and Havassy, 1984). The cultural differences between extremely poor homeless persons and mental health professionals may also contribute (Kuhlman, 1994; Koegel, 1992). Finally, in some cases, psychiatric disorder itself may engender mistrust, as when patients with schizophrenia become paranoid or deny that they have a disorder (Lamb, 1984; Bachrach et al., 1987).

Lack of supports. Providing services for homeless people, with their often fragile systems of social support, is very different from providing them for a typical domiciled population, where a treatment provider can assume that the person is supported by an array of relationships. Furthermore, homeless people lack other supportive factors, such as a permanent place to sleep and live, personal safety, a reasonable diet, and a degree of financial security. Their extremely precarious circumstances should be reflected in treatment and rehabilitation approaches.

Extreme poverty.   The homeless are the poorest of the poor; their resources are inadequate to meet their basic needs. Social welfare in the form of public assistance is based on financial eligibility and provides minimally adequate resources for survival. An intelligent, healthy, and well-organized person may be able to access these resources and sustain a minimal standard of living with supports of this sort. But for many homeless people who are in need of treatment for a psychiatric problem, the challenge can be too great. They may not be able to tolerate the cumbersome procedures for obtaining these resources, or efficiently conserve the small amounts that are received.

Service Design

Three common themes in mental health services for homeless people have emerged in response to these and other shared characteristics: the adoption of a public health perspective, an emphasis on housing, and the need for linkage and integration. We illustrate how these themes influence the delivery of services in the case of homeless people with chronic psychotic disorders such as schizophrenia, to whom we shall refer as the homeless mentally ill. The same themes could be elaborated, however, in relation to services for other subgroups.

Public health perspective.   Service programs for homeless people tend to actively survey the needs of a population, find ways to integrate psychiatric services into the social fabric in unusual locales, and seek out cases in need of treatment (Susser, 1992; Susser et al., 1990). While this approach could benefit any clinical service, it is more essential and is certainly more widely practiced in programs for homeless people, a population with glaring needs, to whom conventional mental health services have been patently unable to deliver effective treatment.

Clinical outreach teams often work with homeless people in public and private shelters, parks, streets, subways, bus and train terminals, and other public spaces. They enter these settings without any invitation from the potential recipients of services who live there. In fact, their presence may be unwelcome to many of these persons. Therefore, they must search for ways to introduce themselves neatly into the social fabric. In one example, a mental health team sought a means to introduce psychiatric services into a transitional residence for homeless mentally ill women, where psychiatric treatment was stigmatized and the presence of the psychiatrist was initially seen as intrusive and threatening. In order to reshape the interaction between the psychiatrist and the community, the clinical team used a weekly Bingo game. Run by the psychiatrist, the Bingo game became a source of amusement and curiosity. Its friendly and non-threatening atmosphere made it the best attended activity in the hotel. Thus, the psychiatrist became an accepted and familiar figure in the community. Soon he was able to initiate psychiatric treatment of women living in the hotel without being feared or resented by residents (Susser, 1992).

Once entry is made into a given community, a mental health team still has to identify people who are in need of treatment and enter into some relation with them. Outreach teams for homeless mentally ill people become skilled at observing people in public spaces and shelters and at identifying the individuals who are most likely to be homeless and mentally ill. The team approaches these people and offers food, clothing, or other assistance as a basis for initial contact. Some individuals accept offers of help relatively easily. Because others may be extremely resistant, repeated contacts may be needed before the person can be persuaded to accept help (Cohen, 1989). The outreach team may conclude that a person is in clear danger through self-neglect or failure to protect herself or himself. In this situation workers may have to use involuntary admission procedures to get a person to treatment, a process that may bring the team into conflict with advocacy or libertarian groups (Cournos, 1989).

Housing.   A second theme is a focus on housing as a primary treatment goal. Because homelessness can cause or exacerbate a broad spectrum of mental problems, housing represents a crucial requisite for optimal treatment. In addition, providing adequate treatment to a person who is literally "on the street" is extremely difficult. It is thus vital to get people housed, and for this purpose to have access to a variety of housing options.

Finding housing in many cases takes priority over other needs, and much of the art of clinical work is directed toward elaborating the patient's feelings about housing and then acting to secure the best available option. Treatment even of severe psychopathology may be postponed if its introduction would disrupt the process of obtaining housing. Treatment of the illness may be postponed if the patient threatens to withdraw because the team insists too strongly on treatment. On the other hand, a mental health team may aggressively pursue treatment of symptoms if this is necessary for the process of housing placement, for example, where severe symptoms prohibit housing placement.

Housing group meetings can provide a forum in which patients discuss their feelings about housing. Information on housing is presented, the skills required to live in each type of housing are specified, and prior experiences are discussed. Thus, group members develop a keener sense of their preferences, their capabilities, and their options before making a choice. For individuals who do not like to attend groups or cannot tolerate them, the same principles can be applied in individual treatment. Patients may be encouraged to visit several potential residences and to reject any and all that make them feel uncomfortable. The program staff then try to identify and discuss the reasons for discomfort. In the process, the patient's housing needs become more clearly defined. The process of adjusting hopes and expectations to the limited options available can be difficult. It is usually helpful to reframe the current options as a beginning rather than an endpoint.

A focus on housing requires close integration with social services. For those who cannot work, public assistance or disability payments are usually a precondition for obtaining housing. The process of securing these benefits can be eased dramatically by clinical programs that establish firm connections with public assistance agencies and other social services. For instance, in a program for mentally ill men in a New York shelter, representatives of the Social Security Administration visit the program for on-site interviews with applicants. In other locations, special arrangements have been made with the U.S. Department of Housing and Urban Development to provide Section 8 rental certificates for homeless persons with mental disabilities (National Resource Center, 1992). When combined with case management, this approach has been quite effective in reducing recurrent homelessness (Center for Mental Health Services, 1994).

Linkage and integration.   A third common theme is the importance of linkages for continuity of care. Specialized services for homeless people are generally time-limited and will transfer care to another team or agency once a person is domiciled. The difficulties of connecting homeless people to other services, and their mobility, underlie the importance of this feature of service delivery.

Most service programs are acutely aware of the need for linkages, but despite this awareness, practical constraints have limited achievements in this area. Many programs are required by their funding agencies to terminate services at the time of, or shortly after, housing placement. In addition, community providers are often reluctant to become involved with formerly homeless patients. In the absence of either a transitional period or a willing agency to "take the baton," effective linkage is unlikely.

The need to develop linkages can be minimized when treatment of the homeless falls under the purview of mobile treatment teams that are an integral part of a comprehensive service system. In this model a mobile treatment team goes out to homeless and other patients in a given community, wherever intervention is needed. They shoulder a long-term commitment to all these patients, for as long as the treatment program is needed. Although it is presently practiced in only a few locations with model mental health services (Cohen, 1990; Diamond et al., 1991; Stein and Test, 1985), this approach is almost certainly superior to the more common use of transitional programs for homeless people within somewhat fragmented service systems.

While categorical federal and other governmental funding has long been the source of service fragmentation, more recent efforts have been focused on the provision of comprehensive services (Drake et al., 1991). Beginning in the early 1990s, the Center for Mental Health Services (Substance Abuse and Mental Health Services Administration) funded the Projects for Assistance in Transition from Homelessness (PATH) Program, which has been successful in providing outreach and case management to homeless mentally ill individuals. To test a variety of service integration strategies, the Center for Mental Health Services subsequently awarded ACCESS (Access to Community Care and Effective Services and Supports) grants to nine states. These strategies range from an innovative voucher system to co-location of services, cross-training of staff, and the use of interagency, multidisciplinary treatment teams (National Resource Center, 1993).

Service Models

The recognition of the special needs of homeless individuals with mental illness has led to the adaptation of traditional models of mental health services. This is perhaps most obvious in the area of outreach, or engagement of the patient. Successful outreach relies on a balance between gentle respect and the application of leverage (Susser et al., 1990; Susser et al., 1992). Persuasive techniques can span across a wide range—from offering incentives to engage the patient in conversation, to limit-setting and insisting on medication compliance as a condition of service.

The high incidence of substance abuse among homeless individuals with mental illness points to the need for special treatment approaches. Mental health and substance abuse services have traditionally been separated and located in different agencies with little interaction (Drake et al., 1991). Treatment programs, particularly residential programs for persons suffering from both disorders, are in short supply. A more realistic way of coping with the various stages of use and addiction in this population may be the creation of ''low-demand'' residences that permit substance use but attempt to limit it (Baumohl, 1989; Osher and Kofoed, 1989).

Many innovative outreach and service programs available today for the homeless mentally ill follow principles initially developed in the Program for Assertive Community Treatment (PACT) model (Chapter 16). Treatment occurs in SRO hotels, halfway houses, transportation centers, Social Security Administration offices, or other places where the patient lives or visits (Dixon et al., 1995). One program for mentally ill men in a New York City shelter builds on PACT principles, but adds features appropriate for this environment. Because cities like New York can offer service-rich but fragmented environments, the Critical Time Intervention (CTI) program places special emphasis on linking patients to existing services as they move from living in a homeless shelter to establishing residence in the community (Susser et al., 1992). It is during such transition periods that individuals who are mentally ill are most vulnerable to dislocations which could result in a return to homelessness. The CTI model posits that special assistance is needed for a period up to nine months, to bridge the transition between the two settings. During this period, the patient remains under the care of the shelter psychiatry team as well as the prospective community providers. The CTI worker focuses on developing a service plan that will outlast his or her involvement; community agencies, families, friends, and others are enlisted to play a role. This approach attempts to mediate conflicts between the community providers and the patients, convincing them that they can find ways to work effectively together over the long term (Susser et al., 1992).

Strategies for the Prevention of Homelessness

Mental health programs for homeless people are essential, but in essence are merely palliative and do not address the basic causes of the problem. Part of the role of the

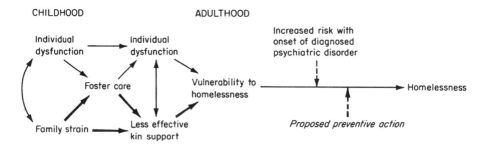

Figure 28–1 A causal model linking childhood foster care and adult homelessness in psychiatric patients. Thicker lines indicate that family strain is hypothesized to have a greater effect than individual dysfunction. In the child, individual dysfunction refers to emotional and behavioral problems, as well as physical disabilities, and may include premorbid signs of psychiatric disorders diagnosed in adulthood. In adulthood, individual dysfunction also includes problems in social adaptation, such as illiteracy, substance use, premarital pregnancy, and less resilience to adverse events without otherwise overt dysfunction.

generic mental health service system is to provide a system of services that prevents homelessness among people with psychiatric problems. Effective mental health service strategies are needed to prevent individuals from falling through the cracks. Mental health services should be evaluated as to the extent to which they actively implement preventive strategies.

Identification of Risk Factors

A first stage in this endeavor is the identification of risk factors. Childhood placement in foster care, for example, is a risk factor for homelessness later in life (Susser et al., 1987, 1991), as is substance abuse co-occurring with mental illness (Belcher, 1989; Drake et al., 1991). If risk profiles can be established, a basis for identifying people at risk can be established and special preventive interventions can be developed in mental health programs.

The types of preventive programs that are likely to be effective depend on the causal pathways that link childhood experience to adult homelessness. Several causal pathways are plausible, and it is likely that each of them occurs to some degree (Susser et al., 1991) (Fig. 28–1). Their relative importance is of no small interest, however. Each of them implies a different strategy for preventive intervention.

Thus, some investigators may believe that weak kin support is the crucial intervening variable in the causal path between disruptive childhood experiences and adult homelessness. They would logically attempt an intervention to strengthen or supplement kin networks. Others may view social disability as the more important intervening variable. They would pursue aggressive rehabilitation to minimize disability. Yet others may emphasize the extreme poverty of these patients and attempt to enhance their ability to compete for jobs or to acquire disability benefits effectively.

The Importance of Housing

Perhaps the most important aspect of prevention is to develop a range of housing options. Supported housing, with varying degrees of supervision to meet the varied needs of disabled persons, is essential to a well-developed mental health service system, and basic to preventing homelessness. Mentally ill people, as others, have preferences about the setting in which they live. If their preferences are ignored, one response is to leave, even to become homeless, rather than stay in an unsatisfactory situation. Unfortunately, a fully developed system of supported housing is not available in most places. Yet even in its absence, it may be possible to reduce significantly the incidence of homelessness among mentally ill people by implementing preventive programs targeted to high-risk groups.

Homelessness prevention approaches may be broadly divided into two types. One approach focuses on providing a specified type of supported housing. Another focuses on services in other areas that may improve patients' ability to remain in housing, such as job training, literacy, social supports, psychiatric treatments, and substance abuse treatments.

Supported housing that is directed toward early intervention to prevent homelessness differs in important ways from what is generally offered by mental health systems. In order to be preventive, the intervention must begin in the early phase of the disorder, at which stage few patients want to live in supervised residences for mentally ill people. Others do not want to be tied to a fixed residence over a long period, preferring to feel free to try various living options, for example to move in with lovers at certain times. What is needed is a model that mixes features of a family home with those of a treatment facility, with three central features. First, it is congregate housing that is not primarily a treatment facility—a person is entitled to live there whether symptomatic or not, and whether in treatment or not. Second, the residence can be used episodically over an indefinite period—a person has the right to return at any time, or to use it as "housing of last resort." Third, there are on-site staff who know the residents personally. Staff can provide treatment or referrals, but their key role is to function as a source of social support.

This housing model may also prove effective in treatment of people already homeless. Some homeless patients with schizophrenia desire housing but will not be tied to a single residence over a long period of time. Others reject the supervised residences that are now available for mentally ill people because they require the patient to assume the identity of a mental patient (Susser, 1992). It is these patients, who cannot accommodate to what is presently offered by the mental health system, who present the greatest difficulty in the clinical care of homeless individuals. Perhaps they also offer the most insight into the deficiencies of our present system of care, and into the type of housing that is needed for effective prevention among patients with disruptive childhood experiences.

HIV Prevention

Finally, while we underscore the need to work toward housing, it is also vitally important that professionals who work with the homeless mentally ill address the need for HIV prevention among their patients. Many in the mental health field have long felt that such activities are not an appropriate or necessary part of their responsibilities (Goldfinger et al., 1994). However, growing evidence suggests that the mentally ill are disproportionately affected by this life-threatening disease (Susser et al., 1993; Empfield et al., 1993; Cournos et al., 1991; Volavka et al., 1991; Sacks et al., 1992). In large part, elevated infection rates may be traced to practices that are directly related to the homeless condition. Early successes in one HIV prevention program, titled "Sex, Games, and Videotapes," suggest that homeless mentally ill men may be able to modify the nature, if not the frequency, of their sexual episodes (Susser et al., 1994). This curriculum combines skills-training methods with clinical approaches and is built around activities that are central to life in the shelter: competitive games, storytelling, and watching videos. Whether through such structured activities or in group and individual counseling, clinicians can play a vital role in identifying risky behaviors and educating patients to protect themselves.

Conclusion

The homeless mentally ill are a diverse population, living in differing conditions and experiencing various routes to homelessness. Many suffer from substance abuse disorders which compound the difficulties in making contact and establishing a treatment relationship. Successful programs serving the homeless mentally ill often have several characteristics: They apply a public health perspective to the development of services; they focus on housing as a primary goal; and they emphasize the development of linkages so as to achieve continuity of care. Drawing from the principles developed in the Programs for Assertive Community Treatment (PACT), these programs have evolved to provide more effective treatment to the homeless mentally ill, reducing frustrations felt by clinicians and patients alike. Ultimately the problem of homelessness will only be solved by methods to identify mentally ill persons at risk of homelessness and to implement appropriate preventive strategies.

References

Bachrach, L.L., Talbott, J.A., and Meyerson, A.T. (1987) The chronic psychiatric patient as a "difficult" patient: a conceptual analysis. *New Directions for Mental Health Services,* 33:35–49.

Ball, F.L.J., and Havassy, B.E. (1984) A survey of the problems and needs of homeless consumers of acute psychiatric services. *Hospital and Community Psychiatry,* 35:917–921.

Bassuk, E.L., and Rosenberg, L. (1988). Why does family homelessness occur? A case control study. *American Journal of Public Health,* 78:783–788.

Bassuk, E.L., Rubin, L., and Lauriat, A.S. (1986) Characteristics of sheltered homeless families. *American Journal of Public Health,* 76:1097–1101.

Bassuk, E.L., Rubin, L. and Lauriat, A. (1984) Is homelessness a mental health problem? *American Journal of Psychiatry,* 141:1546–1550.

Baumohl, J. (1989) Editor's introduction: alcohol, homelessness, and public policy. *Contemporary Drug Problems,* 16:281–300.

Belcher, J.R. (1989) On becoming homeless: a study of chronically mentally ill persons. *Journal of Community Psychology,* 17:173–185.

Breakey, W.R., Fischer, P.J., Kramer, M., Nestadt, G., Romanoski, A.J., Ross, A., Royall, R.M., and Stine, O.C. (1989). Health and mental health problems of homeless men and women in Baltimore. *Journal of the American Medical Association,* 262:1352–1357.

Breakey, W.R., and Fischer, P.J. (1990) Homelessness: the extent of the problem. *Journal of Social Issues,* 46(4):31–47.

Brickner, P.W., Scharer, L.K., Conanan, B., Savarese, M., and Scanlan, B.G. (1990) *Under the Safety Net: The Health and Social Welfare of the Homeless in the United States.* New York: Norton.

Caton, C.L.M., Shrout, P.E., Eagle, P.F., Opler, L.A., and Felix, A. (1994) Correlates of co-disorders in homeless and never homeless indigent schizophrenic men. *Psychological Medicine,* 24:681–88.

Center for Mental Health Services (1994) *Making a Difference: Interim status report of the McKinney Research Demonstration Program for Homeless Adults with Serious Mental Illness.* Rockville, MD: Center for Mental Health Services, U.S. Department of Health and Human Services.

Cohen, C.I. (1993) Poverty and the course of schizophrenia: implications for research and policy. *Hospital and Community Psychiatry,* 44:951–958.

Cohen M.B. (1989) Social work practice with homeless mentally ill people: engaging the client. *Social Work,* 34:505–512.

Cohen N.L. (ed.) (1990) *Psychiatry Takes to the Streets.* New York: Guilford Press.

Cohen, N.L., Putnam, J.F., and Sullivan, A.M. (1984) The mentally ill homeless: isolation and adaption. *Hospital and Community Psychiatry,* 35:922–924.

Cournos, F. (1989) Involuntary medication and the case of Joyce Brown. *Hospital and Community Psychiatry,* 40:736–740.

Cournos, F., Empfield, M., Horwath, E., McKinnon, K., Meyer, I., Schrage, H., Currie, C., and Agosin, B. (1991) HIV seroprevalence among patients admitted to two psychiatric hospitals. *American Journal of Psychiatry,* 148:1225–1230.

Davies, M.A., Munetz M.R., Schultz, S.C., and Bromet, E.J. (1987) Assessing mental illness in SRO shelter residents. *Hospital and Community Psychiatry,* 38:1114–1116.

Diamond, R., Stein, L., and Susser, E. (1991) Essential and nonessential roles for psychiatrists in community mental health centers. *Hospital and Community Psychiatry,* 42:187–189.

Dixon, L.B., Krauss, N., Kernan, E., Lehman, A.F., and DeForge, B.R. (1995) Modifying the PACT model to serve homeless persons with severe mental illness. *Psychiatric Services,* 46:684–688.

Drake, R.E., Osher, F.C., and Wallach, A.M. (1991) Homelessness and dual diagnosis. *American Psychologist,* 46:1149–1158.

Empfield, M., Cournos, F., Meyer, I., McKinnon, K., Horwath, E., Silver, M., Schrage, H., and Herman, R. (1993) HIV seroprevalence among homeless patients admitted to a psychiatric inpatient unit. *American Journal of Psychiatry,* 150:47–52.

Fischer, P.J. (1991) *Alcohol and drug abuse and mental problems among homeless persons: A review of the literature, 1980–1990.* Rockville, MD: Alcohol, Drug Abuse, and Mental Health Administration DHHS Publication No. (ADM) 91–1763 (A).

Fischer, P.J. (1989) Estimating prevalence of alcohol drug and mental health problems in the contemporary homeless population: a review of the literature. *Contemporary Drug Problems,* 16:333–390.

Fischer, P.J. (1992) Victimization and homelessness: cause and effect. *New England Journal of Public Policy,* 8(1):229–246.

Gelberg, L., and Linn, L.S. (1989) Assessing the physical health of homeless adults. *Journal of the American Medical Association,* 262:1973–1979.

Goldfinger, S.M., and Chafetz, L. (1984) Developing a better service delivery system for the homeless mentally ill. In Lamb, H.R. (ed.), *The Homeless Mentally Ill.* Washington, D.C.: American Psychiatric Press.

Goldfinger, S.M., Susser, E., and Roche, B. (1994) *HIV, homelessness, and the severely mentally ill.* Washington, D.C.: Substance Abuse and Mental Health Services Administration.

Hermann, R.C. (1988) Center provides approach to major social ill: homeless urban runaways, "throwaways." *Journal of the American Medical Association,* 260:311–312.

Hollingshead, A.B., and Redlich, F.C. (1958) *Social Class in Mental Illness.* New York: John Wiley and Son.

Institute of Medicine, Committee on Health Care for Homeless People (1988) *Homelessness, Health and Human Needs.* Washington, D.C.: National Academy Press.

Knickman, J.R., and Weitzman, B.C. (1989) A study of homeless families in New York City: Risk assessment models and strategies for prevention. Presented at the 117th Annual Meeting of the American Public Health Association, Chicago, Illinois, October 22–26.

Koegel, P. (1992). Through a different lens: an anthropological perspective on the homeless mentally ill. *Culture, Medicine, and Psychiatry,* 16:1–22.

Koegel, P., and Burnam, A. (1988). Alcoholism among homeless adults in the inner city of Los Angeles. *Archives of General Psychiatry,* 45:1011–1018.

Koegel, P., and Burnam, M.A. (1987) Traditional and nontraditional homeless alcoholics. *Alcohol Health and Research World,* 11(3):28–35.

Koegel, P., Burnam, A., and Farr, R.K. (1988) The prevalence of specific psychiatric disorders among homeless individuals in the inner city of Los Angeles. *Archives of General Psychiatry,* 45:1085–1092.

Kuhlman, T.L. (1994) *Psychology on the Streets: Mental Health Practice with Homeless Persons.* New York: John Wiley and Sons.

Lamb, H.R. (1984) Deinstitutionalization and the homeless mentally ill. *Hospital and Community Psychiatry,* 35:899–907.

Lamb, H.R., Bachrach, L.L., and Kass, F.I. (eds.) (1994) *Treating the homeless mentally ill: A Task Force Report of the American Psychiatric Association.* Washington, D.C.: American Psychiatric Association.

Lehman, A.F., and Cordray, D.S. (1993) Prevalence of alcohol, drug, and mental disorders among the homeless: one more time. *Contemporary Drug Problems,* 20:355–383.

Link, B.G., Andrews, H., and Cullen, F.T. (1992) The violent and illegal behavior of mental patients reconsidered. *American Sociological Review,* 57:275–292.

London, J. (1907). *The Road.* New York: The Macmillan Company.

Mulkern, V., Bradley, V.J., Spence, J.R., Allein, S., and Oldham, J.E. (1985) *Homelessness needs assessment study: Findings and recommendations for the Massachusetts Department of Mental Health.* Boston: Human Services Research Institute.

Mundy, P., Robertson, M., Robertson, J., and Greenblatt, M. (1990) The prevalence of psychotic symptoms in homeless adolescents. *Journal of the American Academy of Child and Adolescent Psychiatry,* 29:724–731.

National Resource Center on Homelessness and Mental Illness (1992) McKinney projects respond to emerging needs. *Access,* 4(4):1–4.

National Resource Center on Homelessness and Mental Illness (1993) ACCESS grantees test services integration strategies. *Access,* 5(4):1–3.

North, C.S., and Smith, E.M. (1992) Post-traumatic stress disorder among homeless men and women. *Hospital and Community Psychiatry,* 43:1010–1016.

Osher, F.C., and Kofoed, L.L. (1989) Treatment of patients with psychiatric and psychoactive substance abuse disorders. *Hospital and Community Psychiatry,* 40:1025–1030.

Piliavin, I., Sosin, M., and Westerfeldt, H. (1988) *Conditions contributing to long-term homelessness: An exploratory study.* Madison: University of Wisconsin Institute for Research on Poverty.

Reich, R., and Siegel L. (1978) The emergence of the Bowery as a psychiatric dumping ground. *Psychiatric Quarterly,* 50:191–201.

Robertson, J.M. (1988) Homeless adolescents: a hidden crisis. *Hospital and Community Psychiatry,* 39:475.

Robertson, M.J., Koegel, P., and Ferguson, L. (1989) Alcohol use and abuse among homeless adolescents in Hollywood. *Contemporary Drug Problems,* 16:415–452.

Rosenheck, R., Leda, C., Meda, S., Thompson, D., and Olson, R.S. (1988) *Progress report on the Veterans Administration's Domiciliary Care for Homeless Veterans Program.* West Haven, Connecticut: West Haven VA Medical Center.

Rossi, P.H., Fisher, G.A., and Willis, G. (1986) *The Condition of the Homeless of Chicago.* Chicago: National Opinion Research Center.

Roth, D., Bean, J., Lust, N., and Saveanu, T. (1985) *Homelessness in Ohio: a Study of People in Need, Statewide Report.* Columbus: Ohio Department of Mental Health, Office of Program Education and Research.

Rotheram-Borus, M.J., Koopman, C., and Ehrhardt, A.A. (1991) Homeless Youths and HIV Infection. *American Psychologist,* 46:1188–1197.

Sacks, M., Dermatis, H., Looser-Ott, S., Burton, W., and Perry, S. (1992) Undetected HIV infection among acutely ill psychiatric inpatients. *American Journal of Psychiatry,* 149: 544–545.

Schutt, R.K. (1988) Boston's homeless, 1986–87: *Change and continuity. Report to the Long Island Shelter.* Boston: University of Massachusetts.

Schutt, R.K., and Garrett, G.R. (1986) *Homeless in Boston in 1985: The view from Long Island.* Boston: University of Massachusetts.

Schutt, R.K., and Garrett, G.R. (1992) *Responding to the Homeless: Policy and Practice.* New York: Plenum Press.

Smith, E.M., North, C.S., and Spitznagel, E.L. (1992) A systematic study of mental illness, substance abuse and treatment in 600 homeless men. *Annals of Clinical Psychiatry,* 4: 111–120.

Smith, E.M., North, C.S., and Spitznagel, E.L. (1993) Alcohol, drugs, and psychiatric comorbidity among homeless women: an epidemiologic study. *Journal of Clinical Psychiatry,* 54(3):82–87.

Snyder, M. (1984) Testimony before a joint hearing of Congressional Subcommittees on Housing and Community Development and Manpower and Housing, quoted by Smith, T.K., and McDaid, E.W. (1987) Homelessness in Pennsylvania: Numbers, needs and services. A report to the Pennsylvania Department of Public Welfare. Philadelphia: The Conservation Company.

Solarz, A.L. (1988) Homelessness: Implications for children and youth. *Social Policy Report*, 3(4):1–16.

Sosin, M., Colson, P., and Grossman, S. (1988) *Homelessness in Chicago: Poverty and Pathology, Social Institutions and Social Change.* Chicago: University of Chicago School of Social Service Administration.

Stein, L.I., and Test, M.A. (1985) The evolution of the Training in Community Living model. *New Directions for Mental Health Services,* 26:7–16.

Susser E. (1992) Working with people who are mentally ill and homeless: the role of a psychiatrist. In Jahiel, R. (ed.), *Homelessness: A Prevention-Oriented Approach,* pp. 207–217. Baltimore: Johns Hopkins University Press.

Susser, E., Conover, S., and Struening, E.L. (1989) Problems of epidemiologic method in assessing the type and extent of mental illness among homeless adults. *Hospital and Community Psychiatry,* 40:261–265.

Susser, E., Goldfinger, S.M., and White, A. (1990) Some clinical approaches to the homeless mentally ill. *Community Mental Health Journal,* 26(5):463–480.

Susser, E., Lin, S.P., Conover, S.A., and Struening, E.L. (1991) Childhood antecedents of homelessness in psychiatric patients. *American Journal of Psychiatry,* 148(8):1026–1030.

Susser, E.S., Moore, R., and Link, B. (1993) Risk factors for homelessness. *American Journal of Epidemiology,* 15:546–556.

Susser, E., Struening, E., and Conover, S. (1987). Childhood experiences of homeless men. *American Journal of Psychiatry,* 144, 1599–1601.

Susser, E., Valencia, E., and Conover, S. (1993) Prevalence of HIV infection among psychiatric patients in a New York City men's shelter. *American Journal of Public Health,* 83:568–570.

Susser, E., Valencia, E., and Goldfinger, S. (1992) Clinical care of the homeless mentally ill: strategies and adaptation. In Lamb, H.R., Bachrach, L., Kass, F. (eds.), *Treating the Homeless Mentally Ill.* Washington, D.C.: American Psychiatric Association.

Susser, E., Valencia, E., and Torres, J. (1994) Sex, games and videotapes: an HIV-prevention intervention for men who are homeless and mentally ill. *Psychosocial Rehabilitation Journal,* 17(4):31–40.

Torrey, E.F. (1994) Violent behavior by individuals with serious mental illness. *Hospital and Community Psychiatry,* 45(7):653–662.

Vernez, G., Burnam, M.A., McGlynn, E.A., Trude, S., and Mittman, B.S. (1988) *Review of California's program for the homeless mentally disabled.* Santa Monica: RAND Corporation.

Volavka, J., Convit, A., Czobor, P., Douyon, R., O'Donnell, J., Ventura, F. (1991). HIV seroprevalence and risk behaviors in psychiatric inpatients. *Psychiatry Research,* 39:109–114.

Weitzman, B.C., Knickman, J.R., and Shinn, M. (1990) Pathways to homelessness among New York City families. *Journal of Social Issues,* 46(4):125–140.

Weitzman, B.C., Knickman, J.R., and Shinn, M. (1992) Predictors of shelter use among low-income families: psychiatric history, substance abuse, and victimization. *American Journal of Public Health,* 82:1547–1550.

Wood, D., Valdez, R.B., Hayashi, T., and Shen, A. (1990). Homeless and housed families in Los Angeles: A study comparing demographic, economic, and family function characteristics. *American Journal of Public Health,* 80(9):1049–1052.

Wright, J.D., and Weber, E. (1987) *Homelessness and Health.* Washington, D.C.: McGraw-Hill.

Zolopa, A.R., Hahn, J.A., Gorter, R., Miranda, J., Wlodarczyk, D., Peterson, J., Pilote, L., and Moss, A.R. (1994) HIV and tuberculosis infection in San Francisco's homeless adults. *Journal of the American Medical Association,* 272:455–461.

Zozus, R.T., and Zax, M. (1991) Perception of childhood: Exploring possible etiological factors in homelessness. *Hospital and Community Psychiatry,* 42:535–537.

29

Patients with HIV Disease

CONSTANTINE G. LYKETSOS
MARC FISHMAN
GLENN J. TREISMAN

The Human Immunodeficiency Virus (HIV) pandemic is associated with a major burden of psychiatric disorders worldwide. To begin with, certain vulnerabilities and behaviors associated with mental illness place individuals at risk for HIV infection, so that increasingly large numbers of patients with mental disorders are becoming infected with the virus. They may be relatively unresponsive to education, likely to continue high-risk HIV behavior, and likely to play a significant role in the continued spread of the disease. The end result for the patient is a terminal infection with considerable medical morbidity. For others, infection with HIV is accompanied by considerable understandable psychological stress related to the incurable nature of the illness and the circumstances in which, in some cases, it was contracted. Furthermore, HIV infection produces brain injury, leading directly to the development of psychiatric syndromes. For all these reasons, there is a strong relationship between HIV infection and psychiatric disorder.

This chapter adopts a public health approach, considering primary, secondary, and tertiary prevention, and outlining a model program to address the problems associated with the HIV pandemic within the community psychiatrists' setting. Although scientific knowledge about HIV and its treatment is constantly changing, the aim is to stress principles and methods which are less affected by new knowledge.

History and Scope of the HIV Pandemic

In 1981 two reports of *pneumocystis carinii* pneumonia and Kaposi's sarcoma, usually diseases of the immunosuppressed, were reported in young men of previously good health (Gotlieb et al., 1981; Masur et al., 1981; Seigal et al., 1981). These were the first reported cases of AIDS, now recognized as the endpoint of a 7- to 10-year infection with HIV, a retrovirus first identified in 1983. HIV transmission occurs by three principal routes: sexual contact; parenteral inoculation of infected body fluids; and the most rapidly growing means of transmission, vertical infection from a mother to her child (between 20 and 30 percent of infected mothers transmit the infection to their children) (Chaisson, 1992).

The pandemic has spread worldwide in distinct patterns (Mann and Chin, 1988): In pattern 1, which predominates in western countries and North Africa, sexual transmission occurs primarily among homosexual and bisexual men. In pattern 2, mostly in sub-Saharan Africa and the Caribbean, sexual transmission through heterosexual contact is the predominant means of spread. In the final pattern, mostly in Eastern Europe and Asia, infection rates are relatively low and are accounted for by exposure to travelers or blood products from other areas.

By 1993, over 340,000 cases of AIDS had been reported in the United States; more than half of new cases occurred in the preceding 5 years (Centers for Disease Control, 1992). By 1990 it was estimated that approximately one million Americans were infected with HIV, most concentrated in major cities on the coasts (Centers for Disease Control, 1990). Worldwide, approximately 10 to 15 million persons are thought to be infected (Chaisson, 1992), and it is estimated that this number may reach 40 million at the height of the pandemic. The worst impact is likely to occur in sub-Saharan Africa, India, and Indochina, where in certain areas as many as 30 percent of the population may eventually die of AIDS (Chaisson, 1992). Thus far, nearly two-thirds of people infected with HIV have died of AIDS, although with time a much larger proportion likely will develop AIDS and die (Centers for Disease Control, 1990).

The Virus, the Disease, and Its Treatment

HIV infection runs a predictable, well-staged course (Bartlett and Finkbeiner, 1991). This begins with a brief mononucleosis-like syndrome soon after the virus has entered the bloodstream (stage 1), followed by a lengthy incubation period with a median duration of 10 years (Munoz et al., 1992). The individual is asymptomatic and the CD4 lymphocyte count declines steadily (stage 2). During these early stages of infection the virus also infects the central nervous system (McArthur, 1992).

As the CD4 count drops below 500 and approaches 200 cells per microliter, the patient develops a variety of symptoms such as weakness, anorexia, fatigue, fever, chills, insomnia, and weight loss. At this time, generalized lymphadenopathy may present and the patient is said to have entered stage 3 of the infection. Once the CD4 count drops below 200 cells per microliter or the patient develops a disease associated with immune deficiency, stage 4 (AIDS) is diagnosed. One of several opportunistic or other infections might develop, and there is high risk for the development of neoplasias, dementia, hematologic decline, and/or a wasting syndrome. Finally, specific consequences of HIV organ infection such as carditis and nephropathy occur at this stage (Bartlett and Finkbeiner, 1991).

Several treatment strategies have been pursued. The first is a vaccine for primary prevention (Picard et al., 1990; Koff and Hoth, 1988). Unfortunately, the ability of a vaccine to stimulate the immune system is greatly reduced, and in addition the virus continues to mutate on a regular basis. Thus it is unlikely that vaccine efforts will yield results for several years (Chaisson, 1992). A second strategy has been that of prophylaxis. Zidovudine (AZT) and Didanocine (DDI) can delay the time of progression to AIDS and may extend overall survival (Chaisson, 1992). There has been greater success in chemoprophylaxis for the prevention of opportunistic infection.

Treatment of the clinical complications of AIDS has met with greater success. Once AIDS has developed, however, survival usually does not extend beyond 18 months to 2 years (Chaisson, 1992). Treatments of HIV-associated dementia with high-dose AZT may be efficacious in slowing progression (McArthur, 1992).

General Psychiatric Aspects

Epidemiologic studies of HIV-infected patients and patients with AIDS have demonstrated a higher than expected rate of recent mental morbidity and a very high lifetime prevalence of mental disorders (Gorman et al., 1991). There is continuing controversy as to whether they occur with different frequencies at different stages of the infection (Lyketsos et al., 1993a).

If considered stage by stage, persons at risk for HIV infection—such as homosexual men and injection drug users—have high lifetime prevalences of substance use disorders, anxiety disorders, mood disorders, and in some cases personality disorders (Gorman et al., 1991; Atkinson et al., 1988; Perry et al., 1989; Perkins et al., 1993). Acute seroconversion is associated with a transient period of a grief-like reaction including depression, anxiety, insomnia, worrying, and ruminations (Huggins et al., 1991). Rarely does this condition last more than 6 months.

Over the ensuing years, while the disease incubates, patients are asymptomatic but report more fearfulness, less hopefulness, more insomnia, and more anorexia than uninfected comparison subjects (Lyketsos et al., 1993a). However, there is no demonstrable increase in the prevalence of specific mental disorders in this stage when compared to at-risk populations (Gorman et al., 1991; Lyketsos et al., 1993a). Six to 18 months before clinical AIDS develops, there is a dramatic increase in depressive and cognitive symptoms (Hoover et al., 1992; McArthur, 1992). Incident cases of major depression, mania, dementia, and delirium occur at this stage; these are directly related to brain infection and possibly to the systemic effects of viral infection and general system decline (Perry, 1990). In late stages of AIDS there is a strong association between HIV dementia and manic episodes (Lyketsos et al., 1993b).

At intake to medical HIV clinics, as many as 50 percent of patients have diagnosable psychiatric morbidity (Chuang, 1992; Lyketsos et al., 1994), in most cases adjustment disorders or major depression. The same disorders commonly occur in psychiatric specialty clinics that care for patients referred to them from medical care providers (O'Dowd and McKegney, 1991; Treisman et al., 1994). In inpatient acute psychiatric wards, HIV-infected psychiatric patients typically suffer from organic mental disorders with mood and cognitive symptoms (Perry, 1994; Nurnberg et al., 1984). Similarly, in inpatient medical wards caring for HIV-infected patients, as many as 50 percent of patients have psychiatric disorders, usually organic syndromes with cognitive and mood symptoms (Johannet and Muskin, 1990; Dilley et al., 1985).

Clinical Presentation

There are three important issues in evaluating HIV-infected patients. The first is the interpretation of complaints such as fatigue, insomnia, anorexia, headache, and preoccupation with signs such as rash and oral thrush. All of these can be attributed to HIV infection itself; however, such complaints can be symptoms of depressive disorders, so that the differential diagnosis becomes quite complex (Lyketsos et al., 1993a). A careful history with special attention to the stage of the patient's HIV disease, prior psychiatric and family history, and the presence or absence of physical signs is informative. In early disease patients, such complaints are closely intertwined with depression and improve if treated as such (Treisman et al., 1993, 1994). In later stage disease, the differentiation is more difficult, but cognitive symptoms, memory loss, and self-attitude change suggest the presence of major depression.

The second major issue is the tendency of patients and providers to seek meaningful explanations for psychiatric symptoms. Depression, anxiety, and hopelessness can be understood as psychological reactions that anybody would have in the context of a debilitating terminal illness. Consequently, such symptoms are often dealt with in a supportive way, not with an intent to cure. This "trap of meaning" can lead clinicians and other care-givers to miss the signs of treatable mental illness (Treisman et al., 1993). Although personal support and meaningful understanding of psychological complaints is extremely important, if these complaints form the recognizable constellations of psychiatric syndromes, they should be treated aggressively with appropriate pharmacologic agents.

The third clinical issue is the complexity of HIV-infected patients. Presentations are typically not straightforward: Most often patients present with a variety of psychiatric problems, requiring a psychiatrist to approach the case from several perspectives (McHugh and Slavney, 1983). They include syndromal disorders (such as major depression), personality disturbances, behavioral disorders (such as substance abuse and paraphilia), and life circumstance disturbances of severe proportions. Examples of the latter include limited resources, multiple personal and other losses, hopelessness, unemployment, and poverty. It is essential to recognize the entire spectrum of disturbances and to treat all of them at once (Treisman et al., 1993).

Specific Disorders

Mood disturbances are the most common complaints of HIV-infected patients (Perry, 1994). The differential diagnosis is broad, including "minor depressions" or subsyndromal major depression, dysthymia, bereavement, adjustment disorders, "organic'' mood disorders, and syndromal major depression. Typical symptoms include depression, anhedonia, neurovegetative change, and cognitive and self-attitude changes (Treisman et al., 1993). Complaints of memory disturbance, forgetfulness, and the belief that death is approaching rapidly are common. Depressed mood may also reflect acute distress in patients with personality disorders (Perkins et al., 1993) and may accompany substance use and withdrawal (Treisman et al., 1993). In the absence of obvious causative organic factors, if a full major depressive syndrome is present, the diagnosis of major depression is most appropriate, even if stressors can account for its existence.

Adjustment disorders are also common in HIV-infected patients, related to stressors which may be multiple, ranging from personal grief on discovering their HIV positivity, to bereavement relating to loss of loved ones from HIV, to bad news of a declining CD4 count, to being socially ostracized. Many HIV-positive patients adjust to these stressors remarkably well within a short period. Thus, even though adjustment disorders may be accompanied by mood disturbances, anxiety, neurovegetative symptoms, and social withdrawal, they tend to be transient and moderate in severity.

Organic mood disorders may have several causes (Perry, 1990). HIV disease and its treatment, substance use, and brain injury from a variety of causes (infection, head trauma, meningitis) are the most common precipitants. Organic syndromes encountered in these patients include delirium, dementia (subcortical), mania, and psychotic disorders. Typically, these disturbances occur late in the course of infection when patients become debilitated, are very vulnerable to the effects of metabolic stressors, and are more likely to have HIV brain infection.

HIV dementia, also known as HIV encephalopathy or the AIDS dementia complex (McArthur, 1992), occurs typically after the CD4 count has dropped below 100 cells per microliter. It portends a poor prognosis, survival being on the order of 6 months.

However, HIV-infected patients often have cognitive impairments early in the progression of the infection. These impairments may not be progressive and may result from prior head trauma and substance use (McArthur, 1992). Thus, while cognitive impairment should be ascertained in early stages of the disease, it does not necessarily imply the presence of HIV dementia.

Mania is being increasingly recognized as a serious complication or associated disorder (Lyketsos et al., 1993b). A distinction can be made between late-onset mania, occurring for the first time after the CD4 count has dropped below 200, and mania that occurs early in the course of the HIV infection. A slight excess prevalence of bipolar disorder has been noted in the early stages of HIV disease (Gorman et al., 1991), and it is possible that manic episodes confer some increased risk of contracting the virus. Late-onset mania, most likely a consequence of HIV-related brain infection of subcortical brain areas, has been described in close association with dementia when the CD4 count has dropped below 100 (Lyketsos et al., 1993b), a condition that leads to significant disability and is hard to treat.

Substance use disorders are highly prevalent in patients with HIV infection. The most commonly abused substances are alcohol, cocaine, and, to a lesser extent, heroin and benzodiazepines. They should be evaluated in all HIV-infected patients because high prevalences are reported in HIV-infected patients whether or not they are injection drug users. The presence of a substance use disorder also complicates the treatment of other psychiatric disorders (Treisman et al., 1993).

Personality disorders, most commonly of the DSM-III-R cluster B, are more prevalent in HIV patients (Perkins et al., 1993). Anti-social, histrionic, and dependent traits are frequently observed (Treisman et al., 1993). Such patients focus on the present rather than the future and the past, seek immediate rewards rather than avoid long-term adverse consequences, and have transient but strong emotions that drive their behavior (Treisman et al., 1993; McHugh and Slavney, 1983).

Although the prevalence of chronic mental disorders, particularly schizophrenia, tends to be low in HIV-infected patients (Perkins et al., 1994), atypical psychosis is frequently observed (Sewell et al., 1994). The main risk factor is a history of stimulant or sedative hypnotic use disorder. There is no relationship between psychosis and HIV stage, anti-retroviral treatment, HIV risk factor, and family history in HIV-infected patients, and there are no significant differences in neuropsychological testing between psychotic and non-psychotic HIV-infected patients (Sewell et al., 1994).

The HIV Pandemic and the Community Psychiatrist

High-Risk Groups

Although still a minority of HIV-infected people, the chronically mentally ill are being infected at increasing rates. Factors that contribute to this include impulsiveness, impaired judgment, self-destructive behavior, poor social skills, hypersexuality, cognitive impairment, poor reality testing, affective instability, depression, intravenous drug use, lack of knowledge about AIDS, and vulnerability to victimization (Lyketsos et al., 1993c; Carmen and Brady, 1990; Kalichman et al., 1994; Baer et al., 1988). High-risk behaviors in the chronically mentally ill are common (Sacks et al., 1992; Cournos et al., 1994). As many as 10 to 20 percent of men report sexual contact with other men, and a similar proportion inject drugs in inner-city settings (Sacks et al., 1990). Between 30 and 50 percent of patients with chronic mental disorders in large cities suffer from comorbid substance use disorders (Chapter 25) (Lyketsos et al., 1993b). More than half of chronically mentally ill women do not use condoms at the time of intercourse, while similar or even higher rates of unprotected intercourse among chronically mentally ill men have been reported consistently (Coverdale and Aruffo, 1992). The chronically mentally ill are quite active sexually; over 80 percent in outpatient mental health settings report sexual activity in the past year (Coverdale and Aruffo, 1992; Carmen and Brady, 1990). One survey in a high-risk urban area found that high-risk behaviors such as prostitution, violent sex, and intercourse under the influence of substances occurred in 20 percent of chronically mental ill patients (Kelly et al., 1992). Similar numbers have frequent anonymous sexual contacts, and 15 percent have been treated for sexually transmitted diseases (Kelly et al., 1992). Recent evidence suggests that most of the sexual activity occurs with other individuals with mental disorders (Kalichman et al., 1994), so that introduction of the HIV pandemic to some clients of a community mental health system might lead to spread of infection within the group in a "point-source" pandemic.

Rates of HIV infection among the chronically mentally ill average 8 percent in those urban areas where HIV disease is highly concentrated. Roughly 5 percent of patients in acute state hospital wards (Cournos et al., 1991), 10 to 12 percent of patients in acute general hospital psychiatric wards (Sacks et al., 1992), and 6 to 7 percent of patients in mental health centers in these areas test positive for HIV (Lyketsos et al., 1993b).

A new population of patients is increasingly presenting for treatment in emergency rooms. These are individuals caught up in the drug epidemic because of premorbid vulnerabilities such as personality disorders, mood disorders, and anxiety disorders. These patients are at very high risk for contracting HIV. This group is also in close contact with correctional services as they frequently are on parole or probation or have histories of arrests or incarcerations.

Both the traditional group of chronically mentally ill and this newer population of patients seen by community psychiatric services will require the close attention of community psychiatrists. Not only will they have special care needs, but they are also the people who will least benefit from public education and thus continue to play a role in the spread of the epidemic. Both groups are resistant to changing their high-risk HIV-related behavior (Carmen and Brady, 1990; Hanson et al., 1992).

The Role of the Community Psychiatrist

Community psychiatrists have important roles in the HIV epidemic (Carmen and Brady, 1990; Cohen, 1990; Treisman et al., 1993). Treating HIV-infected patients presents long-term, complex medical issues, and invariably requires medical management of patients. HIV patients are vulnerable to medical illness, frequently develop "organic" disorders, and are quite susceptible to medication effects. It is essential to recognize the complexities the disease presents and that the care of patients with HIV requires close coordination with a multidisciplinary team. Integration of medical care, psychiatric care, social work service, and nursing care is crucial for success. Addressing the needs of HIV patients adds to the complexity of the multidisciplinary teams in which community psyciatrists are accustomed to working. Patients with HIV are found in diverse settings, so that community psychiatrists may need to follow patients in different locations to ensure continuity of care. In addition to functioning in mental health centers, it is crucial to interface with medical care providers, prison health services, and nursing homes dealing with AIDS patients. Relationships with inpatient psychiatric and medical personnel are needed to provide psychiatric management for HIV patients in these settings.

Goals for community psychiatrists dealing with HIV-infected patients can be considered in terms of primary, secondary, and tertiary prevention.

Primary prevention.   In seronegative patients the presence of high-risk behavior should be ascertained by asking well-defined questions: "How often are you sexually active?", "With whom?", "Do you know this person's past?", "Do you always use condoms?", "Do you have sex when you are high?", "Do you use drugs?", "Do you shoot up?", "Do you share needles?" Such behavior, if present, should be addressed as a high-priority treatment goal. Asking patients alone about high-risk behavior may not be adequate, so that collateral information from family members and other care-providers should be sought, using appropriate care and discretion. Conversely, the serostatus of patients practicing high-risk behavior should be ascertained on a regular basis. This should not be left to primary medical care providers, given the poor compliance that the chronically mentally ill tend to exhibit with their medical care providers.

Mental health centers should be prepared to provide on-site counseling and testing for the HIV virus. This is particularly true if they are located in a high-prevalence area. In low-prevalence areas there should be a clear and simple relationship with an agency such as the Red Cross, which provides on-site counseling and testing and can easily take referrals. Among those who are found to be seropositive, primary prevention activities are best directed at intervening to stop behavior that is likely to transmit the infection. Specific programs found to be useful for this purpose include drop-in groups, condom distribution, and focused education (Carmen and Brady, 1990). Model curricula for HIV education among the chronically mentally ill are available (Goisman et al., 1991). One program has demonstrated some efficacy in reducing high-risk injection drug use in collaboration with a methadone program (Baker et al., 1993).

Secondary prevention.   This has two aspects. The first relates to the community psychiatrist's role in supporting good medical care of patients with mental disorders and HIV infection. Secondary prevention to retard the progression of disease through anti-retroviral treatment, and chemoprophylaxis for opportunistic infection are the most effective treatments for HIV infection, and thus should be pursued aggressively to prolong good-quality life. A community psychiatrist does not assume primary responsibility for patients' medical care, but rather participates by discussing its importance with patients and by encouraging compliance with medical care visits and with medications and preventive regimens. When and if vaccines become available (Koff and Hoth, 1988), community psychiatrists will have an important role in supporting the vaccination of their patients.

The other aspect of secondary prevention is the identification of previously unascertained cases of mental disorder among the HIV-infected. Screening procedures for the identification of psychiatric cases among those who are HIV-infected both in medical clinics and in prisons have been developed (Lyketsos et al., 1994). Health care personnel in medical clinics or correctional facilities can be trained to apply screening procedures for HIV-infected patients that will identify psychiatric cases. They must, of course, be prepared to provide treatment in these instances.

Tertiary prevention.   Treatment of psychiatric complications in HIV-infected patients requires a multifaceted approach (Treisman et al., 1993; Coverdale et al., 1992). Psychiatric diseases and syndromes should be carefully evaluated; behavioral disorders and personality vulnerabilities impacting on patients' presentations and treatment should also be identified and patients' life stories should be addressed, as they tend to be chaotic and have a major effect on treatment. Evaluations should include the patient's psychiatric history, social history, family history, a careful mental status and physical examination, and a review of laboratory studies.

Diagnosis and formulation guide treatment. With regard to major depression, the treatment is usually pharmacologic with adjunctive supportive psychotherapy (Perry, 1994; Treisman et al., 1993; Treisman et al., 1994). Given HIV patients' propensity toward the development of side effects, low-side-effect profile medications are preferred. It is important to give low doses at the start and to carefully monitor patients with blood levels as appropriate. Dosages are best elevated as high as safely tolerated and kept there for at least 4 to 6 weeks before failures are called. Subsequently, if patients do not respond to one medication, augmentation with lithium, thyroid hormone, or fluphenazine should be considered. If the boosting approach fails, then an anti-depressant from a different class should be tried (Treisman et al., 1993). Maintenance treatment should last for at least 6 to 9 months, possibly even longer. Few patients can safely come off anti-depressants without relapse in the HIV setting (Treisman et al., 1993).

Early-onset mania is treated with lithium (Treisman et al., 1993). As HIV disease advances, erratic swings in lithium levels have been observed even where dosing is assured under supervision. In end-stage patients with AIDS and mania, lithium is poorly tolerated; low-dose haloperidol or fluphenazine are preferred and are often used long-term.

For organic mental disorders, treatment of the primary cause is pursued first. If delirium is present with agitation, and disturbing hallucinations, low-dose haloperidol may be used for palliation (Fernandez et al., 1988). In contrast, treatment of dementia is more complicated, as brain injury has occurred, which cannot be reversed. However, there is some evidence that high-dose AZT may slow the progression of the dementia (Schmitt et al., 1989).

Fifteen to 20 percent of HIV-infected patients suffer from comorbid substance use and other mental disorders, the so-called "triple" diagnosis patients (Lyketsos et al., 1994). Addressing substance abuse concurrently with other psychiatric disorders is the most effective approach to ensure the best outcome for both types of conditions (Chapter 25). To provide these services at the same time as addressing other medical conditions requires integration of substance use, psychiatric, and medical services in both inpatient and outpatient settings. Special attention must be paid personality disorders, which frequently lead to relapses of substance use.

Addressing personality vulnerabilities is one of the most complicated aspects of dealing with some HIV-infected patients. As noted, patients may be totally focused on the present, be unable to foresee consequences, and be unable to resist their strong impulses (Treisman et al., 1993). They may engage in "staff splitting," "doctor shopping," and "manipulative behaviors," which need to be recognized and addressed. Patients respond far better to rewards than punishment. They should be provided with firm limits, structure, and behavioral goals that lead to rewards quickly. A team approach with a specific treatment plan that is agreed upon by all members will avoid splitting and abuses of clinic resources.

Dealing with the meaningful consequences of HIV infection is a continuing process. The triad of progressive social ostracism, progressive physical debilitation, and progressive loss of social supports can be devastating to any patient. Grief or mourning and other responses are treated with psychological rather than pharmacological interventions. Psychotherapy should be supportive and encouraging, focusing on the here and now. It combines an opportunity for patients to express their problems openly with the opportunity to receive direct counseling. Pharmacologic intervention can be used for brief intervals when severe persistent sleep disturbance or other anxious feelings arise. Trazodone starting at 25–50 mg at bedtime, titrating up as high as 150 mg as needed, is the safest and most effective agent for this purpose (Treisman et al., 1993). A main goal of psychotherapy in this setting is to combat demoralization and to help patients develop adaptive coping strategies. Practical and detailed help with a maze of governmental and community support services is essential; social work intervention could be crucial to help patients make ends meet. Support groups (both HIV related and otherwise), buddy systems, encouragement of social and family interaction, community-based AIDS advocacy and support organizations, and other similar interventions become important.

A Model Program

The integration needed for success may be accomplished in one of three ways. First, psychiatric and substance use staff may be located in a medical clinic and also provide care in medical wards, chronic care wards, or inpatient psychiatric wards. Alternatively, a mental health center or system might be the primary locus, with medical staff located on site. Finally, all the providers involved—psychiatric, substance use, medical—may develop collaborative agreements through which they might care for each others' patients in their own settings. The approach chosen is best determined by the prevalence of HIV disease in a particular area.

For high-prevalence areas a systematic approach to the HIV pandemic similar to the one represented in Figure 29–1 is indicated (Treisman et al., 1993; Lyketsos et al., 1994). This model provides all the components important to the care of HIV-infected patients in any area. Where HIV infection is less prevalent, mental health centers are still best advised to provide primary, secondary, and tertiary preventive services on site. Where HIV medical clinics are not available, linkages should be pursued with primary-care clinics. In some instances program components will be at the same location, for example, as part of a general hospital or a community health department; in other instances, they may be physically apart.

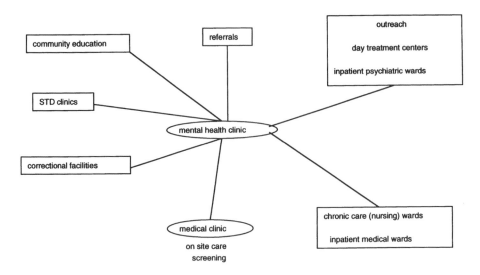

Figure 29–1 Schematic drawing of the proposed model program to address HIV infection in mental health systems.

Within mental health programs, regular screening for high-risk HIV behavior and regular testing for HIV infection should be instituted as medically indicated for newly evaluated patients and for existing patients. In high-prevalence areas, on-site testing and counseling for HIV infection is crucial. Once identified as HIV-positive, patients in all stages of infection are referred to the medical clinic and regularly encouraged to attend. Similarly, mental health staff develop screening procedures for the identification of psychiatric cases among medical clinic patients. With the development of good professional collaboration, medical care providers are more than willing to participate in such a process and are grateful for a psychiatric presence in their clinics (Lyketsos et al., 1994).

In mental health centers these activities can be fostered by specific individuals (psychiatrists or others) who coordinate HIV programs and educate center staff on HIV matters. These staff members also have the role of providing a variety of interventions to address high-risk HIV behaviors in mental health center patients. This is accomplished through the development of educational programs, group sessions, case management, and outreach. The regular focus on patients' behavior by these specialists is likely to impact on their changing these behaviors. Finally, such specialists provide other team members with updated knowledge regarding the pandemic.

In this model, either the psychiatric or the medical clinic may be the principal locus for psychiatric evaluation and treatment. Where patients receive their ongoing psychiatric treatment is determined by the severity of their medical condition. Early-stage patients are best treated within the mental health center, particularly if the HIV specialist spends a lot of time in dealing with their behavior. As their medical conditions worsen, often with an associated decrease in high-risk behaviors, it is more important for them to be receiving medical care. Psychiatrists should consider establishing regular hours in the medical clinic to see patients there on the days they come for medical care. This decreases the burden on patients, who only have to come to one place for both types of treatment, and improves their compliance with care (Lyketsos et al., 1994).

Community psychiatrists should also be accessible for consultation about their outpatients who are admitted to inpatient and day wards. This promotes continuity of care, educates other providers in these settings, and allows for the smooth transition of patients to and from the community mental health program.

It is important to have a quality-improvement system that monitors the progress of the program. A simple system basically identifies patients as they come into the clinic and later charts their course and treatment. Major outcome issues include success in eradicating high-risk behaviors and in achieving compliance with medical and psychiatric treatment. Similarly, regular education is provided to patients and staff about HIV infection.

Screening procedures for psychiatric disorders and HIV infection can also be developed in correctional facilities and other sites of medical and psychiatric care where the volume of HIV infection is steady, although lower.

Summary

This chapter has briefly reviewed several issues on medical and psychiatric aspects of the HIV pandemic. It has focused on the role of community psychiatrists in this pandemic and has proposed a comprehensive model program to address it. The main messages are that HIV infection is widespread and serious and that it is intimately linked with psychiatric disorder. Because of the changing nature of this pandemic in the United States, this relationship between HIV infection and psychiatric disorder is going to become increasingly important both from the public health point of view and also from the point of view of providing psychiatric treatment. Because of the complexities of HIV infection, the serious medical nature of its associated psychiatric complications, the frequent presence of comorbid substance use and other behavioral disorders, and the many treatment sites involved, community psychiatrists must lead the efforts of mental health care systems to address the pandemic. This is particularly true because of accumulating evidence showing the under-recognition of the pandemic in mental health settings.

References

Atkinson, J.H., Grant, I., Kennedy, C.J., Richman, D.D., Spector, S.A., and McCutcheon, J.A. (1988) Prevalence of psychiatric disorders among men infected with Human Immunodeficiency Virus. *Archives of General Psychiatry,* 45:859–864.

Baer, J.W., Dwyer, P.C., and Lewitter-Koehler, S. (1988) Knowledge about AIDS among psychiatric inpatients. *Hospital and Community Psychiatry,* 39:986–988.

Baker, A., Heather, N., Wodak, A., Dixon, J., and Holt, P. (1993) Evaluation of a cognitive-behavioural intervention for HIV prevention among injecting drug users. *AIDS,* 7(2): 247–256.

Bartlett, J.G., and Finkbeiner, A.K. (1991) *The Guide to Living with HIV Infection.* Baltimore: Johns Hopkins Press.

Carmen E., and Brady, S.M. (1990) AIDS risk and prevention for the chronic mentally ill. *Hospital and Community Psychiatry,* 41(6):652–657.

Centers for Disease Control (1992) The second 100,000 cases of AIDS—United States. June 1981–December 1991. *MMWR,* 41:28–29.

Centers for Disease Control (1990) HIV prevalence estimates and AIDS case projections for the United States: Report based upon a workshop. *MMWR,* 39(RR–16):1–31.

Chaisson, R.E. (1992) Epidemiology of Human Immunodeficiency virus infection and Acquired Immunodeficiency Syndrome. In Gorbach, S.L., Bartlett, J.G., Blacklow, N.R. (eds.), *Infectious Diseases,* pp. 907–918. New York: W. B. Saunders Co.

Chuang, E.A. (1992) Psychiatric morbidity in patients with HIV infection. *Canadian Journal of Psychiatry,* 37:109–115.

Cohen, M.A.A. (1990) Biopsychosocial approach to the Human Immunodeficiency Virus pandemic. A clinician's primer. *General Hospital Psychiatry,* 12:98–123.

Cournos, F., Empfield, M., Horwath, E., McKinnon, K., Meyer, I., Schrage, H., Currie, C., and Agosin, B. (1991) HIV seroprevalence among patients admitted to two psychiatric hospitals. *American Journal of Psychiatry,* 148:1125–1130.

Cournos, F., Guido, J.R., Coomaraswamy, S., Meyer-Bahlburg, H., Sugden, R., and Horwath, E. (1994) Sexual activity and risk of HIV infection among patients with schizophrenia. *American Journal of Psychiatry,* 151(2):228–232.

Coverdale, J.H., and Aruffo, J.F. (1992) AIDS and family planning counseling of psychiatrically ill women in community mental health clinics. *Community Mental Health Journal,* 28(1):13–20.

Coverdale, J., Aruffo, J., and Grunebaum, H. (1992) Developing family planning services for female chronic mentally ill outpatients. *Hospital and Community Psychiatry,* 43(5):475–478.

Dilley, J.W., Ochitill, H.N., Perl, M., et al. (1985) Findings in psychiatric consultations with patients with acquired immune deficiency syndrome. *American Journal of Psychiatry,* 142:82–86.

Fernandez, F., Levy, J.K., and Mansell, P.W. (1988) Management of delirium in terminally ill AIDS patients. *International Journal of Psychiatry in Medicine,* 19:165–172.

Goisman, R.M., Kent, A.B., Montgomery, E.C., Cheevers, M.M., and Goldfinger, S.M. (1991) AIDS education for patients with chronic mental illness. *Community Mental Health Journal,* 27(3):189–197.

Gorman, J.M., Kertner, R., Todak, G., Rabkin, J.S., Williams, J.B., Mayer-Bahlburg, H.F., Mayeux, R., Stern, Y., Lange, M., Spitzer, D.J.R., and Ehrhardt, A.A. (1991) Multi-disciplinary baseline assessment of homosexual men with and without Human Immunodeficiency Virus infection. *Archives of General Psychiatry,* 480:120–123.

Gotlieb, M.S., Schroff, R., and Schanker, H.M. (1981) *Pneumocystis carinii* pneumonia and mucosal *candidiasis* in previously healthy homosexual men: evidence of new acquired cellular immunodeficiency. *New England Journal of Medicine,* 305:1425.

Hanson, M., Kramer, T.H., Gross, W., Quintana, J., Li, P.W., and Asher, R. (1992) AIDS awareness and risk behaviors among dually disordered adults. *AIDS Education and Prevention,* 4(1):41–51.

Hoover, D.R., Munoz, A., Saah, A., Phair, J., and Detels, R. (1992) The progression of untreated HIV-1 infection prior to AIDS. *American Journal of Public Health,* 82:1538–1541.

Huggins, J., Elman, N., Baker, C., and Stedman, N. (1991) Affective and behavioral responses of gay and bisexual men to HIV antibody testing. *Social Work,* 36:61–66.

Johannet, C., and Muskin, P.R. (1990) Mood and behavioral disturbances in hospitalized AIDS patients. *Psychosomatics,* 31:55–59.

Kalichman, S.C., Kelly, J.A., Johnson, J.R., and Bulto, M. (1994) Factors associated with risk for HIV infection among chronic mentally ill adults. *American Journal of Psychiatry,* 151(2):221–227.

Kelly, J.A., Murphy, D.A., Bahr, G.R., Brasfield, T.L., Davis, D.R., Hauth, A.C., Morgan, M.G., Stevenson, L.Y., and Eilers, M.K. (1992) AIDS/HIV risk behavior among the chronic mentally ill. *American Journal of Psychiatry,* 149(7):886–889.

Koff, W.C., and Hoth, E.F. (1988) Development and testing of AIDS vaccines. *Science,* 241: 426–431.

Lyketsos, C.G., Hanson, A.L., Fishman, M., and Treisman, G.J. (1994) Screening for psychiatric morbidity in a medical outpatient clinic for HIV infection: the need for a psychiatric presence. *International Journal of Psychiatry in Medicine,* 242(2):115–125.

Lyketsos, C.G., Hoover, D.R., Guccione, M., Wesch, J., Dew, M.A., Bing, E., and Treisman, G.J. (1993a) Depression and its risk factors over the course of HIV infection before AIDS. Presented at the 146th American Psychiatric Association Annual Meeting, May 24. San Francisco, Calif. Abstract 3E.

Lyketsos, C.G., Hanson, A.L., Fishman, M., Rosenblatt, A.R., McHugh, P.R., and Treisman, G.J. (1993b) Manic episode early and late in the course of HIV. *American Journal of Psychiatry,* 150:326–327.

Lyketsos, C.G., Storch, D.D., Lann, H.D., Finn, R., Haber, R., and Meng, R. (1993c) HIV Infection in Maryland public psychiatric facilities: results of an informal survey. *Maryland Medical Journal,* 42(6):571–573.

Mann, J.M., and Chin, J. (1988) AIDS, a global perspective. *New England Journal of Medicine,* 319:302–303.

Masur, H., Michelis, M.A., and Greene, J.B. (1981) An outbreak of community-acquired *Pneumocystis carinii* pneumonia: initial manifestations of cellular immune dysfunction. *New England Journal of Medicine,* 305:1431.

McArthur, J.C. (1992) Neurologic manifestations of Human Immunodeficiency Virus infection. In Asbury, T., McKhann, G., McDonald, J. (eds.), *Diseases of the Nervous System.* New York: Raven Press.

McHugh, P.R., and Slavney, P.R. (1983) *The Perspectives of Psychiatry.* Baltimore: Johns Hopkins University Press.

Munoz, A., Curey, V., Taylor, J.M.G., et al. (1992) Estimation of time since exposure for a prevalent cohort. *Statistics in Medicine.* 11:939–952.

Nurnberg, H.G., Prudic, J., Fiori, M., et al. (1984) Psychopathology complicating acquired immune deficiency syndrome (AIDS). *American Journal of Psychiatry,* 141:95–96.

O'Dowd, M.A., and McKegney, P.T. (1991) Characteristics of patients attending an HIV related psychiatric clinic. *Hospital and Community Psychiatry,* 42:615–619.

Perkins, D.O., Stern, R.A., Golden, R.N., Murphy, C., Naftolowitz, D., Evans, D.L. (1994) Mood disorders in HIV infection: prevalence and risk factors in a nonepicenter of the AIDS pandemic. *American Journal of Psychiatry,* 151:233–236.

Perkins, D.O., Davidson, E.J., Leserman, J., Liao, D., and Evans, D.L. (1993) Personality disorder in patients infected with HIV: a controlled study with implications for clinical care. *American Journal of Psychiatry,* 150:309–315.

Perry, S., Jacobsberg, L.B., and Fishman, B. (1989) Psychiatric diagnosis before serological

testing for the Human Immunodeficiency Virus. *American Journal of Psychiatry,* 147:
89–93.

Perry, S.W. (1994) HIV-related depression. In Price, R.W., Perry, S.W. (eds.), *HIV, AIDS and
the Brain.* New York: Raven Press.

Perry, S. (1990) Organic mental disorders caused by HIV: update on early diagnosis and treatment. *American Journal of Psychiatry,* 147:696–710.

Picard, O., Giral, P., Defer, M.C., et al. (1990) AIDS vaccine therapy: Phase I trial. *Lancet* ii:
179.

Sacks, M.H., Silberstein, C., Weiler, P., and Perry, S. (1990) HIV-related risk factors in acute
psychiatric inpatients. *Hospital and Community Psychiatry,* 41:449–451.

Sacks, M., Dermatis, H., Loosser-Ott, S., and Perry, S. (1992) Seroprevalence of HIV and risk
factors for AIDS in psychiatric inpatients. *Hospital and Community Psychiatry,* 43(7):
736–737.

Schmitt, F.A., Bigley, J.W., McKinnis, R., et al. (1989) Neuropsychological outcome of Zidovudine (AZT) treatment of patients with AIDS and AIDS-related complex. *New England Journal of Medicine,* 319:1573–1578.

Seigal, F.P., Lopez, C., Hammer, H.M., et al. (1981) Severe acquired immunodeficiency in
male homosexuals, manifested by chronic perianal ulcerative *herpes simplex* lesions.
New England Journal of Medicine, 305:1439.

Sewell, D.D., Jeste, D.V., Hampton, T., Atkinson, J., Heaton, R.K., Hesselink, J.R., Wiley, C.,
Thal, L., Chandler, J.L., Grant, I., and the San Diego HIV Neurobehavioral Research
Center (1994) HIV-associated psychosis: a study of 20 cases. *American Journal of
Psychiatry,* 251(2):237–242.

Treisman, G.J., Lyketsos, C.G., Fishman, M., Hanson, A.L., Rosenblatt, A., and McHugh, P.R.
(1993) Psychiatric care for patients with HIV infection. *Psychosomatics,* 34:432–439.

Treisman, G.J., Fishman, M., Lyketsos, C.G., and McHugh, P.R. (1994) Evaluation and treatment of psychiatric disorders associated with HIV infection. In Price, R.W., Perry, S.W.
(eds.), *HIV, AIDS and the Brain.* New York: Raven Press.

INDEX